Evolution of Atopic Dermatitis in the 21st Century

Ichiro Katayama • Hiroyuki Murota
Takahiro Satoh
Editors

Evolution of Atopic Dermatitis in the 21st Century

Springer

Editors
Ichiro Katayama
Department of Dermatology
Integrated Medicine
Graduate School of Medicine
Osaka University
Suita, Osaka, Japan

Hiroyuki Murota
Department of Dermatology
Integrated Medicine
Graduate School of Medicine
Osaka University
Suita, Osaka, Japan

Takahiro Satoh
Department of Dermatology
National Defense Medical College
Tokorosazawa, Saitama, Japan

ISBN 978-981-10-5540-9 ISBN 978-981-10-5541-6 (eBook)
https://doi.org/10.1007/978-981-10-5541-6

Library of Congress Control Number: 2017959195

Printed on acid-free paper

This Springer imprint is published by Springer Nature
The registered company is Springer Nature Singapore Pte Ltd.
The registered company address is: 152 Beach Road, #21-01/04 Gateway East, Singapore 189721, Singapore

Contents

Part VIII Management

Part IX Complications

Part X Clinical Questions

Part I

Introduction

History and Definition

1

Kiyoshi Nishioka

Abstract

History of atopic dermatitis is reviewed. Atopic dermatitis was recognized as a chronic relapsing pruritic skin disease and called differently historically. Neurodermite disseminatus and prurigo diathetique are the distinct concepts leading to that of atopic dermatitis. Sulzburger established the concept of atopic eczema/dermatitis by introducing the concept of atopic hypersensitiveness to this skin disease. His idea was now widely accepted. In 1980 a new phenotype of atopic dermatitis appeared to us and was named adult-type atopic dermatitis. The mechanism and pathogenesis have been investigated extensively to define the real figure of this intractable skin disease.

Keywords

Lichen simplex chronicus disseminatus • Neurodermite disseminatus Prurigo diathetique • Atopic dermatitis

Atopic dermatitis is now one of the most familiar skin diseases among physicians, as well as general population. It is a chronic relapsing pruritic skin disease with characteristic phenotype and persists long to disturb patients' quality of life. In the history of dermatology, this disease might be regarded as one of the severe types of eczema or as different skin diseases. The historical record by Suetonius reported that the first emperor of Roman Empire, Augustus, had been suffering from a chronic itchy skin disease complicated with asthmatic symptoms and rhinitis. This description suggests us atopic predisposition in our modern dermatology [1]. Therefore, we can understand the existence of this intractable skin disease even in the ancient time. However, it was not specifically discussed before the seventeenth

K. Nishioka
Hyogo Medical College, Mukogawacho 1-1, Nishinomiya City 663-8501, Japan
e-mail: knish@hyo-med.ac.jp

I. Katayama et al. (eds.), *Evolution of Atopic Dermatitis in the 21st Century*,
https://doi.org/10.1007/978-981-10-5541-6_1

century. Helmont reported a case complicated with pruritus and asthmatic attacks in 1607 and Trousseau suggested in 1884 that the same etiological factor was working in eczema and asthma [2].

1.1 Atopic Dermatitis in the Nineteenth Century, Lichen-Neurodermatitis-Prurigo

In 1884 a famous dermatologist, Hebra, described chronic severe pruritic skin lesions localized on the neck and cubital and popliteal fossae and proposed the name "mycosis sive eczema flexurarum" to this skin disease [2]. This name did not live long because of failure to demonstrate fungal elements from skin lesions. Vidal categorized this skin disease as "lichen" and named lichen simplex chronicus disseminatus [3] and Blocq and Jacquet as "nevrodermite" and named neurodermite disseminatus [4]. Blocq and Jacquet suggested that neurodermite (neurodermatitis) is a nervous disease in both the somatic and psychiatric senses. They summarized the characteristics of their disease as follows: (1) nervousness including above-normal to unstable emotion, furious, depressive, hysteric, alcoholism, etc., (2) constant itching always preceding the appearance of visible skin lesions, (3) sharp demarcation of the plaque precisely limited to the area of the preceding itching, (4) skin changes arranged concentric zones resembling other dermatoses of nervous origin, (5) absolute dryness of the lesions, and (6) chronicity of its course. They pointed that (7) hypertrophy of the papillae of the cutis was responsible to this skin change.

In 1892 Besnier classified this skin disease into a category of "prurigo" [5] and proposed the name "prurigo diathetique eczemato-lichenienne" [6]. He pointed that it is a distinct skin disease from "prurigo de Hebra (dermatite multiforme prurigineuse chronique)." Prurigo de Hebra shows that itchy urticarial papules appear to turn into seropapules and then to prurigo-papules on the extensor surface of extremities and trunk of children of early infancy. And it does not show lichenification.

1.2 Besnier Presented His Typical Cases

Case 1 was a 19-year-old male farmer who was suffering from infantile eczema since his age of 3 months. Skin lesions were lichenification and diffuse pigmentation distributed to the trunk and extremities and exudated lesions on legs. However, his head, genital area, and scrotum were clear from skin lesions. The lesions exacerbated in winter. He showed "masque eczematique (eczema face)" and cervical lymphadenopathy.

Case 2 was an 18-year-old copper refiner whose eczema started at age 4. His skin lesions were worse in summer but cleared completely in winter. Papules and lichenified plaques appeared on his face and neck and brown pigmentation with white cicatrical flecks on the chest and abdomen.

Case 3 was a 17-year-old tailor who had no skin lesions before his age of 14. The skin lesions started after he stayed in a hotel at Paris and were worse in winter. He had diffuse pigmentation on his trunk and papules on pigmentation at inguinal and

Table 1.1 Synonyms of atopic dermatitis

Diagnostic term	Author
Mycosis sive eczema flexurarum	Hebra (1884)
Lichen simplex chronicus disseminatus	Vidal (1886)
Neurodermite disseminatus	Brocq and Jacquet (1891)
Prurigo diathetique eczemato-lichenienne	Besnier (1892)
Neurodermite diffuse	Brocq (1902)
Prurigo Besnier	Rasch (1903)
Asthma-Ekzem	Jadassohn (1903)
Prurigo asthma	Sabouraud (1912)
Eczema pruriginosum	Unna
Eczema flexurarum	Kaposi
Früeh- und späetexdudatives eczematoid	Rost (1928)
Atopic eczema/atopic dermatitis	Sulzburger (1933)
Constitutional prurigo-eczema	Bonnevie (1939)
Endogenes Ekzem	Korting (1954)
Intrinsic allergic dermatitis	Cooke (1947)

iliac areas. His extremities showed eczematization and lichenification. Inguinal lymphadenopathy was noted.

The characteristic skin change was "eczematization and lichenification" and intense and remittent pruritus with nocturnal paroxysm and seasonal exacerbation. Besnier named "prurigo diathetique eczemato-lichenienne" to this disease as he recognized their intense and remittent itching as constitutional origin [6]. The skin lesions started at early infancy but could start at any age. At infancy skin lesions were non-characteristic and polymorphous, consisting of erythema, urticaria, or pseudo-lichen. They exacerbated by repeated eczematization and then progressed to lichenification. Most of the cases developed emphysema, asthma, hay fever, and gastrointestinal disturbance at silence of the skin lesions.

After Besnier many famous dermatologists reported this skin disease and named it eczema, eczematid, prurigo, etc. (Table 1.1). Although all these authors observed the similar skin symptoms of the patients, they described it with different dermatological terms: lichen, neurodermatitis, and prurigo. This change of medical terms will remind us the discussion on the pathogenesis of this skin disease in the era of descriptive dermatology.

1.3 Atopic Hypersensitiveness and Atopic Dermatitis

In the beginning of the twentieth century, knowledge has been accumulated in the field of immunology and allergology. The concept of atopic hypersensitiveness was introduced by Coca and Cook [7]. Those authors classified hypersensitiveness into two groups, physiological and abnormal hypersensitiveness. Dermatitis venenata and serum sickness were included in the former group and anaphylaxis, hypersensitivity of infection, and atopy in the latter group. They explained that atopic hypersensitiveness was a reaction induced against nonprecipitable substance as well as against precipitable substances. The hypersensitive state has not been shown to be passively transferable to normal individuals with serum except one observation. It could be greatly lessened but not completely removed by suitable injection of active substance. The reaction was characteristic to human and different from anaphylaxis of animals. It was inherited and accompanied with hay fever and asthma [7]. Although minor differences of understanding are present when compared with our recent understandings, Sulzburger applied the concept of atopy to this intractable eczematous disease. He recognized that all the features of atopy could be found in each and every case of atopic dermatitis. He explained that neurodermatitis disseminatus of Brocq and Jacquet was the most classical type of atopic dermatitis and that those of Besnier were its evoluted type. The name "neurodermatitis" was not a proper one because skin disease of nervous origin was misunderstood as the disease of psychiatric origin [8]. An article of *New York Times* in 1954 reported that an aviation engineer was dismissed for 5 months from his job by being diagnosed his skin disease as neurodermatitis that was confused with psychoneurosis [5]. He named "atopic dermatitis" to this skin disease according to the concept of atopic hypersensitiveness and classified into three stages: (1) infantile eczema of atopic type, i.e., atopic eczema, (2) atopic dermatitis of childhood, and (3) atopic dermatitis in the adolescent and young adult. He used the terms atopic eczema for the infantile cases and atopic dermatitis for the lichenified cases [9, 10]. Skin symptoms of atopic eczema are non-characteristic and polymorphous ones, consisting of papulovesicular rash, exudative erythema, or sometimes wheal. They spread from cheeks to trunk and extremities. Patients in childhood stage show papulation rather than exudation. Lichenified lesions appear on cubital and popliteal fossae, the neck, and wrists accompanying with intense pruritus. Atopic dermatitis in adolescence and young adult shows gray to dark pigmented lichenified lesions on the face, neck, and cubital fossae with occasional oozing, weeping, and crusting. The patients show dry skin with intense itching. The cases in adolescent and young adult correspond to neurodermite disseminatus of Blocq and Jacquet and prurigo diathetique of Besnier. And infantile eczema is the forerunner of atopic dermatitis. Patients have high rate of family history of atopic manifestation and personal history of atopic diseases and infantile eczema [9].

Hill and Sulzburger demonstrated relationship between atopens, allergens, and regains, IgE antibodies [8]. Positive skin test by food materials was more common in infantile cases, and rate of the positive skin test with environmental materials was increasing with their age. Significance of food allergens in atopic dermatitis has already been discussed among researchers in those days. Oral challenge of food materials responsible for the positive skin test did not induce exacerbation of atopic dermatitis [11]. Role of food allergens has been insisted by pediatric researchers even until recently; however, its significance has already been discussed at the beginning of history of atopic dermatitis.

1.4 Atopic Dermatitis in the 1980s

The term "atopic dermatitis" was accepted worldwide after the World War II. We have had only limited cases of adolescent and young adult cases at that time. Almost all of the cases with atopic dermatitis were limited in children, and the severity of the disease was also limited. Especially almost all cases were easily treated with mild topical corticosteroid.

The situation around atopic dermatitis has changed in the 1980s in Japan. Numbers of adult cases with atopic dermatitis were increased [12, 13]. Age distribution pattern of atopic dermatitis has changed much between 1975 and 1985. The age distribution pattern of patients with atopic dermatitis in outpatient clinic of Kitasato University Hospital showed a sharp peak at age 1–2 and a gentle slope to the increasing age in 1975. In contrast two peaks were observed in 1985, a sharp peak at age 1–2 and second sharp high peak at age 15–25. Atopic dermatitis in 1975 was the disease of childhood. It became the disease of adolescence and young adult in addition to those of childhood in 1985. Such adult patients showed peculiar skin symptoms in addition to the classical symptoms of atopic dermatitis: (1) red face with frequent swelling and oozing (Fig. 1.1), (2) rippled pattern pigmentation on the neck [14], and (3) erythrodermic skin on trunk and extremities with (4) occasional swelling of lower extremities. Their skin manifestation was different from that described by Besnier and that by Sulzburger for atopic dermatitis in adolescent and young adult. Therefore, we called this condition as "adult

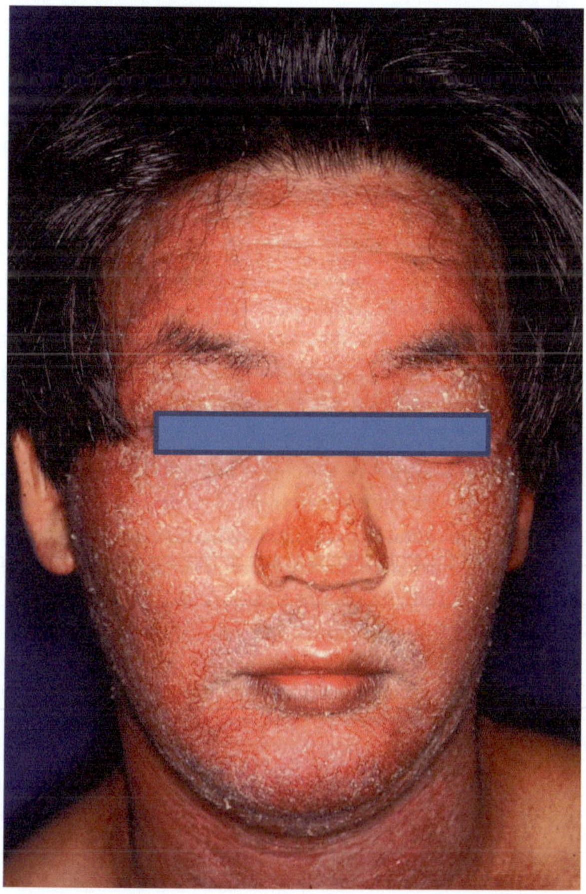

Fig. 1.1 Red face of adult-type atopic dermatitis. Swelling and oozing

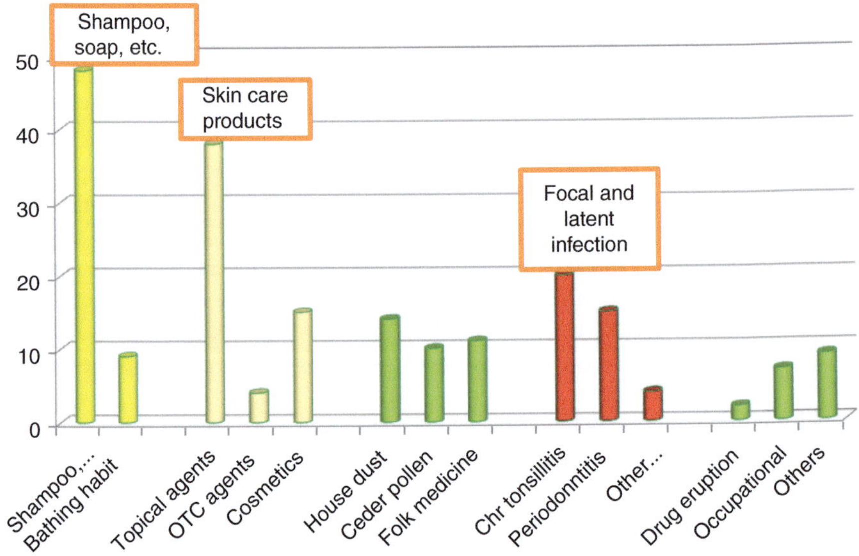

Fig. 1.2 Aggravating factor of atopic dermatitis. Factors detected in 102 patients with adult-type atopic dermatitis (Adapted from Allergy & Immunity 2001) [16]

type atopic dermatitis" to study its pathogenesis [12, 15]. Thirty-nine percent of our 64 patients started their skin symptoms within 6 months after birth and 28% at 1–4 years of age. Seventy-five percent of them had the onset before 10 years of age. The course of their skin symptom was classified into three groups; 75% of our cases started their skin symptom at their early infancy. (1) Skin symptoms persisted and progressed gradually to other parts of the body in 56% of cases, (2) 19% of them cleared skin symptom for years and then redeveloped after their adolescence, and (3) the rest (25%) had no skin troubles before their adolescence and their skin symptoms started after adolescent and adult age. Their skin symptoms were highly resistant to the conventional topical corticosteroid therapy. In these patients, we recognized the significance of irritant and allergic substances in their daily life. Those substances stimulated their skin to induce inflammatory reaction as well as to enhance and modulate their immune response. We have analyzed the exacerbating factors of those cases [16]. We found shampoo and soap, topical agents including skin care products and cosmetics, and focal and latent infections such as tonsillitis, odontoradiculitis, etc., as important exacerbating factors of these severe cases of adult-type atopic dermatitis (Fig. 1.2). The focal and latent infections modulated their immune conditions to enhance the inflammatory reaction. Those factors intermingled with each other to induce the skin condition. It was not unusual that multiple exacerbating factors were detected in a single case. Their skin symptoms were not improved by removing a single exacerbating factor. Careful effort to remove such factors from their daily life resulted in improvement of their symptoms dramatically [17].

1.5 Atopic Dermatitis in the Twenty-First Century

Increment of severe cases with atopic dermatitis forced the researchers to concentrate their efforts to elucidate the pathogenesis of atopic dermatitis: discovery of model animals, production of transgenic and knockout mouse as model animals, barrier dysfunction, cytokines profile, and so on [18–25]. These findings are leading us to establish a new concept of atopic dermatitis.

Skin diseases in general can be affected by environmental factors. Atopic dermatitis is one of the typical diseases influenced much by our living environment. Our severe cases with atopic dermatitis could be attributed to the environmental change in our modern life. Modulated immune response can affect severity of the disease and force to change into different expression pattern of atopic dermatitis. Therapeutic agents may also modify figure of the disease. Atopic dermatitis is evolving with times. New concept of atopic dermatitis may be proposed in very near future as well as the new name of this interesting skin disease.

References

1. Mier PD. Earliest description of the atopic dermatitis. Br J Dermatol. 1975;92:359.
2. Masuda T. Atopic dermatitis. In: Kitamura K, et al., editors. Japanese compendia of dermatology, Eczema and related diseases, vol. 3. Tokyo: Kanehara Pbl Co; 1967. p. 301–401.
3. Vidal E. Du lichen (lichen, prurigo, strophulus). Ann Dermatol Syph. 1886;7:133–54.
4. Brocq L, Jacquet L. Notes pour server a l'histoire des nevrodermites. Ann Dermatol Syphil. 1891;3:97–122, 193–208.
5. Willan R. Prurigo. On cutaneous diseases, vol. 1. London: Johnson J; 1808. p. 67–104.
6. Besnier ME. Premiere note et observations preliminaries pour server d'introduction a l'etude des prurigos diathesiques. Ann Dermatol Syph. 1892;3:634–47.
7. Coca AF, Cooke RA. On the classification of the phenomena of hypersensitiveness. J Immunol. 1922;3:163–82.
8. Bear RL. The development of the concept of atopic dermatitis. In: Bear RL, editor. Atopic dermatitis. New York: New York University Press; 1955. p. 1–9.
9. Hill LW, Sulzburger MB. Evolution of atopic dermatitis. Arch Derm Syphilol. 1935;32:451–63.
10. Sulzburger MB. Atopic dermatitis: its clinical and histologic picture. In: Bear RL, editor. Atopic dermatitis. New York: New York University Press; 1955. p. 11–42.
11. Rostenberg A Jr. Atopic dermatitis: a discussion of certain theories concerning its pathogenesis. In: Bear RL, editor. Atopic dermatitis. New York: New York University Press; 1955. p. 57–80.
12. Nishioka K, Mukai H, Kamimura K, Horiuchi Y, Itoh A, Noguchi T, Nishiyama S. Clinical course of severe cases with adult type atopic dermatitis. Jpn J Dermatol. 1988;98:873–7.
13. Nishioka K. Adult type atopic dermatitis. Clin Dermatol. 1991;33:413–8.
14. Mukai H, Nishioka K, Kamimura K, Katayama I, Nishiyama S. Poikiloderma-like lesions on the neck in atopic dermatitis: a histopathological study. J Dermatol. 1990;17:85–91.
15. Nishioka K. Atopic eczema of adult type in Japan. Austral J Dermatol. 1996;37:S7–9.
16. Nishioka K. Potent infection as the exacerbating factors of severe cases with atopic dermatitis of adult type. Allergy Immun. 2001;8:65–9.
17. Katayama I, Taniguchi H, Matsunaga T, Yokozeki H, Nishioka K. Evaluation of non-steroidal ointment therapy for adult type atopic dermatitis: inquiry analysis on clinical effect. J Dermatol Sci. 1997;14:37–44.

18. Soumelis V, Reche PA, Kanzler H, Yuan W, Edward G, Homey B, et al. Human epithelial cells trigger dendritic cell mediated allergic inflammation by producing TSLP. Nat Immunol. 2002;37:673–80.
19. Novak N, Bieber T, Leung DYM. Immune mechanisms leading to atopic dermatitis. J Allergy Clin Immunol. 2003;112:S128–39.
20. Smith FJD, Irvine AD, Terron-Kwiatkowski A, Sandilands A, Campbell LE, Zhao Y, et al. Loss-of-function mutations in the gene encoding filaggrin cause ichthyosis vulgaris. Nat Genet. 2006;36:337–42.
21. Cork MJ, Robinson DA, Vasilopoulos Y, Ferguson A, Moustafa M, MacGowwan A, Duff GW, et al. New perspectives on epidermal barrier dysfunction in atopic dermatitis: gene-environment interactions. J Allergy Clin Immunol. 2006;118:3–21.
22. Irvine AD, McLean WHI, Leung DYM. Filaggrin mutations associated with skin and allergic diseases. N Engl J Med. 2011;365:1315–27.
23. Bieber T. Atopic dermatitis. N Engl J Med. 2008;358:1438–94.
24. Kubo A, Nagao K, Amagai M. Epidermal barrier dysfunction and cutaneous sensitization in atopic dermatitis. J Clin Invest. 2012;122:440–7.
25. Kabashima K. New concept of the pathogenesis of atopic dermatitis: interplay among the barrier, allergy and pruritus as a trinity. J Dermatol Sci. 2013;70:3–11.

Part II

Epidemiology

Epidemiology of Atopic Dermatitis in Japan

2

Takumi Takizawa, Akihiro Morikawa,
and Hirokazu Arakawa

Abstract

Atopic dermatitis (AD) is a common, chronic, and eczematous skin disease. The prevalence of AD is increasing worldwide and varies among countries. AD prevalence in regions with different climates even within a country is different. A number of genetic mutations have been implicated in the development of AD. Mutations in the filaggrin gene and its frequencies are different between different populations. A wide range in AD prevalence and a rapid increase in prevalence strongly indicate that environmental factors play crucial roles in development of AD. Epigenetics might be key to understanding genetic-environmental interactions in this disease.

Keywords

Epidemiology • Children • Environmental factors • Climate

2.1 Introduction

Atopic dermatitis (AD) is a common, chronic, and eczematous skin disease. Skin and general symptoms caused by AD such as intense itching, sleep disturbance, irritability, and appearance cast an enormous burden on affected individuals and their families and consequently on society [1]. In addition, AD is frequently associated with other allergic diseases.

The prevalence of AD is increasing worldwide [2, 3], though it varies among countries and within a country. AD is most prevalent in infants and gradually

T. Takizawa, M.D., Ph.D. (✉) • A. Morikawa, M.D., Ph.D. • H. Arakawa, M.D., Ph.D.
Department of Pediatrics, Gunma University Graduate School of Medicine,
3-35-22 Showa, Gunma 371 8511, Japan
e-mail: takizawt@gunma-u.ac.jp; morikawa@gunma-u.ac.jp

I. Katayama et al. (eds.), *Evolution of Atopic Dermatitis in the 21st Century*,
https://doi.org/10.1007/978-981-10-5541-6_2

decreases with age. Nevertheless, prevalence has been recently increasing in most age groups. AD is a multifactorial disease. Onset and natural history of AD likely involve a number of genetic and epigenetic factors as well as a wide range of known and unknown environmental factors relating to industrialized lifestyle and climate. The complex interactions between genetic susceptibility and environmental factors may underlie the development of AD.

In this chapter, we would like to review epidemiological studies of AD and discuss characteristic features of the disease epidemiology. This will provide us with further insights into the disease.

2.2 Global Variations in Prevalence of AD Symptoms in Children

A seminal investigation of the global AD prevalence is the international study of asthma and allergies in childhood (ISAAC) phase I [4]. This questionnaire-based survey was carried out from 1994 to 1996 and covered 256,410 children aged 6–7 years in 90 cities and 458,623 children aged 13–14 years in 153 cities in 53 countries. Although the global average prevalence of eczema symptoms was 7.3% and 7.4% in 6–7- and 13–14-year-olds, respectively, wide variations were found between countries (Fig. 2.1). For instance, the prevalence was higher in Northern Europe and Oceania and lower in Asia and Eastern Europe. ISAAC phase III was performed from 2001 to 2003 and covered 60 countries [5]. The overall global prevalence was 6.1% and 8.8% in 6–7- and 13–14-year-olds, respectively. The lowest prevalence was 2.7% in India, and the highest was 22.5% in Ecuador. In some countries, such as Panama, Singapore, and Thailand, the prevalence increased from phase I to phase III in the 6–7-year-old group. Only Russia and Georgia saw a significant decrease in this age group. Global prevalence for 13–14-year-olds increased by 1.4% from phases I to III (Fig. 2.2). It is worth noting in countries that showed higher prevalence in phase I—the UK, New Zealand, and Sweden—prevalence decreased in phase III, while it increased in some Asian countries that had relatively lower prevalence in phase I, such as Indonesia, South Korea, and Singapore (Fig. 2.2).

There have been several studies concerning the prevalence of AD in Japanese populations (Table 2.1) [6]. The prevalence is widely different among studies (Table 2.1) and ranges from 3.85 to 24.3% in age 6–10 years and 3.85 to 17.3% in age 12–13 years. The wide variations of the reported prevalence of AD are due at least in part to the fact that epidemiological studies of AD are influenced by a variety of factors, including year of survey, region, and methods of investigation [7]. A nationwide prevalence survey performed in Japan from 2000 to 2002 showed 11.8% in age 6–7 years [8] (Table 2.1). Prevalence in Tokyo obtained by the ISAAC core written questionnaire was 10.9–19.6% in 6–14-year-old schoolchildren (Table 2.1) [9]. A web-based study performed in 2012 showed 13.0% average prevalence in 6–12-year-olds [10]. In contrast to children, there are not many surveys of AD

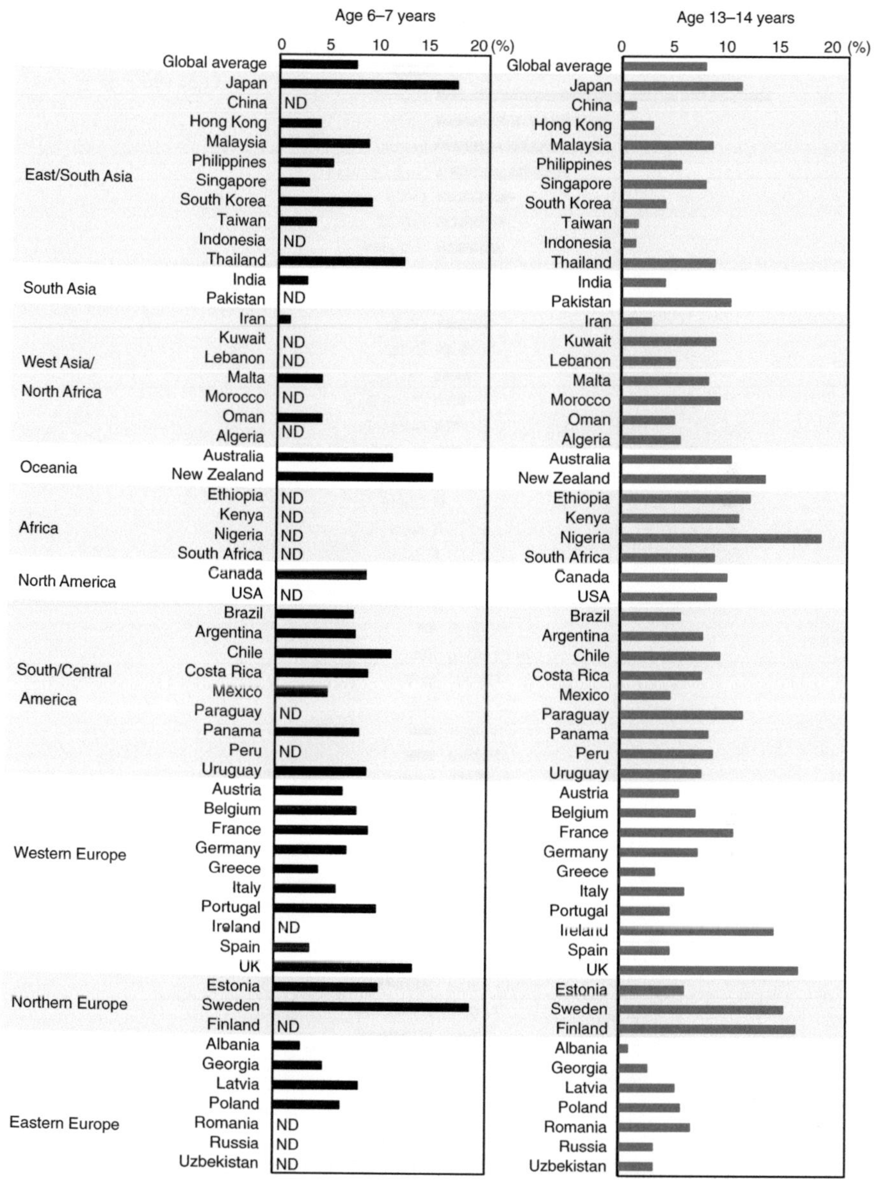

Fig. 2.1 The global AD prevalence is based on the international study of asthma and allergies in childhood (ISAAC) phase I [4]

prevalence in adult populations. There was one in Japan that was a survey of students and employees at two universities. Prevalence ranged from 9.4% for participants in their 20s to 2.5% for participants in their 60s [11] (Fig. 2.3).

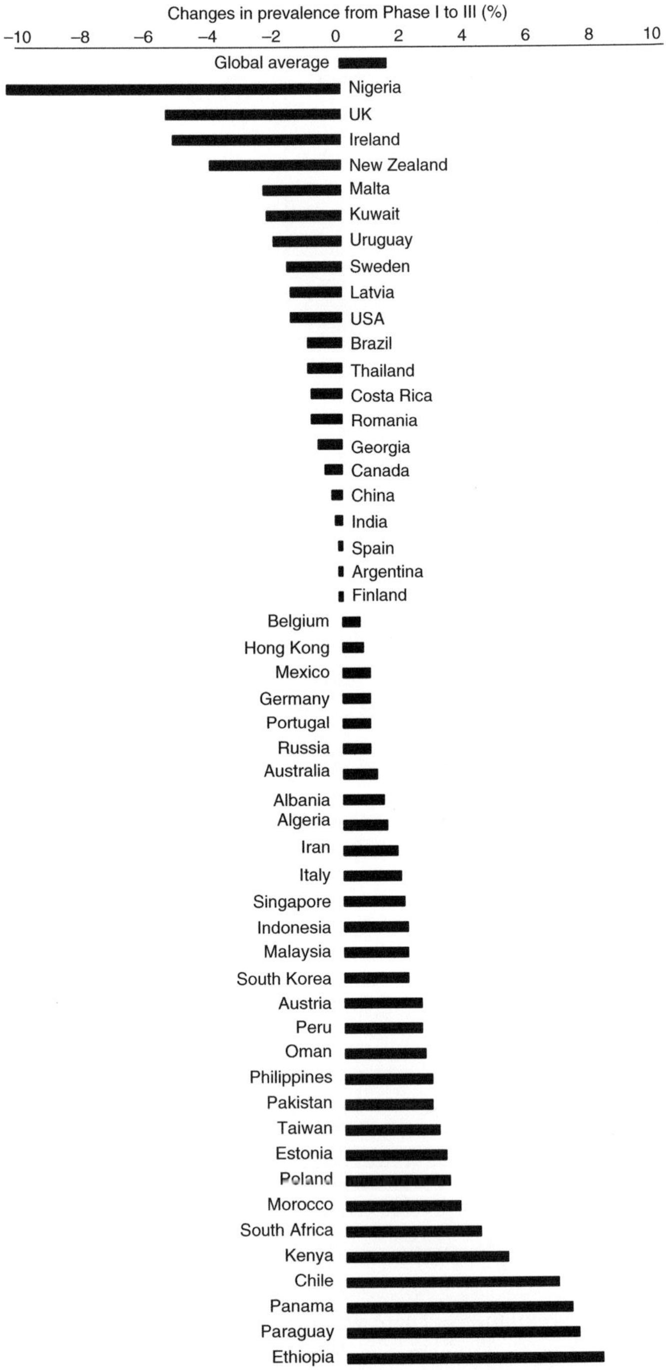

Fig. 2.2 Changes in AD prevalence at age 13–14 years from phase I to III of ISAAC. The numbers were calculated from available data from phases I and III of the study [4, 5]

Table 2.1 AD prevalence as determined by Japanese studies

		6–10 years (%)	12–13 years (%)	14–15 years (%)
1981–1983	Aichi	3.85		1.96
1990	Osaka, questionnaire	19	9.2	9.0
1992	West Japan (11 prefectures, questionnaire)	17.3		
1993	Hirosaki	9	9.2	
1993	Hamamatsu	24.3		
1995	Nagasaki	8.0		
1996	Ibaragi	7.6		
1992–1997	Hiroshima, Asa area	13.7		
2001	Hiroshima	10.9		
2001	Maebashi	9.9		
2002	Isahaya	10.1		
2002	West Japan (11 prefectures, questionnaire)	13.8		
2000–2002	All Japan, eight cities	11.8	10.6	
2005	Tokyo	19.6 (6 years old)	13.6 (12 years old)	10.9 (14 years old)
2012	Web-based study	13.0		

Data are adapted from references [9, 10, 23]

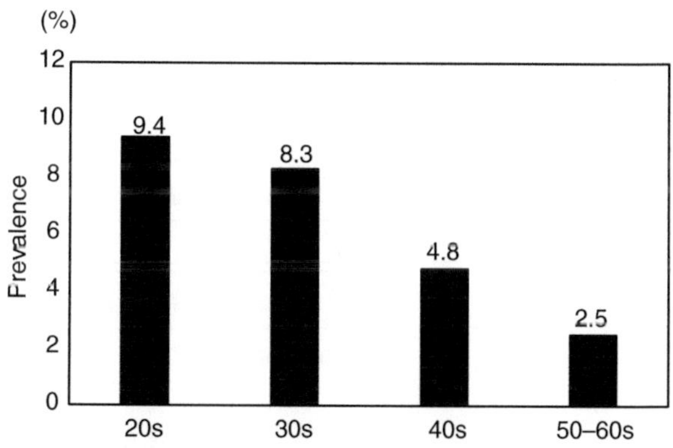

Fig. 2.3 AD prevalence in a Japanese adult population [11]

2.3 The Prevalence of AD Differs Within a Country

Variations in AD prevalence are observed not only between countries but also within countries. This is evident in the ISAAC phase III study [5] (Fig. 2.4) and in Japanese domestic studies (Table 2.1). A number of studies show that the geography and climate influence the development of allergic diseases. Weiland et al. [12] studied AD prevalence in 12 countries in Western Europe and found that it was positively associated with latitude and negatively associated with mean annual outdoor temperature. Different prevalence in regions with distinct climates was also observed within Japan.

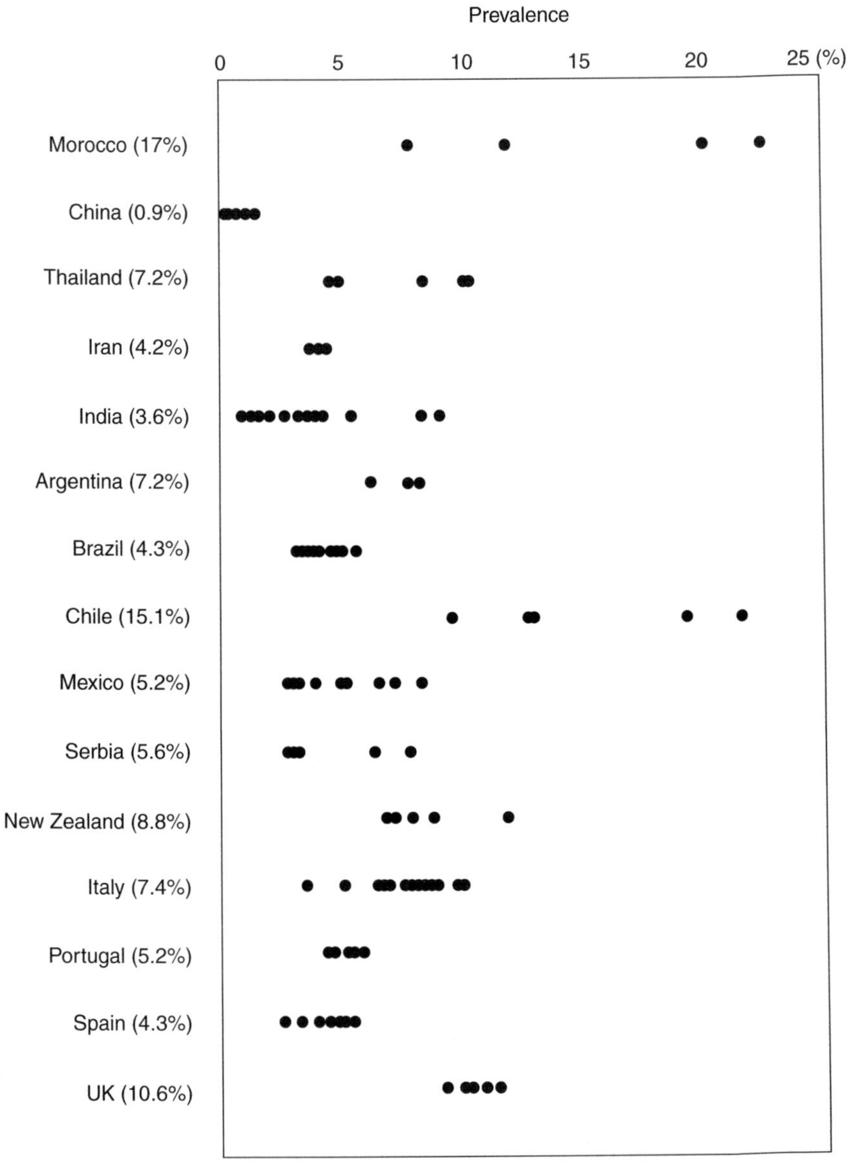

Fig. 2.4 Diversified AD prevalence within countries. Each *black dot* represents a center or a region that participated in the ISAAC study in each country. Countries with more than three centers are depicted. Data were adapted from [5]

While average prevalence of childhood AD in mainland Japan is 12–13%, it drops by half on Ishigaki Island, which is remotely located in a subtropical area of Japan [13] (Fig. 2.5). The comparatively lower rate was also observed in another remote subtropical island, Ogasawara [14] (Fig. 2.5). In Ogasawara, AD prevalence in preschool,

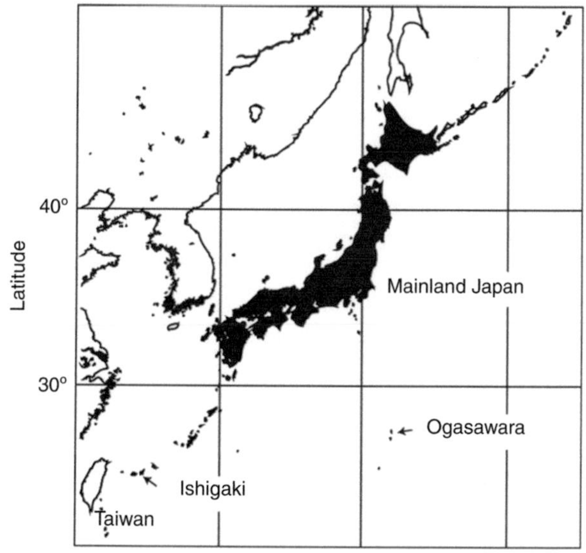

Fig. 2.5 A map of Japan. Ogasawara and Ishigaki islands are located at a similar latitude to Taiwan

elementary school, and junior high school students combined was 4.3%; individual age-group prevalences were 7.1% for preschool, 2.8% for elementary school, and 2.3% for junior high school. The prevalence of AD was evidently lower in Ogasawara Island than in mainland Japan. Both islands are at a similar latitude to Taiwan, where prevalence is also lower than Japan (Fig. 2.1). The lower prevalence in these subtropical islands is consistent with observations in Western Europe [12]. Nevertheless, the possibility cannot be excluded that the lower prevalence in these subtropical islands may be attributed to not only climate conditions such as higher temperature and humidity but also different lifestyles of children there compared to children from other regions of Japan. On the islands, children spend shorter amounts of time inside watching TV and more time exercising outside instead [14].

2.4 The Natural History of Atopic Dermatitis

In general, most children who suffer from AD start presenting skin symptoms within the first months of life. Around 60% of children will outgrow the disease or become free from symptoms before puberty [15–17]. A significant number of patients will sequentially develop other allergic diseases such as allergic rhinitis and asthma. In fact, AD increases the risk of developing asthma to ~50% and the risk of developing allergic rhinitis to as much as 75% [18–20]. This typical sequence of development of allergic diseases during childhood is called "atopic march" [21, 22]. Futamura et al. reported that among 27,389 children aged 6–14 years, 14.0%, 41.6%, and 31.3% of children had symptoms of asthma, allergic rhino-conjunctivitis, and atopic dermatitis, respectively. While 43.1% of the children in this study had more than one of the symptoms during the past 12 months, 2.2% had all three symptoms.

AD affects up to ~20% of children during infancy and early childhood [9, 23]. Understanding of occurrence and progression of infantile atopic dermatitis is based on a cohort study of infants aged 4 months to 3 years reported by the Health and Labour Science Research, from 2006 to 2008, in the cities of Yokohama, Chiba, and Fukuoka. The report shows that 16.2% of ordinary infants who received a medical examination at 4 months of age developed atopic dermatitis. Atopic dermatitis regressed in 50% of the 4-month-old patients before the age of 18 months, indicating an extremely dynamic progression of atopic dermatitis in infancy [24].

AD affects 2–10% of adults (Fig. 2.3) [9, 23], which is much lower than the rates in children (7–19%) (Table 2.1). A hospital-based investigation showed that the number of AD patients gradually decreases from childhood to adolescence and abruptly drops in the fourth decade of life. After that, the prevalence again gradually decreases with age (Fig. 2.6) [23, 25]. A caveat of this data is that investigation took

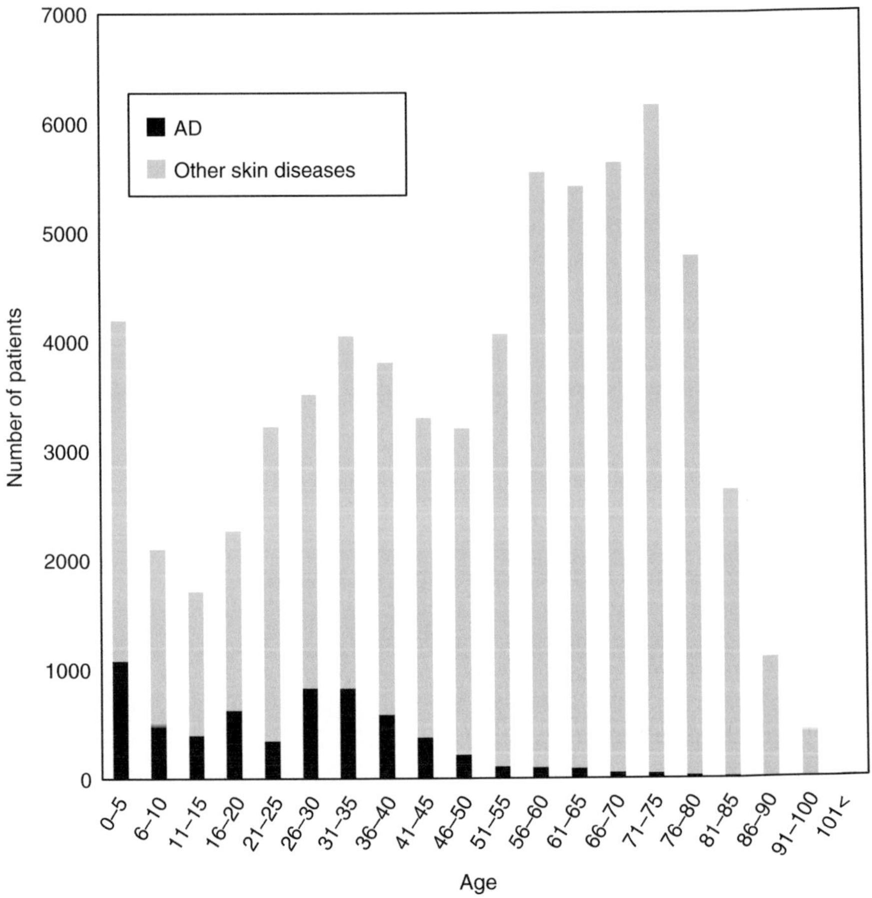

Fig. 2.6 Age distribution of patients in dermatology clinics in Japan [25]. Among 67,448 patients, 6733 were diagnosed with AD

place at clinics or hospitals. Diagnosis was based on direct examination, and therefore it was more reliable than questionnaire-based study, but the reported prevalence is open to influence by behavioral factors; also, the total number of patients who visited hospitals and clinics is inconsistent between age groups (Fig. 2.6).

2.5 Genetic Factors Associated with Childhood Atopic Dermatitis

A number of studies have demonstrated that there is a strong genetic predisposition for AD. Studies in twins clearly imply the presence of genetic effects in the development of AD and allergic diseases [26]. For instance, the pairwise concordance rate of AD in monozygotic twins was significantly higher (72%) than in dizygotic twins (23%) [27]. In addition to twin studies, genetic linkage analysis and association studies have also revealed the genetic background of AD. A notable example is the profilaggrin/filaggrin gene (FLG) [28]. Loss-of-function mutations in FLG account for 40% of the total mutations in AD patients [29]. FLG mutations are found in 10–50% patients with AD [28, 30, 31] and found in 9% of the normal population [29, 31]. The mutation is much more frequent (~50%) in European patients with moderate to severe AD than in Chinese patients (27%) [29]. In Japan, FLG mutations were found in about 27% of AD patients, while the same mutations are found in 3.7% of the general population [32, 33]. In addition to varying frequencies, FLG mutations have a wide spectrum. Mutations found in European AD patients are not common in Japanese patients. Mutations in Japanese patients are different from those of Chinese patients [34]. FLG mutations are likely specific to each population. The different genetic background between different populations might partly account for differences in prevalence between countries. FLG is the most influential gene for developing AD within those identified so far. Nevertheless, the frequency of FLG mutations in mild to moderate AD patients (~15%) is not as high as that in moderate to severe patients (~50%) [35]. This seems to indicate that FLG deficiency alone does not sufficiently explain genetic predisposition toward the disease and that other important genetic or nongenetic factors are involved in disease onset.

2.6 Environmental Factors Associated with Atopic Dermatitis

The fact that the prevalence of AD has sharply increased in modern times implies that nongenetic factors play a major role in AD pathogenesis [6]. A nationwide survey of 28,348 Japanese children using the ISSAC questionnaire found that overall prevalence of AD is 13% in 6–12-year-old children. A higher prevalence of AD is associated with birth during fall or winter, duration of exclusive breastfeeding for at least 6 months, and ownership of a pet from infancy, whereas lower prevalence is associated with a high annual household income and two or more siblings [10]. In addition, climate factors, cold and dry air, microbe exposure, better hygiene, farming environment, broad spectrum antibiotics, urban living, a Western diet, air pollution and tobacco smoke [36], and hard water [37] have all been implicated in the development of AD. Protective factors include UV light, maternal contact with farm animals, consumption of unprocessed milk, helminth infection during pregnancy, high levels of endotoxin exposure in early life, and contact with dogs [36]. Meta-analysis pointed out fairly consistent protective effects of dog exposure in early life, with inconsistent effects for cats [38]. It remains unknown what causes this difference. Nevertheless, it is worth pointing out that children with FLG mutations have a greater risk for AD than those without, when exposed to cats [36].

A mechanism that can bridge a gap between environmental factors and genetic response is epigenetics [39]. Epigenetics is molecular modifications that alter functions of genes without altering DNA sequences [7]. Increasing numbers of studies show emerging links between epigenetics and allergic diseases [39–41]. There is accumulating evidence that epigenetic changes such as DNA methylation, histone modifications, and microRNA activity in response to environmental factors contribute to the pathogenesis of AD [29, 42]. Studying epigenetic mechanisms will help us to understand some aspects of AD epidemiology.

Conclusion

AD is a paradigmatic complex disorder involving gene-gene and gene-environment interactions. Therefore, it is difficult to comprehend global epidemiology. Specifically, differences in AD prevalence between countries and within a country showcase the complex etiology of the disease. Accumulating comprehensive knowledge in epidemiology will provide us with insights into the disease process that will help us target effective treatment modalities.

References

1. Takeuchi S, Esaki H, Furusyo N, Hayashida S, Yamamura K, Tsuji G, et al. Incidence, serum IgE and TARC/CCL17 levels in atopic dermatitis associated with other allergic diseases: an update from the Ishigaki cohort. Acta Derm Venereol. 2015;95(4):480–4. doi:10.2340/00015555-1989.
2. Williams HC. Is the prevalence of atopic dermatitis increasing? Clin Exp Dermatol. 1992;17(6):385–91.
3. Takeuchi M, Ueda H. Increase of adult atopic dermatitis (AD) in recent Japan. Environ Dermatol. 2000;7:133–6.
4. Williams H, Robertson C, Stewart A, Ait-Khaled N, Anabwani G, Anderson R, et al. Worldwide variations in the prevalence of symptoms of atopic eczema in the International Study of Asthma and Allergies in Childhood. J Allergy Clin Immunol. 1999;103(1 Pt 1):125–38.
5. Odhiambo JA, Williams HC, Clayton TO, Robertson CF, Asher MI, Group IPTS. Global variations in prevalence of eczema symptoms in children from ISAAC Phase Three. J Allergy Clin Immunol. 2009;124(6):1251–1258. e23. doi:10.1016/j.jaci.2009.10.009.
6. Takeuchi S, Esaki H, Furue M. Epidemiology of atopic dermatitis in Japan. J Dermatol. 2014;41(3):200–4. doi:10.1111/1346-8138.12331.
7. Williams HC. Epidemiology of atopic dermatitis. Clin Exp Dermatol. 2000;25(7):522–9.
8. Katayama I, Kohno Y, Akiyama K, Aihara M, Kondo N, Saeki H, et al. Japanese guideline for atopic dermatitis 2014. Allergol Int. 2014;63(3):377–98. doi:10.2332/allergolint.14-RAI-0769.

9. Futamura M, Ohya Y, Akashi M, Adachi Y, Odajima H, Akiyama K, et al. Age-related prevalence of allergic diseases in Tokyo school children. Allergol Int. 2011;60(4):509–15. doi:10.2332/allergolint.10-OA-0293.
10. Sasaki M, Yoshida K, Adachi Y, Furukawa M, Itazawa T, Odajima H, et al. Environmental factors associated with childhood eczema: findings from a national web-based survey. Allergol Int. 2016;65(4):420–4. doi:10.1016/j.alit.2016.03.007.
11. Saeki H, Oiso N, Honma M, Iizuka H, Kawada A, Tamaki K. Prevalence of atopic dermatitis in Japanese adults and community validation of the U.K. diagnostic criteria. J Dermatol Sci. 2009;55(2):140–1. doi:10.1016/j.jdermsci.2009.04.004.
12. Weiland SK, Husing A, Strachan DP, Rzehak P, Pearce N, Group IPOS. Climate and the prevalence of symptoms of asthma, allergic rhinitis, and atopic eczema in children. Occup Environ Med. 2004;61(7):609–15.
13. Hamada M, Furusyo N, Urabe K, Morita K, Nakahara T, Kinukawa N, et al. Prevalence of atopic dermatitis and serum IgE values in nursery school children in Ishigaki Island, Okinawa. Jpn J Dermatol. 2005;32(4):248–55.
14. Okada Y, Kumagai H, Morikawa Y, Akasawa A. Epidemiology of pediatric allergic diseases in the Ogasawara Islands. Allergol Int. 2016;65(1):37–43. doi:10.1016/j.alit.2015.06.010.
15. Garmhausen D, Hagemann T, Bieber T, Dimitriou I, Fimmers R, Diepgen T, et al. Characterization of different courses of atopic dermatitis in adolescent and adult patients. Allergy. 2013;68(4):498–506. doi:10.1111/all.12112.
16. Bieber T. Atopic dermatitis. N Engl J Med. 2008;358(14):1483–94. doi:10.1056/NEJMra074081.
17. Rystedt I. Long term follow-up in atopic dermatitis. Acta Derm Venereol Suppl (Stockh). 1985;114:117–20.
18. van der Hulst AE, Klip H, Brand PL. Risk of developing asthma in young children with atopic eczema: a systematic review. J Allergy Clin Immunol. 2007;120(3):565–9. doi:10.1016/j.jaci.2007.05.042.
19. Thomsen SF. Epidemiology and natural history of atopic diseases. Eur Clin Respir J. 2015;2 doi:10.3402/ecrj.v2.24642.
20. Spergel JM, Paller AS. Atopic dermatitis and the atopic march. J Allergy Clin Immunol. 2003;112(6 Suppl):S118–27. doi:10.1016/j.jaci.2003.09.033.
21. Dharmage SC, Lowe AJ, Matheson MC, Burgess JA, Allen KJ, Abramson MJ. Atopic dermatitis and the atopic march revisited. Allergy. 2014;69(1):17–27. doi:10.1111/all.12268.
22. Spergel JM. From atopic dermatitis to asthma: the atopic march. Ann Allergy Asthma Immunol. 2010;105(2):99–106; quiz 7–9, 17. doi:10.1016/j.anai.2009.10.002.
23. Furue M, Chiba T, Takeuchi S. Current status of atopic dermatitis in Japan. Asia Pac Allergy 2011;1(2):64–72. doi:10.5415/apallergy.2011.1.2.64.
24. Kohno Y. Identification of causative and exacerbation factors of atopic dermatitis and studies for improvement of living environment to prevent the development and exacerbation of symptoms. Reports of Research on Allergic Disease and Immunology. Ministry of Health, Labour and Welfare of Japan 2006–2007. 2008:173–7.
25. Furue M, Yamazaki S, Jimbow K, Tsuchida T, Amagai M, Tanaka T, et al. Prevalence of dermatological disorders in Japan: a nationwide, cross-sectional, seasonal, multicenter, hospital-based study. J Dermatol. 2011;38(4):310–20. doi:10.1111/j.1346-8138.2011.01209.x.
26. Thomsen SF. The contribution of twin studies to the understanding of the aetiology of asthma and atopic diseases. Eur Clin Respir J. 2015;2:27803. doi:10.3402/ecrj.v2.27803.
27. Schultz LF. Atopic dermatitis: a genetic-epidemiologic study in a population-based twin sample. J Am Acad Dermatol. 1993;28(5 Pt 1):719–23.
28. Palmer CN, Irvine AD, Terron-Kwiatkowski A, Zhao Y, Liao H, Lee SP, et al. Common loss-of-function variants of the epidermal barrier protein filaggrin are a major predisposing factor for atopic dermatitis. Nat Genet. 2006;38(4):441–6. doi:10.1038/ng1767.
29. Kim JE, Kim JS, Cho DH, Park HJ. Molecular mechanisms of cutaneous inflammatory disorder: atopic dermatitis. Int J Mol Sci. 2016;17(8):E1234. doi:10.3390/ijms17081234.
30. Leung DY. Our evolving understanding of the functional role of filaggrin in atopic dermatitis. J Allergy Clin Immunol. 2009;124(3):494–5. doi:10.1016/j.jaci.2009.07.041.

31. Henderson J, Northstone K, Lee SP, Liao H, Zhao Y, Pembrey M, et al. The burden of disease associated with filaggrin mutations: a population-based, longitudinal birth cohort study. J Allergy Clin Immunol. 2008;121(4):872–877. e9. doi:10.1016/j.jaci.2008.01.026.
32. Nemoto-Hasebe I, Akiyama M, Nomura T, Sandilands A, McLean WH, Shimizu H. FLG mutation p.Lys4021X in the C-terminal imperfect filaggrin repeat in Japanese patients with atopic eczema. Br J Dermatol. 2009;161(6):1387–90. doi:10.1111/j.1365-2133.2009.09406.x.
33. Osawa R, Akiyama M, Shimizu H. Filaggrin gene defects and the risk of developing allergic disorders. Allergol Int. 2011;60(1):1–9. doi:10.2332/allergolint.10-RAI-0270.
34. Akiyama M. FLG mutations in ichthyosis vulgaris and atopic eczema: spectrum of mutations and population genetics. Br J Dermatol. 2010;162(3):472–7. doi:10.1111/j.1365-2133.2009.09582.x.
35. Brown SJ, McLean WH. Eczema genetics: current state of knowledge and future goals. J Invest Dermatol. 2009;129(3):543–52. doi:10.1038/jid.2008.413.
36. Flohr C, Mann J. New insights into the epidemiology of childhood atopic dermatitis. Allergy. 2014;69(1):3–16. doi:10.1111/all.12270.
37. Perkin MR, Craven J, Logan K, Strachan D, Marrs T, Radulovic S, et al. Association between domestic water hardness, chlorine, and atopic dermatitis risk in early life: a population-based cross-sectional study. J Allergy Clin Immunol. 2016;138(2):509–16. doi:10.1016/j.jaci.2016.03.031.
38. Langan SM, Flohr C, Williams HC. The role of furry pets in eczema: a systematic review. Arch Dermatol. 2007;143(12):1570–7. doi:10.1001/archderm.143.12.1570.
39. Sabounchi S, Bollyky J, Nadeau K. Review of environmental impact on the epigenetic regulation of atopic diseases. Curr Allergy Asthma Rep. 2015;15(6):33. doi:10.1007/s11882-015-0533-1.
40. Tan TH, Ellis JA, Saffery R, Allen KJ. The role of genetics and environment in the rise of childhood food allergy. Clin Exp Allergy. 2012;42(1):20–9. doi:10.1111/j.1365-2222.2011.03823.x.
41. Liang Y, Chang C, Lu Q. The genetics and epigenetics of atopic dermatitis-filaggrin and other polymorphisms. Clin Rev Allergy Immunol. 2016;51(3):315–28. doi:10.1007/s12016-015-8508-5.
42. Bin L, Leung DY. Genetic and epigenetic studies of atopic dermatitis. Allergy Asthma Clin Immunol. 2016;12:52. doi:10.1186/s13223-016-0158-5.

Epidemiology of Childhood AD in Asian Countries

3

Yasuyuki Sumikawa

Abstract

There have been many reported studies regarding the prevalence of childhood atopic dermatitis in Asia. The first large-scale worldwide investigation was the ISAAC Phase I study reported by Williams et al., who reported that the prevalence of atopic dermatitis in Asian countries, except for Japan, is lower than that of European countries. Moreover, they showed that symptoms of atopic eczema exhibit wide variations in prevalence both within and between countries inhabited by similar ethnic groups; they thus suggested that environmental factors may be critical for disease expression. These factors may be partially explained by "hygiene hypothesis," which suggests that infections, especially during childhood, can protect against allergic diseases. This indicates that the clean environment in developed countries promotes the increase of allergic diseases such as atopic dermatitis.

In recent years, Asian countries have been rapidly developing. The aim of this chapter it is to report the transition of prevalence of atopic dermatitis among children (age 6–15 years) in Asian countries. The previously reported data indicate that the prevalence rate in the Asia-Pacific region is high and increasing, in the Eastern Mediterranean area is low and increasing, and in the South Asia region is low and has not changed.

Keywords

Atopic dermatitis • Prevalence • Childhood • Asia

Y. Sumikawa
Department of Dermatology, School of Medicine, Sapporo Medical University, 060-8556 S1W16, Chuo-ku, Sapporo city, Hokkaido, Japan
e-mail: y.sumikawa@sapmed.ac.jp

I. Katayama et al. (eds.), *Evolution of Atopic Dermatitis in the 21st Century*, https://doi.org/10.1007/978-981-10-5541-6_3

3.1 Introduction

There have been many reported studies regarding the prevalence of childhood atopic dermatitis in Asia. The first large-scale worldwide investigation was the ISAAC Phase I study reported by Williams et al., who reported that the prevalence of atopic dermatitis in Asian countries, except for Japan, is lower than that in European countries [1]. Moreover, they showed that symptoms of atopic eczema exhibit wide variations in prevalence both within and between countries inhabited by similar ethnic groups; they thus suggested that environmental factors may be critical for disease expression. These factors may be partially explained by Strachan's "hygiene hypothesis," which suggests that infections, especially during childhood, can protect against allergic diseases [2]. This indicates that the clean environment in developed countries promotes the increased prevalence of allergic diseases such as atopic dermatitis. The ISAAC Phase I study showed that the prevalence of atopic dermatitis in Japan is higher than that in other countries; this may be explained by the hygiene hypothesis.

In recent years, Asian countries have been rapidly developing. The aim of this chapter it is to report the transition of prevalence of atopic dermatitis among children (age 6–15 years) in Asian countries. The prevalence has been reported in three ways: lifetime prevalence rate, 12-month prevalence rate, and prevalence rate of physician-diagnosed eczema. To allow for comparison between studies, the 12-month prevalence rate and prevalence rate of physician-diagnosed of eczema were applied in this review because these rates exclude infantile eczema.

3.2 Prevalence of Atopic Dermatitis in Asian Countries

3.2.1 China

Some studies have reported the prevalence of atopic dermatitis in China. For instance, the ISAAC Phase I study reported a prevalence rate in 1995 of 1.2% among children aged 13–14 years [1]. The ISAAC Phase III study reported a rate of 0.9% in 2001 in the same age group [3]. In addition, Wang et al. reported prevalence rates in the same age group of 1.3% in 1994–1995 and 2.2% in 2001 [4]. A 2016 report showed that the prevalence rate was 10.39% among children aged 6–7 years in many parts of China [5]. The prevalence rate of our survey in Yixing (between Nanjing and Shanghai), China, in 2005 was 2.63% among children in this age group [6]. In particular, in Lhasa (the central city of Tibet), the prevalence rate was 0%. A similar result (0.2%) was reported in the ISAAC Phase III study in 2001. These data suggest that the environment of Tibet may provide clues regarding the prevention of atopic dermatitis.

The above data indicate that until around 2005, the prevalence of atopic dermatitis in China was very low, but increased rapidly from 2005 to 2016. This timeline is consistent with the rapid development of the economy of China over the same period, suggesting that factors associated with the rapid economic growth may have contributed to the increase in the prevalence of atopic dermatitis. However, China includes peoples of various racial backgrounds, socioeconomic statuses, and customs and has a variable climate. Thus, to better understand the increasing prevalence of atopic dermatitis, there is a need for more investigations among the same group or groups.

3.2.2 Taiwan

There are several studies that have investigated the prevalence of atopic dermatitis in Taiwan. The ISAAC Phase I study reported prevalence rates in 1995 of 3.5% and 1.4% among children aged 6–7 and 13–14 years, respectively [1]. In contrast, the ISAAC Phase III study reported rates in 2001–2002 of 7.5% and 4.2% among the same age groups, respectively [3]. Furthermore, Lee et al. reported that rates among children aged 12–15 years were 2.4% in 1995–1996 and 4.0% in 2001 [7]. They suggested that the increase was due to changes in the indoor environment, such as temperature and humidity, but that these factors were not major contributors to the observed increase. Additionally, Liao et al. reported prevalence rates of 1.1% in 1987, 1.9% in 1994, and 3.4% in 2002 among children aged 6–15 years, representing an increase of 3.05-fold over the previous 15 years [8]. They suggested that the increased prevalence of atopic eczema may be due to a decline in breast-feeding, the early introduction of weaning foods, and the widespread use of food additives. They also reported that atopic dermatitis is more prevalent in higher social classes and that rapid urbanization, including a more westernized lifestyle and a higher standard of living and education, may explain the rapid increase of atopic dermatitis. Finally, Yan et al. reported prevalence rates in 1994–1995 and 2001–2002 of 1.4% and 4.1%, respectively [9], in children aged 13–14 years, thus showing the same tendency toward an increasing prevalence rate between 1994 and 2002. However, more recent data regarding the prevalence rate are unavailable;, thus, there is a need for further investigations.

3.2.3 Korea

There are several studies that have investigated the prevalence of atopic dermatitis in Korea. The ISAAC Phase I study reported prevalence rates in 1995 of 8.8% and 3.8% among children aged 6–7 and 13–14 years, respectively [1]. The ISAAC Phase III study reported rates in 2001 of 11.3% and 5.7% in the same age groups, respectively [3]. Moreover, Oh et al. reported prevalence rates among children aged 6–12 years of 7.3% in 1994–1995 and 10.7% in 2001–2002 and among children aged 12–15 years of 3.5% and 6.1%, respectively [10]. In contrast, the same study reported the prevalence rate of food allergy was not significantly different from 1995 to 2000, indicating a poor correlation between the prevalence of atopic dermatitis and that of food allergy. Furthermore, in 1994–1995, Kim et al. reported prevalence rates of atopic dermatitis of 17.5% for urban, 9.6% for rural, and 4.0% for industrial areas among children aged 6–8 years; among children aged 10–12 years, these rates were 6.7%, 6.5%, and 3.5%, respectively [11]. The total prevalence rate for children aged 16–18 years was 6.0%. Using national statistics, including hospital- and clinic-based clinical information, Yu et al. reported that the prevalence rates from 2003 to 2008 decreased from 4.2 to 4.0%, respectively [12]. These data suggest that the prevalence rate in Korea peaked after 2008. In contrast, Kim et al. reported prevalence rates in 2009 on Jeju Island (off the coast of Korea) of 11.9% among children aged 6–9 years and 7.5% among those aged 9–12 years, with a total prevalence rate of 9.5% [13]. Moreover, Hong et al. reported prevalence rates in 2010 of 16.7% and 14.5% among children aged 7–9 and 10–13 years, respectively, and that the treatment frequency was 13.2% and 11.4%, respectively [14]. The lower treatment rates suggest that atopic dermatitis patients, especially those with mild disease, do not visit the hospitals or the clinics for treatment. This illustrates that medical institution-based surveys may have a limitation in that they may underestimate the prevalence rate of atopic dermatitis.

3.2.4 Singapore

In Singapore, controversial findings regarding the prevalence of atopic dermatitis have been reported. The ISAAC Phase I reported prevalence rates in 1995 of 2.8% and 3.4% among children aged 6–7 and 13–14 years, respectively [1]. In contrast, the ISAAC Phase III study reported rates of 8.9% and 9.2% among the same age groups, respectively [3]. Tay et al. reported rates of 22.7%, 17.9%, and 21.5% in children aged 7, 12, and 16 years, respectively [15]. They also reported high prevalence rates of allergic rhinitis and asthma. They concluded that the reason for the high prevalence rate of atopic dermatitis may be the rapid urbanization of the city state of Singapore, its westernized lifestyle, and a high standard of living and education. Goh et al. reported prevalence rates in 1994 of 8.8% and 9.5% among children aged 6–12 and 12–15 years, respectively [16]. In contrast, Wang et al. reported prevalence rates in 2001 of 11.0% and 11.6% in the same age groups, respectively [17], indicating that the prevalence rate in Singapore was increasing. As a more recent rate has not been reported, there is a need for further investigations.

3.2.5 Malaysia

Only one study regarding the prevalence of atopic dermatitis has been reported in Malaysia. The ISAAC Phase I study reported prevalence rates in 1995 of 8.5% and 8.0% among children aged 6–7 and 13–14 years, respectively [1]. The ISAAC Phase III study reported rates in 2001–2002 of 12.6% and 9.9% among the same age groups, respectively [3]. In addition, Quah et al. reported rates in 1995 of 14.0% and 12.1% among the same age groups, respectively; they also reported rates in 2001 of 17.6% and 13.4%, respectively. They discussed that, except for atopic dermatitis, there were no major changes in the symptoms of asthma and allergic diseases in this community between 1995 and 2001. This indicates that air pollution, which induces asthma, may not be important for inducing atopic dermatitis.

3.2.6 Thailand

There are several studies that have investigated the prevalence of atopic dermatitis in Thailand. For instance, the ISAAC Phase I study reported prevalence rates in 1995 of 11.9% and 8.2% among children aged 6–7 and 13–14 years, respectively [1]. In contrast, the ISAAC Phase III study reported rates of 15.6% and 9.9% among the same age groups, respectively, indicating that the prevalence rate in Singapore increased over this period [3]. As a more recent rate has not been reported, there is a need for further investigations.

3.2.7 India

There are few studies reporting the prevalence of atopic dermatitis in India. The ISAAC Phase I study reported prevalence rates in 1997 of 2.7% and 3.8% among children aged 6–7 and 13–14 years, respectively [1]. The ISAAC Phase III study reported rates in 2001–2003 among the same age groups, respectively [3]; however, because of an expansive national territory with various climate and customs, the variability of the prevalence rate in each city is very large. For example, prevalence rates in 2001–2003 among children aged 6–7 years ranged from 0.9% to 6.2%. In addition, Grills et al. reported a prevalence rate of dermatological disease in north India of 9.2% among all ages [18], though the rate among children was not reported. Interestingly, their report also showed a high prevalence rate of both atopic dermatitis and skin infectious disease. This result disagrees with the hygiene hypothesis. However, in India, owing to the scarce data, it is difficult to evaluate trends regarding the prevalence of atopic dermatitis, thus more nationwide investigations are needed.

3.2.8 Iran

There are few studies reporting the prevalence of atopic dermatitis in Iran. The ISAAC Phase I study reported prevalence rates in 1997 of 1.1% and 2.6% among children aged 6–7 and 13–14 years, respectively [1]. The ISAAC Phase III study reported rates of 3.2% and 4.2% in 2001–2003 among the same age groups, respectively [3]. Furthermore, Farajzadeh et al. reported rates in 2009–2010 of 13.5% and 8.3% among children aged 2–7 and 7–12 years, respectively [19]; however, this survey was conducted in Kerman, a desert area, where a low prevalence was expected. In other non-desert areas of Iran, the prevalence rate was 2.1% among children aged 6–12 years in Shahrekord (a city in southwest Iran) and 3.9% among children aged 7–11 years in Ahwaz (a city in southern Iran). These data suggest that prevalence was high in the desert area. The authors provided the following explanation. First, Kerman has a special geographic condition as it is located near Kavir Loot, one of the largest desert areas in Iran. In addition, Kerman has dry, sunny, and hot weather in contrast to the hot and humid weather of Ahwaz. Second, low humidity has a demonstrated effect on exacerbating and provoking atopic dermatitis. In contrast, indoor relative humidity is negatively associated with eczema symptoms. Third, furthermore, the ethnic origin of the population of Kerman is mainly Persian, whereas in Ahwaz, it is mainly Semitic.

3.2.9 Kuwait

Only one study regarding the prevalence of atopic dermatitis has been reported in Kuwait. Based on the ISAAC study, Owayed et al. reported prevalence rates of in 1995–1996 and 2001–2002 of 11.3% and 12.8%, respectively, among children aged 13–14 years, suggesting that the prevalence rate was high and did not increase [20].

3.3 The Prevalence of Atopic Dermatitis in Asian Regions

The ISAAC study reported prevalence rates for each region in Asia as detailed below.

3.3.1 Asia-Pacific Region

In the Asia-Pacific region, the ISAAC Phase I study reported a prevalence rate for atopic dermatitis in 1997 of 8.2% and 4.6% among children aged 6–7 and 13–14 years, respectively [1]. The ISAAC Phase III study reported rates of 10.1% and 5.3% among the same age groups, respectively [3].

3.3.2 Eastern Mediterranean Region

In the Eastern Mediterranean region, the ISAAC Phase I study reported prevalence rates for atopic dermatitis in 1997 of 2.9% and 6.5% among children aged 6–7 and 13–14 years, respectively [1]. The ISAAC Phase III study reported rates in 2001–2003 of 4.8% and 6.3% among the same age groups, respectively [3].

3.3.3 South Asia Region

In the South Asia region, the ISAAC Phase I study reported prevalence rates of atopic dermatitis in 1997 of 2.7% and 3.6% among children aged 6–7 and 13–14 years, respectively [1]. The ISAAC Phase III study reported rates of 3.0% and 3.8% among the same age groups, respectively [3].

The above data indicate that the prevalence rate in the Asia-Pacific region is high and increasing, in the Eastern Mediterranean area is low and increasing, and in the South Asia region is low and has not changed.

3.3.4 Tibet

The prevalence rate of atopic dermatitis is very low in Tibet (0–0.2%) [3, 6], suggesting that the Tibetan environment includes factors that help avoid development of atopic dermatitis. We have previously investigated and reported the prevalence of atopic dermatitis and evaluated skin barrier function by measurement of trans-epidermal water loss (TEWL) and capacitance in Chinese and Japanese school students. In addition, we conducted a survey regarding bathing customs, as these might influence the prevalence of atopic dermatitis symptoms as well as skin barrier function. We found that the values of TEWL, bath frequency, and prevalence of atopic dermatitis in Lhasa were 6.78 L/m^3/h, 2.2/month, and 0%, respectively. The corresponding values were 7.35 L/m^3/h, 6.4/week, and 2.63%, respectively, in Yixing and 10.3 L/m^3/h, 7.7/week, and 4.26%, respectively, in Nishinomiya [6].

3.4 Skin Barrier Function and Atopic Dermatitis

Two hypotheses have been proposed concerning the mechanism underlying degradation of the skin barrier function that is clinically observed in atopic dermatitis. The "inside-outside" hypothesis is that inflammation in skin destroys the stratum corneum and decreases barrier function [21]. On the other hand, the "outside-inside" hypothesis is that xeroderma exists first and leads to decreased barrier function of the skin, thus exacerbating inflammatory skin diseases such as atopic dermatitis [22]. According to the outside-inside hypothesis, it has been reported that mouse keratinocytes, obtained from skin that had undergone physical destruction of the barrier function, secrete cytokines such as tumor necrosis factor-α, which induces inflammation [23]. Based on this hypothesis, evaluation of the barrier function of the stratum corneum has been tried as an approach to analyze the condition of a patient with atopic dermatitis.

However, noninvasive methods such as those used to measure TEWL or capacitance to evaluate skin barrier function are commonly used [24]. An increase in TEWL has been observed in atopic dermatitis patients with skin eruptions as well as those with normal skin [25]. On the other hand, it has been reported that capacitance decreases in atopic dermatitis patients with xerosis but not in those without clinical xerosis [26]. This suggests that capacitance can be used to evaluate the presence of clinical xerosis. A previous report showed that TEWL and capacitance are related to the clinical score of atopic dermatitis [27]. These reports support that methods used to measure TEWL and capacitance are useful to analyze the condition of atopic dermatitis patients.

A previous report showed high TEWL and low capacitance in atopic dermatitis patients compared to healthy volunteers in the dorsum manus, medial forearm, and back [28]. Accordingly, in a study conducted by us, we measured TEWL and capacitance only at the medial forearm. When comparing first graders of Nishinomiya, Japan; Yixing, China; and Lhasa, Tibet, we revealed the tendency for TEWL to increase with the prevalence of atopic dermatitis. Moreover, there was a relationship between the increased TEWL induced by skin barrier dysfunction and the onset or aggravation of atopic dermatitis. However, owing to the low TEWL, skin barrier function seems to have been preserved, and there were no first graders with atopic dermatitis among those in Lhasa. Generally, in Japan it was thought that atopic dermatitis is exacerbated in winter because of drying; nevertheless, Tibet is always dry, but there were no students with atopic dermatitis.

Accordingly, living in a dry environment per se might not be essential for the onset of atopic dermatitis but might be an exacerbation factor. Previously, it was thought that the recommended conditions for measurement of TEWL and capacitance should be a temperature lower than 22 °C and humidity from 40 to 60% [29]. However, our previous study was limited in that it was impossible to control for environmental conditions; notwithstanding, this study established data for comparison in future investigations in which we can observe changes by measuring TEWL and capacitance annually.

3.5 Factors Concerning Development of Atopic Dermatitis

3.5.1 Socioeconomic Conditions

The worldwide prevalence of atopic dermatitis varies by country and age group, with a higher prevalence in wealthy developed nations compared to poorer developing nations. In Asia, it seems that the prevalence rate increases in proportion to the per capita gross domestic product.

McFadden postulates the "hapten-atopy" hypothesis wherein increased hapten and irritant chemical exposure during periods when there is already a natural tendency to T helper cell-2 immunological bias (such as occurs during maternal pregnancy and the first year of life) contributes to the subsequent development of atopic disease in the children [30]. He reports that between 1959 and 1976, there was a 250% global increase in the sale of toiletries, most of which was in industrialized countries, which also experienced a large increase in atopic diseases. These results suggest that habits regarding toiletry use may promote atopic dermatitis in industrialized and developed countries. In addition, this may explain the increase in the prevalence rate in accordance with per capita gross domestic product.

3.5.2 Climate

Atopic dermatitis also seems to be influenced by climate. However, it is controversial whether high or low temperature and whether high or low humidity is the exacerbating factor. Generally, low temperature and low humidity promote dry skin, which is essential for development of atopic dermatitis. In Japan, atopic dermatitis is exacerbated among most people in winter. Uenishi et al. examined the seasonal exacerbation of atopic dermatitis using a questionnaire in patients visiting an outpatient clinic [31]. They showed that the overall incidence of exacerbation in spring, summer, autumn, and winter were 25%, 19%, 11%, and 36%, respectively. However, Masuda reported in 1967 that the incidence of exacerbation in spring, summer, autumn, and winter was 22%, 38%, 13%, and 34%, respectively [32], thus showing a discrepancy in the summer rate. Uenishi et al. explained this discrepancy by a change of attitude toward the more frequent use of soap for bathing. This indicated that the high prevalence of atopic dermatitis in southeastern Asia will decrease in accordance with improvements in living standards, such as improved bathing habits.

On the other hand, in Tibet, which has cold and dry conditions, the prevalence of atopic dermatitis is very low. To test the hypothesis that skin barrier function and bathing habits influence the prevalence of atopic dermatitis, a study examined skin barrier function, bathing frequency, and prevalence of atopic dermatitis among children in Lhasa, Yixing, and Nishinomiya [6]. Surprisingly, as reported above, bathing frequency was lowest in Lhasa, yet the skin barrier function evaluated by TEWL was highest in Lhasa. At face value, these data indicate that bathing worsens rather than improves the prevalence of atopic dermatitis.

This apparent discrepancy can be explained on the basis of climate as follows. In hot and humid conditions, frequent bathing prevents development of atopic dermatitis by washing away sweat. In contrast, in cold and dry conditions, frequent bathing further dries the skin and induces atopic dermatitis. As bathing habits in Asian countries have not been well investigated, further research is needed.

3.5.3 House Dust Mites

House dust mites are well known as an exacerbating factor for atopic dermatitis. House dust mites increase when humidity rises above 60%, but do not survive in humidity below 50% [33]. In Lhasa, where the humidity was below 50%, no house dust mites were detected in the living room. This may help to explain why the prevalence of atopic dermatitis in Lhasa is very low. However, other reports refute this hypothesis. For example, Farajzadeh et al. reported that the prevalence rate of atopic dermatitis in desert areas is higher than that in high humidity areas [19]. Moreover, Parthasaradhi et al. reported that the prevalence rate of atopic dermatitis in Saudi Arabia, which is primarily a desert area, was 8.3%, which is relatively high [34]. These reports indicate that atopic dermatitis can develop in low humidity conditions, where house dust mites do not live. This further suggests that house dust mites are not necessary for development of atopic dermatitis.

Conclusion

These epidemiological data suggest various environmental causes of atopic dermatitis. Further research will be the key to resolve the various questions surrounding atopic dermatitis.

References

1. Williams H, Robertson C, Stewart A, Ait-Khaled N, Anabwani G, Anderson R, et al. Worldwide variations in the prevalence of symptoms of atopic eczema in the International Study of Asthma and Allergies in Childhood. J Allergy Clin Immunol. 1999;103(1 Pt 1):125–38. S0091674999000139 [pii]
2. Strachan DP. Family size, infection and atopy: the first decade of the "hygiene hypothesis". Thorax. 2000;55(Suppl 1):S2–10.
3. Odhiambo JA, Williams HC, Clayton TO, Robertson CF, Asher MI. Global variations in prevalence of eczema symptoms in children from ISAAC Phase Three. J Allergy Clin Immunol. 2009;124(6):1251–8 e23. doi:10.1016/j.jaci.2009.10.009. S0091-6749(09)01535-8 [pii]
4. Wang HY, Zheng JP, Zhong NS. Time trends in the prevalence of asthma and allergic diseases over 7 years among adolescents in Guangzhou city. Zhonghua Yi Xue Za Zhi. 2006;86(15):1014–20.
5. Guo Y, Li P, Tang J, Han X, Zou X, Xu G, et al. Prevalence of atopic dermatitis in Chinese children aged 1–7 ys. Sci Rep. 2016;6:29751. doi:10.1038/srep29751. srep29751 [pii]
6. Sumikawa Y, Ueki Y, Miyoshi A, Cheng L, Yin M, Shi HB, et al. Survey of atopic dermatitis and skin barrier functions in Japanese and Chinese school students. Arerugi. 2007;56(10):1270–5. 056101270e [pii]
7. Lee YL, Li CW, Sung FC, Guo YL. Increasing prevalence of atopic eczema in Taiwanese adolescents from 1995 to 2001. Clin Exp Allergy. 2007;37(4):543–51. doi:10.1111/j.1365-2222.2007.02690.x. CEA2690 [pii]
8. Liao PF, Sun HL, Lu KH, Lue KH. Prevalence of childhood allergic diseases in central Taiwan over the past 15 years. Pediatr Neonatol. 2009;50(1):18–25. doi:10.1016/S1875-9572(09)60025-5. S1875-9572(09)60025-5 [pii]
9. Yan DC, Ou LS, Tsai TL, Wu WF, Huang JL. Prevalence and severity of symptoms of asthma, rhinitis, and eczema in 13- to 14-year-old children in Taipei, Taiwan. Ann Allergy Asthma Immunol. 2005;95(6):579–85. doi:10.1016/S1081-1206(10)61022-8. S1081-1206(10)61022-8 [pii]
10. Oh JW, Pyun BY, Choung JT, Ahn KM, Kim CH, Song SW, et al. Epidemiological change of atopic dermatitis and food allergy in school-aged children in Korea between 1995 and 2000. J Korean Med Sci. 2004;19(5):716–23. doi:10.3346/jkms.2004.19.5.716. 200410716 [pii]
11. Kim CW, Park CJ, Kim JW, Koo DW, Kim KW, Kim TY. Prevalence of atopic dermatitis in Korea. Acta Derm Venereol. 2000;80(5):353–6.
12. Yu JS, Lee CJ, Lee HS, Kim J, Han Y, Ahn K, et al. Prevalence of atopic dermatitis in Korea: analysis by using national statistics. J Korean Med Sci. 2012;27(6):681–5. doi:10.3346/jkms.2012.27.6.681.
13. Kim DS, Lee JH, Lee KH, Lee MG. Prevalence and severity of atopic dermatitis in Jeju Island: a cross-sectional study of 4,028 Korean elementary schoolchildren by physical examination utilizing the three-item severity score. Acta Derm Venereol. 2012;92(5):472–4. doi:10.2340/00015555-1410.
14. Hong S, Son DK, Lim WR, Kim SH, Kim H, Yum HY, et al. The prevalence of atopic dermatitis, asthma, and allergic rhinitis and the comorbidity of allergic diseases in children. Environ Health Toxicol. 2012;27:e2012006. doi:10.5620/eht.2012.27.e2012006.
15. Tay YK, Kong KH, Khoo L, Goh CL, Giam YC. The prevalence and descriptive epidemiology of atopic dermatitis in Singapore school children. Br J Dermatol. 2002;146(1):101–6. 4566 [pii]
16. Goh DY, Chew FT, Quek SC, Lee BW. Prevalence and severity of asthma, rhinitis, and eczema in Singapore school children. Arch Dis Child. 1996;74(2):131–5.
17. Wang XS, Tan TN, Shek LP, Chng SY, Hia CP, Ong NB, et al. The prevalence of asthma and allergies in Singapore; data from two ISAAC surveys seven years apart. Arch Dis Child. 2004;89(5):423–6.

18. Grills N, Grills C, Spelman T, Stoove M, Hellard M, El-Hayek C, et al. Prevalence survey of dermatological conditions in mountainous north India. Int J Dermatol. 2012;51(5):579–87. doi:10.1111/j.1365-4632.2011.05131.x.
19. Farajzadeh S, Esfandiarpour I, Sedaghatmanesh M, Saviz M. Epidemiology and clinical features of atopic dermatitis in Kerman, a desert area of Iran. Ann Dermatol. 2014;26(1):26–34. doi:10.5021/ad.2014.26.1.26.
20. Owayed A, Behbehani N, Al-Momen J. Changing prevalence of asthma and allergic diseases among Kuwaiti children. An ISAAC Study (Phase III). Med Princ Pract. 2008;17(4):284–9. doi:10.1159/000129607. 000129607 [pii]
21. Leung DY. Atopic dermatitis: new insights and opportunities for therapeutic intervention. J Allergy Clin Immunol. 2000;105(5):860–76. doi:10.1067/mai.2000.106484. S0091-6749(00)80006-8 [pii]
22. Elias PM, Wood LC, Feingold KR. Epidermal pathogenesis of inflammatory dermatoses. Am J Contact Dermat. 1999;10(3):119–26. S1046199X99000160 [pii]
23. Wood LC, Jackson SM, Elias PM, Grunfeld C, Feingold KR. Cutaneous barrier perturbation stimulates cytokine production in the epidermis of mice. J Clin Invest. 1992;90(2):482–7. doi:10.1172/JCI115884.
24. Tagami H. Atopic dermatitis and skin barrier function. Arerugi. 2005;54(5):445–50. 054050445e [pii]
25. Werner Y, Lindberg M. Transepidermal water loss in dry and clinically normal skin in patients with atopic dermatitis. Acta Derm Venereol. 1985;65(2):102–5.
26. Werner Y. The water content of the stratum corneum in patients with atopic dermatitis. Measurement with the Corneometer CM 420. Acta Derm Venereol. 1986;66(4):281–4.
27. Kim DW, Park JY, Na GY, Lee SJ, Lee WJ. Correlation of clinical features and skin barrier function in adolescent and adult patients with atopic dermatitis. Int J Dermatol. 2006;45(6):698–701. doi:10.1111/j.1365-4632.2005.02644.x. IJD2644 [pii]
28. Loden M, Olsson H, Axell T, Linde YW. Friction, capacitance and transepidermal water loss (TEWL) in dry atopic and normal skin. Br J Dermatol. 1992;126(2):137–41.
29. Pinnagoda J, Tupker RA, Agner T, Serup J. Guidelines for transepidermal water loss (TEWL) measurement. A report from the Standardization Group of the European Society of Contact Dermatitis. Contact Dermatitis. 1990;22(3):164–78.
30. McFadden JP, Basketter DA, Dearman RJ, Puangpet P, Kimber I. The hapten-atopy hypothesis III: the potential role of airborne chemicals. Br J Dermatol. 2014;170(1):45–51. doi:10.1111/bjd.12602.
31. Uenishi T, Sugiura H, Uehara M. Changes in the seasonal dependence of atopic dermatitis in Japan. J Dermatol. 2001;28(5):244–7.
32. Masuda T. Atopic dermatitis. Nihon-Hifuka-Zensho. Kanehara Shuppan Co: Tokyo; 1967.
33. Brandt RL, Arlian LG. Mortality of house dust mites, Dermatophagoides farinae and D. pteronyssinus, exposed to dehydrating conditions or selected pesticides. J Med Entomol. 1976;13(3):327–31.
34. Parthasaradhi A, Al Gufai AF. The pattern of skin diseases in Hail Region, Saudi Arabia. Ann Saudi Med. 1998;18(6):558–61. 18-558 [pii]

Retrospective Cohort Study of Adolescent Atopic Dermatitis

4

Akiko Kijima, Hiroyuki Murota, and Ichiro Katayama

Abstract

Epidemiological studies in Japanese children determined that the prevalence of atopic dermatitis (AD) in Japan increased through the late twentieth century, but has been declining in recent years. However, more recent evidence has revealed an increasing number of adolescent and adult subjects with AD. Many adult subjects with AD take a protracted clinical course through childhood. Furthermore, AD may develop or recur at any age. Thus, morbidity of all age ranges should be considered for estimating the prevalence of AD. Although data obtained from a prospective cohort study is reliable for determining the lifetime prevalence of AD, it takes many years to acquire the data. In contrast, a retrospective study has the advantage of a short study period while still providing a rough estimate of the lifetime prevalence of AD. Moreover, the latest demographic estimate of Japan released in 2016 showed a decreasing trend, with a total population of around 130 million people. A large change in the population would affect the result of any longitudinal epidemiological survey, and as a result, we should continue to update prevalence estimates. This chapter reviews recent studies on the prevalence of AD in Japan.

Keywords

Atopic dermatitis • Prevalence • Adolescent • Allergic march

A. Kijima (✉) • H. Murota • I. Katayama
Department of Dermatology, Osaka University, Suita, Osaka, Japan
e-mail: harukiyutosaki@gmail.com

I. Katayama et al. (eds.), *Evolution of Atopic Dermatitis in the 21st Century*,
https://doi.org/10.1007/978-981-10-5541-6_4

4.1 Current Prevalence of Atopic Dermatitis (AD) Worldwide

AD is a chronic inflammatory skin disorder that can impair quality of life. The incidence of AD is generally considered to be increasing worldwide [1]. To evaluate recent trends in the childhood allergy epidemic, it is necessary to compare sequential data using identical, simple, validated questionnaires involving children of the same age and region sampled in the same way. The International Study of Asthma and Allergies in Childhood (ISAAC) was implemented for this purpose. ISAAC Phase 1 was conducted from 1992 to 1998, and ISAAC Phase 2 was conducted from 1999 to 2004 [2]. According to these studies, the prevalence of AD plateaued at 10–20% in developed countries; however, the prevalence is lower, but continues to increase, in many developing countries.

4.2 Japanese Subjects Presenting with AD at Dermatology Clinics

In Japan, AD became a very commonly diagnosed skin disease from the 1950s through the 1970s. In the Branch Hospital of the University of Tokyo, the incidence of AD in first-visit patients was 5.6% in 1967, 8.7% in 1976, 7.7% in 1986, and 10.1% in 1996 [3]. Similarly, an outpatient dermatology clinic of Kitasato University reported a marked increase in the overall number of adult patients with atopic eczema from 1975 to 1985 and an increase in the ratio of patients 10–30 years old [4]. Since these reports, the number of cases with adolescent- and adult-type atopic eczema has continued to rise [5, 6].

4.3 Prospective Studies on the Prevalence of Childhood AD in Japan

Studies in elementary school children have suggested that the prevalence of AD was increasing in the late twentieth century, but has been plateauing or decreasing more recently. The incidence of AD in Japanese elementary school children was approximately 3% in 1981–1983, but increased to approximately 6–7% in the 1990s [7]. A questionnaire survey was given 15 times from 1975 to 2006 for all children attending public elementary schools in Osaka Prefecture, with the number of subjects ranging from 460,000 to 900,000 and aged 7–12 years. In this study, the lifetime prevalence of AD increased from 15% in 1985 to 24% by 1993 and then decreased to 22.9% by 1997 [8, 9]. A survey investigating 37,036 elementary school children showed a decrease in the prevalence of AD from 1982 to 2002 [10]. A research team at the Japanese Ministry of Health, Labor, and Welfare examined

48,072 children living in Asahikawa, Iwate, Tokyo, Gifu, Osaka, Hiroshima, Kochi, and Fukuoka from 2000 to 2002. They reported that the national average prevalence of AD was 12.8% in individuals aged 4 months, 9.8% in those aged 18 months, 13.2% in those aged 3 years, 11.8% in those aged 6–7 years, 10.6% in those aged 12–13 years, and 8.2% in those aged 18 years [11]. In an examination of 27,196 children aged 6–14 years old living in Tokyo in 2005, the prevalence of AD ranged from 10.9 to 19.6%.

While the prevalence decreased with increasing age, older children were more likely to have severe symptoms [12]. In a large-scale, population-based survey of allergic diseases among school children aged 7–15 years living in Kyoto City, the prevalence of AD was 4.2% in 1996 and 5.6% in 2006 [13]. Among those currently suffering from AD, the number of severe cases increased from 38.2 to 44.5%, while the number of mild cases decreased from 25.6 to 17.0%. Prevalence of a past history of AD also increased in 2006, resulting in an increase in lifetime prevalence from 10.1 to 13.6%. These data suggest that even though mild dermatitis appears to be on the decline in recent years, dermatitis severity actually becomes exacerbated with increasing age.

4.4 A Retrospective Study on Adolescent AD in Japan

To investigate the factors influencing adolescent AD, a retrospective study was conducted for 3321 first-grade students at Osaka University in 2011 [14]. The lifetime prevalence of AD was 16.5%. Family history of AD and comorbid atopic diseases (asthma and/or allergic rhinitis) was a significant risk factor in the development of AD (Table 4.1). Improvement in AD symptoms and the recurrence of AD both peaked during adolescence (Fig. 4.1). AD onset peaked within the first 12 months, BA peaked in early childhood, and AR developed constantly from early childhood to adolescence. There were two peaks of improvement in AD, one observed in early childhood and one in adolescence. There was one peak of improvement in early adolescence in BA and in late adolescence in AR. Having early onset AD or being female increased the likelihood that AD symptoms would improve. Xerosis, seasonal changes, and sweating were the most important factors hindering improvement of AD symptoms (Table 4.2).

There have been a number of studies on the prevalence of childhood AD in Japan; however, most of these studies analyzed a limited period from infancy to late childhood and/or to early adolescence. Managing AD in adolescence is important for improved long-term prognosis. For this reason, further studies conducted from childhood through adulthood are needed to investigate the prevalence of AD, determine risk factors for recurrence, and prevent the shift toward severe AD in adulthood.

Table 4.1 Association of personal and family histories with the prevalence of each atopic disease analyzed by multivariate logistic regression analysis

	AD (*n* = 547)			BA (*n* = 329)			AR (*n* = 1186)		
	%[a]	OR	(95% CI)	%[b]	OR	(95%CI)	%[c]	OR	(95% CI)
Personal history									
AD				44.4	**3.59*****	**(2.77–4.66)**	24.3	**1.81*****	**(1.49–2.21)**
BA	26.7	**3.59*****	**(2.76–4.65)**				16.4	**2.24*****	**(1.75–2.86)**
AR	52.7	**1.81*****	**(1.48–2.21)**	59.0	**2.25*****	**(1.77–2.88)**			
FA	22.9	**5.22*****	**(3.89–7.01)**	23.4	**2.96*****	**(2.13–4.13)**	11.3	**1.75*****	**(1.31–2.34)**
Family history									
AD									
P	10.4	**2.76*****	**(1.72–4.42)**	7.3			4.1	**0.61*****	**(0.37–0.99)**
M	13.8	**3.85*****	**(2.50–5.93)**	9.5	**1.79*****	**(1.30–2.47)**	7.2	**1.61*****	**(1.03–2.52)**
S	39.0	**3.39*****	**(2.64–4.32)**	30.9			21.3		
O	2.5	2.40	(0.99–5.87)	2.3			1.3		
BA									
P	6.2			12.3	**4.22*****	**(2.54–7.04)**	4.4		
M	5.9			10.5	**3.62*****	**(2.10–6.23)**	5.2	**1.75***	**(1.03–2.97)**
S	14.9			23.2	**2.49*****	**(1.70–3.67)**	10.5		
O	4.5	**2.19*****	**(1.09–4.38)**	7.3	**5.15*****	**(2.71–9.81)**	2.9		
AR									
P	32.9			33.6	1.29	(0.96–1.73)	39.9	**2.46*****	**(2.01–3.02)**
M	40.2	1.28	(1.01–1.63)	43.6	**1.37*****	**(1.04–1.80)**	50.1	**2.77*****	**(2.29–3.36)**
S	45.8			45.5			52.6	**2.43*****	**(2.02–2.93)**
O	2.0			3.2			2.4	**5.01*****	**(1.04–12.54)**

Reuse from reference [14] with permission from the Japanese Society of Allergology

AD atopic dermatitis, *BA* bronchial asthma, *AR* allergic rhinitis, *FA* food allergy, *P* paternal, *M* maternal, *S* siblings, *O* others

*$P < 0.05$, **$P < 0.01$, ***$P < 0.001$

[a]Denominator of the ratio is 547

[b]Denominator of the ratio is 329

[c]Denominator of the ratio is 1186

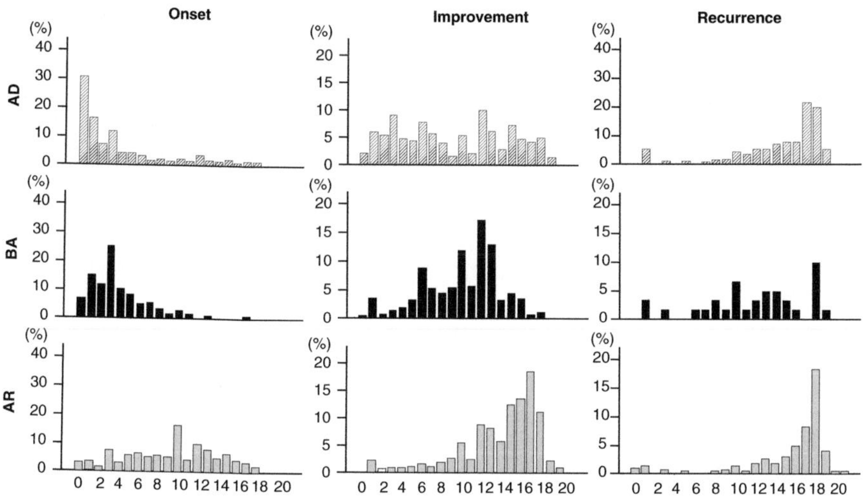

Fig. 4.1 Clinical course of allergic diseases. Clinical course (onset, improvement, and recurrence) of atopic dermatitis (AD; *upper*), bronchial asthma (BA; *middle*), and allergic rhinitis (AR; *lower*) was demonstrated. All three atopic diseases presented a peak of recurrence in adolescence. This figure was reused from reference [14] with permission from the Japanese Society of Allergology

Table 4.2 Risk factor link to *improvement* and *recurrence* of atopic dermatitis (AD)

	Covariate	OR	(95% CI)	*p*
Improvement (yes/no)	Sex (male/female)	0.40	(0.24–0.65)	<0.001
	Onset age	0.94	(0.94–0.90)	0.006
	Aggravating factor			
	Xerosis	0.58	(0.37–0.91)	0.019
	Seasonal turning points	0.51	(0.32–0.82)	0.005
	Sweating	0.70	(0.44–1.09)	0.116
Recurrence (yes/no)	Aggravating factor			
	Psychological stress	4.80	(2.96–7.81)	<0.001
	Sleep	3.03	(1.38–6.67)	0.006

Reuse from reference [14] with permission from the Japanese Society of Allergology
AD atopic dermatitis

References

1. Williams HC. Is the prevalence of atopic dermatitis increasing? Clin Exp Dermatol. 1992;17:385–91.
2. Asher MI, Montefort S, Bjorksten B, et al. Worldwide time trends in the prevalence of symptoms of asthma, allergic rhinoconjunctivitis, and eczema in childhood: ISAAC Phases One and Three repeat multicountry cross-sectional surveys. Lancet. 2006;368:733–43.
3. Furue M. History of atopic dermatitis. Chugai-igakusya. 1998:1–19.
4. Nishioka K. Atopic eczema of adult type in Japan. Australas J Dermatol. 1996;37:S7–9.

5. Ministry of Health and Welfare. Annual report of the research group on allergy. Epidemiological study of allergic diseases. Tokyo: Ministry of Health and Welfare; 1993.
6. Sugiura H, Umemoto N, Deguchi H, et al. Prevalence of childhood and adolescent atopic dermatitis in a Japanese population: comparison with the disease frequency examined 20 years ago. Acta Derm Venereol. 1998;78:293–4.
7. Takeuchi M, Ueda H. Increase of atopic dermatitis (AD) in recent Japan. Environ Dermatol. 2000;7:133–6.
8. Yura A, Shimizu T. Trends in the prevalence of atopic dermatitis in school children: longitudinal study in Osaka Prefecture, Japan, from 1985 to 1997. Br J Dermatol. 2001;145:966–73.
9. Yura A, Shimizu T. Trends of allergic symptoms in school children: large-scale long-term consecutive cross-sectional studies in Osaka Prefecture Japan. Pediatr Allergy Immunol. 2011;22:631–7.
10. Nishima S, Ota K, Okazaki K, Kanatani M, et al. A study on the prevalence of allergic dieseases in school children in western districts of Japan. Jpn J Pediatr Allergy Clin Immunol. 2013;27:149–69.
11. Yamamoto S. Prevalence and exacerbation factors of atopic dermatitis. Skin Allergy Front. 2003;1:85–90.
12. Futamura M, Ohya Y, Akashi M, et al. Age-related prevalence of allergic diseases in Tokyo school children. Allergol Int. 2011;60:509–15.
13. Kusunoki T, Morimoto T, Nishikomori R, et al. Changing prevalence and severity of childhood allergic diseases in kyoto, Japan, from 1996 to 2006. Allergol Int. 2009;58:543–8.
14. Kijima A, Murota H, Takahashi A, et al. Prevalence and impact of past history of food allergy in atopic dermatitis. Allergol Int. 2013;62:105–12.

Part III

Genetics

Genome-Wide Association Study for Atopic Dermatitis in the Japanese Population

5

Mayumi Tamari and Tomomitsu Hirota

Abstract

Atopic dermatitis (AD) is a chronic inflammatory skin disease in which there are considerable genetic contributions. Genome-wide association studies (GWASs) provide an unbiased method to identify the genetic factors of human diseases and phenotypes comprehensively. Although it is well known that loss-of-function mutations in *FLG* are the most significant genetic risk factor for AD, recent GWASs, immunochip analyses, and meta-analyses of GWASs have identified a number of loci associated with AD. Candidate genes identified by GWASs of AD are involved in skin barrier functions and innate and adaptive immune responses. Those findings imply a substantial overlap of genetic components with other autoimmune and inflammatory diseases. Genetic variants may influence molecular phenotypes, including RNA expression and stability, transcription factor binding, DNA methylation, histone modifications, and protein levels. Understanding the functional links between susceptibility variants and phenotypic traits is crucial to improve our knowledge of AD. Further interdisciplinary research is necessary for translation of the genetics of AD into clinical practice.

Keywords

Atopic dermatitis • Genome-wide association study • Immunochip analysis Meta-analysis • Genetic variants

M. Tamari, M.D., Ph.D. (✉)
Professor, The Jikei University School of Medicine, Research Center for Medical Science, Core Research Facilities for Basic Science (Molecular Genetics),
3-25-8, Nishi-shinbashi, Minato-ku, Tokyo 105-8461, Japan
e-mail: mayumitamari@jikei.ac.jp

T. Hirota
Laboratory for Respiratory and Allergic Diseases, Center for Integrative Medical Sciences, Institute of Physical and Chemical Research (RIKEN),
1-7-22 Suehiro, Tsurumi-ku, Yokohama, Kanagawa 230-0045, Japan

I. Katayama et al. (eds.), *Evolution of Atopic Dermatitis in the 21st Century*,
https://doi.org/10.1007/978-981-10-5541-6_5

5.1 Introduction

Atopic dermatitis (AD) is a chronic inflammatory skin disease in which there is a considerable genetic component [1]. Genome-wide association studies (GWASs) provide an unbiased method to identify the genetic factors of human diseases and phenotypes comprehensively [2]. Imputation is a statistical method used to infer untyped genotypes by employing a reference panel of extensively genotyped individuals [3]. Imputation is useful to combine data from GWASs performed using different platforms for meta-analysis, provides a high-resolution overview of association results, and increases the statistical power to identify associated loci. Recent developments in high-throughput genotyping and imputation technologies have made it possible to identify disease susceptibility loci convincingly. Although it is well known that loss-of-function mutations in *FLG* (encoding filaggrin) are the most significant genetic risk factor for AD [4], recent GWASs, immunochip analyses, and meta-analyses of GWASs have identified a number of loci associated with AD (Table 5.1) and have improved our understanding of its pathogenesis.

5.2 Genome-Wide Association Studies of Atopic Dermatitis in European and Chinese Populations

The first GWAS for AD was reported in 2009. The study analyzed 939 cases and 975 controls as well as 270 complete nuclear families with two affected siblings [5]. Genetic variants that showed associations with AD in both discovery set were examined in two independent replication populations totaling 2637 cases and 3957 controls. The GWAS found that rs7927894 located 38 kb downstream of *C11orf30* (11q13.5) was associated with AD ($P = 7.6 \times 10^{-10}$). The locus had been reported to be a susceptibility locus for Crohn's disease, which shares many pathophysiological features with AD such as recurrent inflammation of the epithelium, defective barrier function, and dysfunction of innate immune responses against infections.

In a Chinese Han population, a GWAS of AD was conducted using 1012 cases and 1362 controls followed by a replication set of 3624 cases and 12,197 controls [6]. It also conducted a replication study using 1806 cases and 3256 controls from Germany. The GWAS identified novel two loci, *TMEM232/SLC25A46* (5q22.1) and *TNFRSF6B/ZGPAT* (20q13.33), and found an association of a common variant, rs3126085 in the *FLG* locus, with AD at genome-wide significance levels. The association at the *TNFRSF6B/ZGPAT* locus was replicated in the German sample. *TNFRSF6B* (also called *DCR3*) encodes a TNF receptor superfamily gene that plays a suppressive role in FasL- and LIGHT-mediated cell death. Interestingly, LIGHT is a target for airway remodeling in asthma [14] and binds the herpes virus entry mediator (TNFRSF14) [15].

A genome-wide association meta-analysis using 5606 cases and 20,565 controls from 16 population-based studies was reported in 2011 [7]. The study was followed

Table 5.1 Susceptibility loci of atopic dermatitis identified by GWAS, Immunochip analysis, and GWAS meta-analyses

Chromosome	Locus	Population	Reference
11q13.5	*C11ORF30/LRRC32 (GARP)*	European	[5]
1p21.3	*FLG*	Chinese Han	[6]
5q22.1	*TMEM232/SLC25A46*		
20q13.33	*TNFRSF6B/ZGPAT*		
11q13.1	*OVOL1*	European	[9]
19p13.2	*ACTL9*		
5q31.1	*KIF3A/RAD50/IL13*		
2q12	*IL1RL1/IL18R1/IL18RAP*	Japanese	[10]
3p21.33	*GLB1*		
3q13.2	*CCDC80*		
6p21.3	*The MHC region*		
7p22	*CARD11*		
10q21.2	*ZNF365*		
11p15.4	*OR10A3/NLRP10*		
20q13	*CYP24A1/PFDN4*		
4q27	*IL2/IL21*	European	[26]
11p13	*PRR5L*		
16p13.13	*CLEC16A/DEXI*		
17q21.32	*ZNF652*		
1q21.3	*IL6R*	European	[29]
13q21.31	*PCDH9*	Korean	[30]
2q24.3	*XIRP2*	European	[31]
9p21.3	*DMRTA1*		
14q13.2	*PPP2R3C*	Multi-ancestry[a]	[32]
11q24.3	*–/ETS1*		
1q21.2	*C1orf51/MRPS21*		
8q21.13	*MIR5708/ZBTB10*		
10p15.1	*IL15RA/IL2RA*		
5p13.2	*IL7R/CAPSL*		
2p25.1	*LINC00299/–*		
2p16.1	*PUS10*		
17q21.2	*STAT3*		
3p21.1	*SFMBT1/RFT1*		
2p13.3	*CD207/VAX2*		

[a]European, African, Japanese, and Latino ancestry

by one with 5419 cases and 19,833 controls from 14 studies that finally identified a total of three novel loci that reached genome-wide significance, *OVOL1* (11q13.1), *ACTL9* (19p13.2), and *KIF3A* (5q31.1). Interestingly *OVOL1* and *ACTL9* are implicated in epidermal proliferation and differentiation, and *KIF3A* is located in the cytokine cluster region at 5q31.1 containing *IL13*.

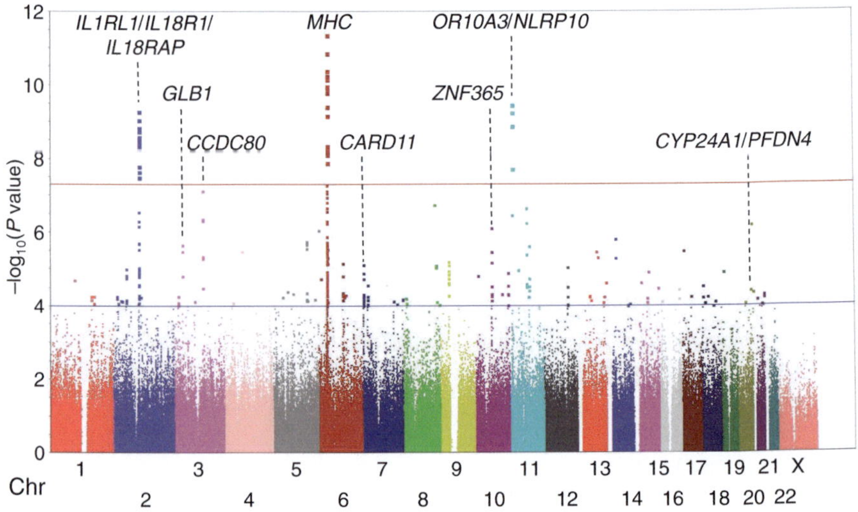

Fig. 5.1 Manhattan plot showing the P values from the GWAS of AD in the Japanese population

5.3 Genome-Wide Association Studies of Atopic Dermatitis in the Japanese Population

In 2012, a GWAS of AD in the Japanese population using a total of 1472 cases and 7971 controls was published, followed by a replication study with an additional 1856 cases and 7021 controls [8]. The study investigated 606,164 SNP loci and identified a total of 8 novel susceptibility loci for AD: *IL1RL1/IL18R1/IL18RAP* (2q12), the *HLA* region (6p21.3), *OR10A3/NLRP10* (11p15.4), *GLB1* (3p21.33), *CCDC80* (3q13.2), *CARD11* (7p22), *ZNF365* (10q21.2), and *CYP24A1/PFDN4* (20q13) (Fig. 5.1). The study also replicated the associations of the *FLG*, *C11orf30*, *OVOL1*, *TNFRSF6B/ZGPAT*, *TMEM232/SLC25A46*, *ACTL9*, and *KIF3A/IL13* loci in prior GWASs for AD. All cases were recruited from hospitals in Japan, and the mean ages of the cases in the discovery and replication study were 28.6 and 33.0, respectively. Candidate genes identified by the GWAS suggested important roles for skin barrier functions, adaptive immune responses, IL-1 family signaling, regulatory T cells, and the vitamin D pathway in the pathogenesis of AD.

5.3.1 *IL1RL1/IL18R1/IL18RAP*

The 2q12 locus contains genes *IL1RL1*, *IL18R1*, and *IL18RAP*, which encode the receptors of IL-1 family cytokines that play crucial roles in the skin. IL1RL1, a component of the IL-33 receptor, is highly expressed in Th2 cells and mast cells. The levels of IL-33 expression are increased in inflamed skin tissue of subjects with AD, and it has been suggested that IL-33 produced in the damaged tissues of AD induces Th2-type inflammation [16].

5.3.2 The HLA Region

The HLA region contains hundreds of immune system genes, and the locus often shows the strongest association for most autoimmune diseases. Generally, seropositive diseases are associated with HLA class II, and seronegative diseases are associated with HLA class I [17]. The most significant association with AD in the GWAS was observed at rs176095 in the HLA class III region ($P = 8.38 \times 10^{-20}$). After logistic regression analysis of the HLA region, there were two independent association signals in the HLA class I and III regions. The HLA region shows significant associations with asthma [18] and peanuts allergy [19]. Recent studies have reported the involvement of autoimmunity in the pathophysiology of AD, and IgE antibodies against keratinocytes and endothelial cells have been identified in severe AD. However, further studies are necessary to elucidate the involvement of autoimmunity in chronic inflammation in subjects with AD.

5.3.3 *OR10A3/NLRP10*

The region at 11p15.4 contains two genes, *NLRP10* and *OR10A3*. *OR10A3* encodes an olfactory receptor family gene. NALP proteins sense both microbial and danger signals, and *NLRP10* encodes a NALP family protein that lacks the leucine-rich repeat region. NLRP10 is highly expressed in the skin and plays a role in immune responses against invasive bacteria. A recent study using a mouse model of contact hypersensitivity has shown that NLRP10 is involved in T cell-mediated skin inflammation and plays a role in epidermal keratinocytes [20].

5.3.4 *GLB1*

GLB1 encodes β-galactosidase-1, but the involvement of the enzyme in allergic inflammation remains unclear. The 3p21.33 locus is located adjacent to the *CCR4* gene, which encodes a chemokine receptor for CCL22 and CCL17 (also called TARC). Interestingly, TSLP derived from keratinocytes induces dendritic cells to produce TARC, and skin-specific recruitment of T cells during inflammation is mediated by CCR4. TARC is produced by endothelial cells, keratinocytes, and fibroblasts and plays an important role in AD, bullous pemphigoid, and mycosis fungoides [21]. Serum TARC levels are associated with the disease activity of AD [21].

5.3.5 *CCDC80*

The 3q13.2 locus includes *CCDC80*, which encodes a protein associated with the induction of peroxisome proliferator-activated receptor γ (PPARγ) and C/EBPα. A recent study has shown that PPARγ agonists suppress the maturation and migration of dendritic cells and decrease TSLP expression in the skin in a mouse model of AD [22]. C/EBPα is expressed in basal keratinocytes and upregulated in terminal differentiation of keratinocytes [23].

5.3.6 *CARD11*

The 3p21.33 locus contains *CARD11*, which encodes CARMA1. CARMA1 regulates T cell receptor/NF-kB signaling and controls completion of Th17 differentiation [24]. Interestingly, mice homozygous for the CARMA1 mutation develop AD with high levels of serum IgE. Sézary syndrome is an erythrodermic form of cutaneous T cell lymphoma characterized by scaling and itching [25]. Sézary cells, circulating atypical T lymphocytes, show a Th2 cytokine profile, activating *CCR4* and *CARD11* mutations in nearly one-third of patients. Overlap of the target genes would be helpful to unveil details of shared etiologies.

5.3.7 *ZNF365*

The 10q21.2 locus includes three genes, *ZNF365*, *ADO*, and *EGR2*. The most associated variant, rs10995251, is located within *ZNF365*. Although the region shows a suggestive association with AD in the Chinese population ($P = 1.1 \times 10^{-7}$), it is associated with AD at the genome-wide significance level in the Japanese population ($P = 5.9 \times 10^{-20}$). The locus is also associated with Vogt-Koyanagi-Harada syndrome, which is a multisystem autoimmune disorder affecting pigmented tissues in the ocular, integumentary, auditory, and central nervous systems [26]. Regulatory T cells control the maintenance of immune tolerance and protect the body from harmful immune responses to antigens. It is recognized that dysregulation of Tregs is responsible for the development of a number of immune-mediated diseases. A recent study has shown that induced Tregs characteristically express both LAG3 and EGR2 [27], and EGR2 is involved in the negative regulation of T cell proliferation and inflammation [28].

5.3.8 *CYP24A1/PFDN4*

The 20q13 locus contains *CYP24A1* and *PFDN4*. *PFDN4* encodes a subunit of a molecular chaperone complex, prefoldin. *CYP24A1* encodes 1,25-dihydroxyvitamin D3 (1,25$(OH)_2$D3) 24-hydroxylase, a mitochondrial cytochrome P450 superfamily enzyme that initiates the degradation of the physiologically active form of vitamin D3 by hydroxylation of the side chain [29]. The active form of vitamin D3, 1,25$(OH)_2$D3 is synthesized in the skin systemically after its exposure to sunlight. Since local 1,25$(OH)_2$D3 synthesis activates innate immune responses, sun exposure is an important environmental factor in immune function. A recent study has shown an association between vitamin D deficiency and the severity of AD [30].

5.4 Immunochip Analysis for Atopic Dermatitis

The Immunochip array is an Illumina Infinium SNP array that was designed by researchers investigating 11 distinct inflammatory and autoimmune diseases in 2009. The chip covers a total of 195,806 SNPs and 718 small insertion-deletions, and the top 2000 associated variants for each disease are included. High-density genotyping study using the Immunochip array identified a total of four novel susceptibility loci for AD in 2013: *IL2/IL21* (4q27), *PRR5L* (11p13), *CLEC16A/DEXI* (16p13.13), and *ZNF652* (17q21.32) [9]. A total of 2425 German subjects with AD and 5449 controls were assessed, and a validation study with 7196 cases and 15,480 controls was conducted using populations from Germany, Ireland, Japan, and China. The *IL2* locus is located near the *IL21* gene. IL-2 is required for T cell activation and proliferation and regulates the proliferation and survival of regulatory T cells. Cyclosporin A is an inhibitor of calcineurin, which suppresses IL-2 production [31]. Interestingly, recent studies have shown associations of *IL2RA* and *IL21* with immune-mediated diseases [17]. *CLEC16A* encodes a member of the C-type lectin domain containing family, and *CLEC16A* variants are associated with multiple immune-mediated diseases such as celiac disease, Crohn's disease, and alopecia areata [32]. A recent study has shown that CLEC16A modulates thymic epithelial cell autophagy and alters T cell selection and reactivity [32]. In the Japanese population, a total of three loci, *PRR5L*, *CLEC16A/DEXI*, and *ZNF652*, were replicated.

5.5 Recent Genome-Wide Association Studies of Atopic Dermatitis in Other Populations

A recent study focused on a total of 318 markers associated with any inflammatory trait obtained from a public GWAS database and assessed associations with AD in a three-step approach using 7130 AD cases and 9253 controls [10]. A functional nonsynonymous variant in *IL6R* (rs2228145, Asp358Ala), which determines the balance between the membrane bound (IL-6R) and soluble forms (sIL-6R), was significantly associated with AD. Interestingly the study also identified increased serum levels of sIL-6R and their influence on the prognosis and persistence of AD.

A GWAS of recalcitrant AD, which is defined as moderate-to-severe AD with allergic sensitization, in Korean children was reported in 2015 [11]. Genetic variants on 13q21.31 were associated with recalcitrant AD at genome-wide significance levels. The closest gene, *protocadherin 9* (*PCDH9*), is located more than 1 Mb from those related variants. In the GWAS, four loci, *NBAS* (2p24.3), *THEMIS* (6q22.33), *GATA3* (10p14), and *SCAPER* (15q24.3), showed P values $<1 \times 10^{-6}$.

A GWAS for AD using an imputed data set consisting of more than 1.6 million variants was reported in 2015 [12]. The GWAS assessed 924 tertiary care cases and 5506 population-based controls, followed by an independent replication of 1383 cases and 1728 controls in the German population. Finally, two novel susceptibility loci were identified in the combined analysis: *XIRP2* (2q24.3) and *DMRTA1* (9p21.3). However, the functions of *XIRP2* and *DMRTA1* remain unknown.

5.6 Multi-ancestry Genome-Wide Association Study for Atopic Dermatitis

GWAS meta-analyses for common diseases using large sample sizes have recently been conducted. Collaborative studies consisting of a number of cohorts ensure sufficient statistical power and reveal disease susceptibility loci. A multi-ancestry genome-wide association study for AD using 21,000 cases and 95,000 controls of European, African, Japanese, and Latino ancestry was reported in 2015 [13]. A replication study of the GWAS was conducted using 32,059 cases and 228,628 controls from 18 studies, and a total of 11 novel loci of AD were finally identified.

Among the 11 novel loci, *MIR5708/ZBTB10* (8q21.13) was associated with asthma, and *ETS1* (11q24.3), *IL15RA/IL2RA* (10p15.1), *MIR5708/ZBTB10* (8q21.13), and *LINC00299* (2p25.1) were associated with self-reported allergy [33]. The study indicated that 15 of the 36 reported psoriasis-associated variants were associated with AD ($P < 0.05$), and 10 variants showed the same direction of association. The GWAS revealed that two loci, *CCDC80/CD200R1L* (3q13.2) and *OR10A3/NLRP10* (11p15.4), might be Japanese-specific signals.

Furthermore, the functional annotations of the associated variants were reviewed in ENCODE consortium [34] and Roadmap Epigenomics Consortium data [35], and their expression quantitative trait loci (eQTL) effects were evaluated in the MuTHER database [36]. The AD associations of DNase I hypersensitivity regions were strongly enriched compared with the rest of the genome, particularly in Th0, Th1, and Th17 cells, at genome-wide significance levels. Interestingly, the most significant *cis* eQTLs were identified at 2p13.3 (rs4852714 and rs6723629) and eQTLs for CD207 (langerin) in the skin. rs4852714 is also located in open chromatin regions with histone marks, suggesting roles for promoter or enhancer activity in lymphoblastoid cell lines. Langerin is highly expressed in Langerhans cells and Langerin$^+$ dermal dendritic cells and has antiviral and antifungal effects [37].

The majority of the novel loci in this study harbor genes with functional annotations involved in autoimmunity. PPP2R3C regulates B cell maturation and survival, and dysregulation of PPP2R3C leads to autoimmunity in mice. The most significantly associated variant at 5p13.2 (rs10214237) is located 4 kb downstream of *IL7R*, which is in strong linkage disequilibrium with an *IL7R* missense variant, rs6897932 ($r^2 = 0.94$). It has already been reported that the risk allele enhances IL-7 bioavailability [38], and IL-7 transgenic mice show the AD-like features of severe dermatitis with pruritus and elevated serum IgE [39]. Hyper IgE syndrome (HIES) is characterized by AD with high serum IgE levels, and those patients show impaired Th17 function and suffer from recurrent staphylococcal infections. A recent study has shown that dominant negative mutations at the DNA binding site of the *STAT3* gene cause HIES [40]. In this GWAS, common variants at the *STAT3* locus (17q21.2) were associated with AD. Interestingly, a related genetic variant (rs5892724) at the *MIR5708/ZBTB10* locus (8q21.13) is located in open chromatin and affects a *STAT3* binding site [41]. *ETS1*, a plausible candidate gene at 11q24.3, plays roles in Th17 and B cell functions and in keratinocyte differentiation. A recent study has shown that ETS1 is a crucial regulator of ILC2 expansion and cytokine production [42].

Candidate genes at novel loci suggest roles for autoimmune regulation in the pathogenesis of AD, and the findings of this study imply a substantial overlap of genetic components with other autoimmune and inflammatory diseases.

5.7 Overlapping Loci Between Atopic Dermatitis and Other Diseases

5.7.1 Psoriasis

AD and psoriasis are common inflammatory diseases affecting the skin that show mutually exclusive clinical characteristics and different immune mechanisms. A recent study using GWAS data has demonstrated that AD and psoriasis have distinct genetic mechanisms in shared pathways involving immune responses and epidermal differentiation [43]. Intriguingly, the influence of genetic factors shows opposite effects in the pathways. Characterization of shared and opposing mechanisms will improve our knowledge of the pathogenesis of inflammatory skin diseases.

5.7.2 Atopic March

The term atopic march refers to the typical progression of allergic disorders that often begin in early childhood. In most cases, the first sign of the history is the development of AD in an infant. A recent multistage GWAS revealed seven loci involved in the atopic march [44]. The study assessed 2428 cases of infantile eczema followed by childhood asthma and 17,034 controls from 12 populations and identified seven loci: *FLG* (1q21.3), *IL4/KIF3A* (5q31.1), *AP5B1/OVOL1* (11q13.1), *C11orf30/LRRC32* (11q13.5), *IKZF3* (17q21), *EFHC1* (6p12.3), and *TMTC2/SLC6A15* (17q21). *EFHC1* and *TMTC2/SLC6A15* are associated with the combined eczema plus asthma phenotype and had never been previously reported as susceptibility loci for allergic disease. The study also suggested a strong contribution of AD genes to the atopic march.

5.8 Epigenetic Analysis of Serum IgE Concentrations

IgE plays an important role in atopic inflammation. Cytosine methylation is generally associated with transcriptional silencing, and perturbations of DNA methylation patterns are often found in disease [45]. A recent study investigated epigenetic associations between serum IgE concentrations and DNA methylation by using Illumina HumanMethylation27 arrays, which assess CpG loci within proximal promoter regions of 14,475 genes [46]. The study identified associations between IgE and low methylation at a total of 36 loci with a meta-analysis false discovery rate $<10^{-4}$. Annotated genes in several loci such as *IL5RA*, *PGR2*, *PGR3*, and *GATA1* encode characteristic proteins of eosinophils. The most significant association was observed within an island of CpG, cg01998785, and adjacent to *LPCAT2*, which encodes lysophosphatidylcholine acetyltransferase 2. That enzyme functions in production of PAF in inflammatory cells. This study implies the presence of new therapeutically tractable pathways involving IgE production.

5.9 Perspectives

5.9.1 Rare Variant Association Studies

Since rare variants are not included in conventional arrays for GWAS, their contributions to AD susceptibility remain unclear. There are several methodologies for rare variant association studies: whole-genome sequencing, whole-exome sequencing, targeted sequencing of candidate genes, and exome arrays. Recent targeted gene sequencing studies have found rare coding genetic variants with strong effects on phenotype variation such as LDL and HDL cholesterol levels. However, a number of rare variant association studies have reported that most variants have modest-to-small effects on the variability of phenotypes [47].

5.9.2 Skin Microbiota and Immunity

Physical and immune skin barriers are maintained by interactions of keratinocytes, immune cells, and microbes under healthy conditions and also under wounding or infection [48]. Several potential mechanisms have been suggested for the influence of the skin microbiota on the initiation or amplification of skin diseases. Genetic components of patients may enhance sensing or translocation of the microbiota. Skin microbes such as *S. aureus* and *C. albicans* may contribute to tissue damage and inflammation in the context of infection. The antimicrobial function of keratinocytes, which are stimulated by IL-17 produced by skin commensal-specific T cells, could enhance skin immunity. Candidate genes identified in GWASs suggest roles for keratinocytes and Th17 cells in the pathogenesis of AD.

5.9.3 Functional Investigation of Susceptibility Loci

Genetic variants might influence molecular phenotypes, including RNA expression and stability, transcription factor binding, DNA methylation, histone modifications, and protein levels. The functional links between susceptibility variants and phenotypic traits are crucial to improve our knowledge of AD. To investigate how these genetic variants influence the pathophysiology of the disease is required for understanding the disease mechanism and utilization of the findings for prevention or treatment.

Expression quantitative trait loci are commonly used to investigate the effects of genetic variants on gene expression. To interpret susceptibility loci identified by GWAS, the Genotype-Tissue Expression (GTEx) project was launched to establish a database showing the relationship between genetic variants and gene expression in human tissues, including the skin (http://www.gtexportal.org/) [49].

The Encyclopedia of DNA Elements (ENCODE) project was launched in 2003 to identify functional elements in the human genome sequence. The NIH Roadmap Epigenomics Program, which builds on the ENCODE project, has shown the crucial role of epigenomic information for improving our knowledge of gene regulation, cellular differentiation, and human disease (http://www.roadmapepigenomics.org). A recent study has shown that trait- and disease-associated variants are enriched in tissue-specific epigenetic marks [50]. The database is a powerful tool to interpret the molecular mechanisms of human diseases.

Although recent studies identified interindividual variability of immune responses, those studies assessed only a few factors. To improve our understanding of the variability of immune responses in human pathologies more comprehensively, the Human Functional Genomics Project (HFGP) was launched in 2013 (http://www.humanfunctionalgenomics.org) [51]. The project combines "omics" techniques with rigorous phenotyping of immune responses in healthy and diseased subjects. The HFGP database will be a valuable tool for functional genomic studies of human immune-mediated disorders.

Conclusions

There are two major hypotheses regarding the mechanism of AD, abnormalities of the skin barrier and skin inflammation due to dysregulation of immune responses. Intriguingly, candidate genes of AD suggested by GWAS are involved in skin barrier functions and innate and adaptive immune responses. There are great differences in clinical phenotypes of AD among individuals. Since the definition of the phenotype is crucial for genetic studies, deep phenotyping and genotyping studies are needed, and further interdisciplinary research is necessary for translation of the genetics of AD into clinical practice.

References

1. Weidinger S, Novak N. Atopic dermatitis. Lancet. 2016;387:1109–22. doi:10.1016/S0140-6736(15)00149-X.
2. Manolio TA. Genomewide association studies and assessment of the risk of disease. N Engl J Med. 2010;363:166–76. doi:10.1056/NEJMra0905980.
3. Marchini J, Howie B. Genotype imputation for genome-wide association studies. Nat Rev Genet. 2010;11:499–511. doi:10.1038/nrg2796.
4. Irvine AD, McLean WH, Leung DY. Filaggrin mutations associated with skin and allergic diseases. N Engl J Med. 2011;365:1315–27. doi:10.1056/NEJMra1011040.
5. Esparza-Gordillo J, Weidinger S, Fölster-Holst R, Bauerfeind A, Ruschendorf F, Patone G, et al. A common variant on chromosome 11q13 is associated with atopic dermatitis. Nat Genet. 2009;41:596–601. doi:10.1038/ng.347.

6. Sun LD, Xiao FL, Li Y, Zhou WM, Tang HY, Tang XF, et al. Genome-wide association study identifies two new susceptibility loci for atopic dermatitis in the Chinese Han population. Nat Genet. 2011;43:690–4. doi:10.1038/ng.851.
7. Paternoster L, Standl M, Chen CM, Ramasamy A, Bønnelykke K, Duijts L, et al. Meta-analysis of genome-wide association studies identifies three new risk loci for atopic dermatitis. Nat Genet. 2011;44:187–92. doi:10.1038/ng.1017.
8. Hirota T, Takahashi A, Kubo M, Tsunoda T, Tomita K, Sakashita M, et al. Genome-wide association study identifies eight new susceptibility loci for atopic dermatitis in the Japanese population. Nat Genet. 2012;44:1222–6. doi:10.1038/ng.2438.
9. Ellinghaus D, Baurecht H, Esparza-Gordillo J, Rodríguez E, Matanovic A, Marenholz I, et al. High-density genotyping study identifies four new susceptibility loci for atopic dermatitis. Nat Genet. 2013;45:808–12. doi:10.1038/ng.2642.
10. Esparza-Gordillo J, Schaarschmidt H, Liang L, Cookson W, Bauerfeind A, Lee-Kirsch MA, et al. A functional IL-6 receptor (IL6R) variant is a risk factor for persistent atopic dermatitis. J Allergy Clin Immunol. 2013;132:371–7. doi:10.1016/j.jaci.2013.01.057.
11. Kim KW, Myers RA, Lee JH, Igartua C, Lee KE, Kim YH, et al. Genome-wide association study of recalcitrant atopic dermatitis in Korean children. J Allergy Clin Immunol. 2015;136:678–684.e4. doi:10.1016/j.jaci.2015.03.030.
12. Schaarschmidt H, Ellinghaus D, Rodríguez E, Kretschmer A, Baurecht H, Lipinski S, et al. A genome-wide association study reveals 2 new susceptibility loci for atopic dermatitis. J Allergy Clin Immunol. 2015;136:802–6. doi:10.1016/j.jaci.2015.01.047.
13. Paternoster L, Standl M, Waage J, Baurecht H, Hotze M, Strachan DP, et al. Multi-ancestry genome-wide association study of 21,000 cases and 95,000 controls identifies new risk loci for atopic dermatitis. Nat Genet. 2015;47:1449–56. doi:10.1038/ng.3424.
14. Doherty TA, Soroosh P, Khorram N, Fukuyama S, Rosenthal P, Cho JY, et al. The tumor necrosis factor family member LIGHT is a target for asthmatic airway remodeling. Nat Med. 2011;17:596–603. doi:10.1038/nm.2356.
15. Montgomery RI, Warner MS, Lum BJ, Spear PG. Herpes simplex virus-1 entry into cells mediated by a novel member of the TNF/NGF receptor family. Cell. 1996;87:427–36.
16. Liew FY, Pitman NI, McInnes IB. Disease-associated functions of IL-33: the new kid in the IL-1 family. Nat Rev Immunol. 2010;10:103–10. doi:10.1038/nri2692.
17. Parkes M, Cortes A, van Heel DA, Brown MA. Genetic insights into common pathways and complex relationships among immune-mediated diseases. Nat Rev Genet. 2013;14:661–73. doi:10.1038/nrg3502.
18. Hirota T, Takahashi A, Kubo M, Tsunoda T, Tomita K, Doi S, et al. Genome-wide association study identifies three new susceptibility loci for adult asthma in the Japanese population. Nat Genet. 2011;43:893–6. doi:10.1038/ng.887.
19. Hong X, Hao K, Ladd-Acosta C, Hansen KD, Tsai HJ, Liu X, et al. Genome-wide association study identifies peanut allergy-specific loci and evidence of epigenetic mediation in US children. Nat Commun. 2015;6:6304. doi:10.1038/ncomms7304.
20. Damm A, Giebeler N, Zamek J, Zigrino P, Kufer TA. Epidermal NLRP10 contributes to contact hypersensitivity responses in mice. Eur J Immunol. 2016;46:1959–69. doi:10.1002/eji.201646401.
21. Saeki H, Tamaki K. Thymus and activation regulated chemokine (TARC)/CCL17 and skin diseases. J Dermatol Sci. 2006;43:75–84.
22. Jung K, Tanaka A, Fujita H, Matsuda A, Oida K, Karasawa K, et al. Peroxisome proliferator-activated receptor γ-mediated suppression of dendritic cell function prevents the onset of atopic dermatitis in NC/Tnd mice. J Allergy Clin Immunol. 2011;127:420–429.e1–6. doi:10.1016/j.jaci.2010.10.043.
23. Lopez RG, Garcia-Silva S, Moore SJ, Bereshchenko O, Martinez-Cruz AB, Ermakova O, et al. C/EBPalpha and beta couple interfollicular keratinocyte proliferation arrest to commitment and terminal differentiation. Nat Cell Biol. 2009;11:1181–90. doi:10.1038/ncb1960.
24. Molinero LL, Cubre A, Mora-Solano C, Wang Y, Alegre ML. T cell receptor/CARMA1/NF-κB signaling controls T-helper (Th) 17 differentiation. Proc Natl Acad Sci U S A. 2012;109:18529–34. doi:10.1073/pnas.1204557109.

25. Wang L, Ni X, Covington KR, Yang BY, Shiu J, Zhang X, et al. Genomic profiling of Sézary syndrome identifies alterations of key T cell signaling and differentiation genes. Nat Genet. 2015;47:1426–34. doi:10.1038/ng.3444.
26. Hou S, Du L, Lei B, Pang CP, Zhang M, Zhuang W, et al. Genome-wide association analysis of Vogt-Koyanagi-Harada syndrome identifies two new susceptibility loci at 1p31.2 and 10q21.3. Nat Genet. 2014;46:1007–11. doi:10.1038/ng.3061.
27. Okamura T, Fujio K, Sumitomo S, Yamamoto K. Roles of LAG3 and EGR2 in regulatory T cells. Ann Rheum Dis. 2012;71:i96–100. doi:10.1136/annrheumdis-2011-200588.
28. Safford M, Collins S, Lutz MA, Allen A, Huang CT, Kowalski J, et al. Egr-2 and Egr-3 are negative regulators of T cell activation. Nat Immunol. 2005;6:472–80.
29. Hart PH, Gorman S, Finlay-Jones JJ. Modulation of the immune system by UV radiation: more than just the effects of vitamin D? Nat Rev Immunol. 2011;11:584–96. doi:10.1038/nri3045.
30. Peroni DG, Piacentini GL, Cametti E, Chinellato I, Boner AL. Correlation between serum 25-hydroxyvitamin D levels and severity of atopic dermatitis in children. Br J Dermatol. 2011;164:1078–82. doi:10.1111/j.1365-2133.2010.10147.x.
31. Haeck IM, Knol MJ, Ten Berge O, van Velsen SG, de Bruin-Weller MS, Bruijnzeel-Koomen CA. Enteric-coated mycophenolate sodium versus cyclosporin A as long-term treatment in adult patients with severe atopic dermatitis: a randomized controlled trial. J Am Acad Dermatol. 2011;64:1074–84. doi:10.1016/j.jaad.2010.04.027.
32. Schuster C, Gerold KD, Schober K, Probst L, Boerner K, Kim MJ, et al. The autoimmunity-associated gene CLEC16A modulates thymic epithelial cell autophagy and alters T cell selection. Immunity. 2015;42:942–52. doi:10.1016/j.immuni.2015.04.011.
33. Hinds DA, McMahon G, Kiefer AK, Do CB, Eriksson N, Evans DM, et al. A genome-wide association meta-analysis of self-reported allergy identifies shared and allergy-specific susceptibility loci. Nat Genet. 2013;45:907–11. doi:10.1038/ng.2686.
34. ENCODE Project Consortium. An integrated encyclopedia of DNA elements in the human genome. Nature. 2012;489:57–74. doi:10.1038/nature11247.
35. Bernstein BE, Stamatoyannopoulos JA, Costello JF, Ren B, Milosavljevic A, Meissner A, et al. The NIH Roadmap Epigenomics Mapping Consortium. Nat Biotechnol. 2010;28:1045–8. doi:10.1038/nbt1010-1045.
36. Grundberg E, Small KS, Hedman ÅK, Nica AC, Buil A, Keildson S, et al. Mapping cis- and trans-regulatory effects across multiple tissues in twins. Nat Genet. 2012;44:1084–9. doi:10.1038/ng.2394.
37. de Jong MA, Geijtenbeek TB. Langerhans cells in innate defense against pathogens. Trends Immunol. 2010;31:452–9. doi:10.1016/j.it.2010.08.002.
38. Lundström W, Highfill S, Walsh ST, Beq S, Morse E, Kockum I, et al. Soluble IL7Rα potentiates IL-7 bioactivity and promotes autoimmunity. Proc Natl Acad Sci U S A. 2013;110:E1761–70. doi:10.1073/pnas.1222303110.
39. Uehira M, Matsuda H, Nakamura A, Nishimoto H. Immunologic abnormalities exhibited in IL-7 transgenic mice with dermatitis. J Invest Dermatol. 1998;110:740–5.
40. Minegishi Y, Saito M, Tsuchiya S, Tsuge I, Takada H, Hara T, et al. Dominant-negative mutations in the DNA-binding domain of STAT3 cause hyper-IgE syndrome. Nature. 2007;448:1058–62.
41. Stritesky GL, Jameson SC, Hogquist KA. Selection of self-reactive T cells in the thymus. Annu Rev Immunol. 2012;30:95–114. doi:10.1146/annurev-immunol-020711-075035.
42. Zook EC, Ramirez K, Guo X, van der Voort G, Sigvardsson M, Svensson EC, et al. The ETS1 transcription factor is required for the development and cytokine-induced expansion of ILC2. J Exp Med. 2016;213:687–96. doi:10.1084/jem.20150851.
43. Baurecht H, Hotze M, Brand S, Büning C, Cormican P, Corvin A, et al. Genome-wide comparative analysis of atopic dermatitis and psoriasis gives insight into opposing genetic mechanisms. Am J Hum Genet. 2015;96:104–20. doi:10.1016/j.ajhg.2014.12.004.
44. Marenholz I, Esparza-Gordillo J, Rüschendorf F, Bauerfeind A, Strachan DP, Spycher BD, et al. Meta-analysis identifies seven susceptibility loci involved in the atopic march. Nat Commun. 2015;6:8804. doi:10.1038/ncomms9804.

45. Schübeler D. Function and information content of DNA methylation. Nature. 2015;517:321–6. doi:10.1038/nature14192.
46. Liang L, Willis-Owen SA, Laprise C, Wong KC, Davies GA, Hudson TJ, et al. An epigenome-wide association study of total serum immunoglobulin E concentration. Nature. 2015;520:670–4. doi:10.1038/nature14125.
47. Auer PL, Lettre G. Rare variant association studies: considerations, challenges and opportunities. Genome Med. 2015;7:16. doi:10.1186/s13073-015-0138-2.
48. Belkaid Y, Segre JA. Dialogue between skin microbiota and immunity. Science. 2014;346:954–9. doi:10.1126/science.1260144.
49. GTEx Consortium. The Genotype-Tissue Expression (GTEx) project. Nat Genet. 2013;45:580–5. doi:10.1038/ng.2653.
50. Roadmap Epigenomics Consortium, Kundaje A, Meuleman W, Ernst J, Bilenky M, Yen A, Heravi-Moussavi A, et al. Integrative analysis of 111 reference human epigenomes. Nature. 2015;518:317–30. doi:10.1038/nature14248.
51. Netea MG, Joosten LA, Li Y, Kumar V, Oosting M, Smeekens S, et al. Understanding human immune function using the resources from the Human Functional Genomics Project. Nat Med. 2016;22:831–3. doi:10.1038/nm.4140.

Part IV

Etiopathology of AD From Japanese Studies

Skin Barrier Function in Atopic Dermatitis

6

Hiroyuki Murota, Kosuke Yamaga, and Ichiro Katayama

Abstract

Recent approaches to explore the pathogenic etiologies of atopic dermatitis using molecular genetic techniques have revealed underlying abnormalities in skin barrier function. Primary cutaneous barrier function is maintained by several physiological factors, including proper skin permeability that is regulated by both the stratum corneum barrier and the tight junction barrier and innate immune response of secretion from both the skin and skin appendages. The corneocyte lipid envelope and natural moisturizing factors derived from filaggrin prevent skin dryness and function in pathogen control. Epidermal tight junctions are composed of claudin-1, which comprises a water barrier correlated with its expression level. Secretions, such as sebum and sweat, contribute to decrease the impact of environmental stimuli (e.g., antigens, detergents, proteases, heat, and mechanical stimuli) to maintain the moistness of the stratum corneum and to regulate temperature. Disruption or dysfunction of these mechanisms impairs skin homeostasis and allows the invasion of pathogens from outside. Development of internal inflammation causes external barrier disruption in turn. This vicious cycle contributes to the chronic inflammation of atopic dermatitis. Appropriate guidance with a main focus on barrier restoration will restrain recurrence of the symptoms. This chapter reviews the barrier function of skin in atopic dermatitis.

Keywords

Atopic dermatitis • Barrier • Filaggrin • Tight junction • Claudins • Stratum corneum • Anti-microbial peptides • Corneocyte lipid envelope

H. Murota (✉) • K. Yamaga • I. Katayama
Dermatology, Department of Integrated Medicine, Graduate School of Medicine, Osaka University, 2-2, Yamadaoka, Suita-shi, Osaka 565-0871, Japan
e-mail: h-murota@derma.med.osaka-u.ac.jp

I. Katayama et al. (eds.), *Evolution of Atopic Dermatitis in the 21st Century*,
https://doi.org/10.1007/978-981-10-5541-6_6

6.1 The Outline of Barrier Dysfunction in Atopic Dermatitis

Previously, barrier dysfunction, such as abnormally increased permeability and higher susceptibility to infection of the skin, was confirmed in atopic dermatitis and thought to be a result of allergic inflammation. More recent evidence, such as (i) a positive correlation between increased permeability of skin and disease severity of atopic dermatitis [1], (ii) impaired barrier function in non-lesional skin of atopic dermatitis patients [2], and (iii) efficacy of proper care for improving skin barrier (e.g., showering, application of moisturizers) to reduce severity of disease [3–5], indicated that these abnormalities in skin barrier observed in atopic dermatitis patients are not a result, but a cause, of this disease.

6.2 The Factor Influencing Permeability of Normal Skin

The stratum corneum, which covers the surface of the epidermis, is one of the elements that has a major influence on the permeability of the skin, protects against environmental dryness by preventing water evaporation from the inside of the body, and also plays an antibacterial role and contributes to the normal microbial flora simultaneously [6].

Corneocytes are flat anuclear cells, are the major component of the stratum corneum, and are surrounded by the corneocyte lipid envelope, showing a major lamella structure consisting of ceramide and cholesterol unesterified fatty acid (Fig. 6.1). The hydrophobic properties of the corneocyte lipid envelope prevent leakage of water from inside to outside [7]. Lamellar granules in the granular layer of the epidermis provide components of the lipid envelope and also participate in supplying enzymes that are required for the synthesis of ceramide and fatty acids (Fig. 6.1). Concurrently, proteases or protease inhibitors derived from lamella granules degrade corneodesmosomes, and subsequently, old corneocytes will be peeled off in order (Fig. 6.1). Antibacterial peptides are also supplied to the corneocyte lipid envelope via lamella granules.

6.3 Genetic Abnormalities in Barrier Dysfunction

The identification of genetic abnormalities in expression of serine proteases, serine protease inhibitors, or filaggrin in the stratum corneum has promoted the understanding of the hereditary predisposition of atopic dermatitis. The mechanisms of barrier dysfunction found in Netherton syndrome, which shows excess activity of serine protease, provided us with useful information for understanding the factors that influence atopic predisposition.

In Netherton syndrome, excess activation of serine protease, resulting from a loss-of-function mutation Glu420Lys (single-nucleotide polymorphism [SNP]) in the serine protease inhibitor *Kazal type 5* (*SPINK5*) (disease specificity of this mutation remains questionable), causes an excessive activation of serine proteases

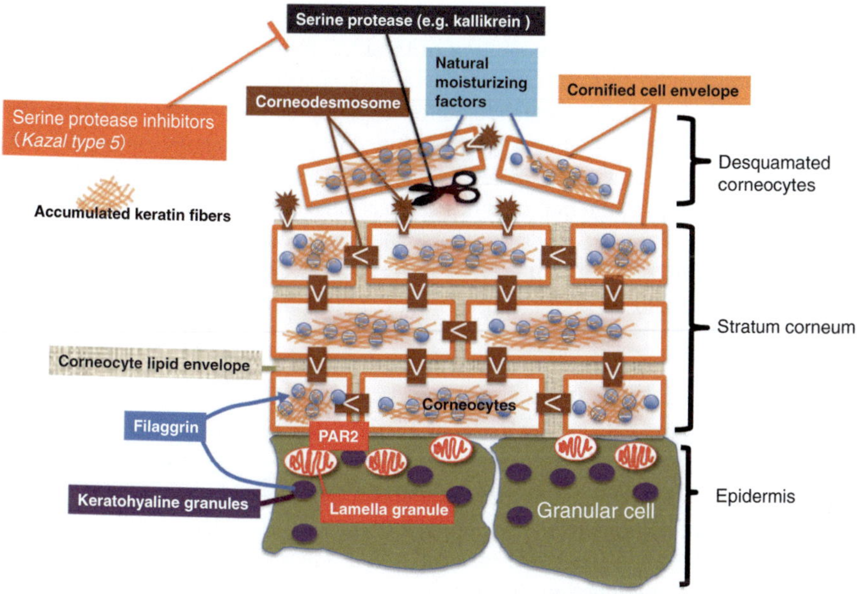

Fig. 6.1 Scheme of a cornified layer barrier: the lamella granules and the keratohyalin granules in the epidermis play important roles in the formation of a mature stratum corneum. The corneocytes are surrounded by a cornified cell envelope, and the keratin fiber is bundled with filaggrin. Filaggrin is degraded into a natural moisturizing factor. A firm barrier is formed via adherence between corneocytes and corneodesmosomes. Serine proteases break down the corneodesmosome, and old corneocytes will be detached

in the stratum corneum and leads to extravagant degradation of both corneodesmosome and lipid processing enzymes [8, 9] (Fig. 6.1). Aberrant degradation of these molecules involved in stabilization of the stratum corneum leads to development of skin phenotypes similar to atopic dermatitis, which is characterized by fragile stratum corneum with abnormally increased permeability [8].

Netherton syndrome is considered a disease that should be excluded from atopic dermatitis according to criteria for atopic dermatitis created by the Japanese Dermatological Association [10]. Additionally accelerated activation of serine protease inhibits secretion of lamella granules via activation of plasminogen activator type 2 receptor (PAR2), leading to barrier dysfunction [11].

Evidence of the close relationship between the etiology of atopic dermatitis and the loss-of-function mutation in filament-aggregating protein (filaggrin [FLG]) suggests that both structural and functional abnormalities of the stratum corneum may be the basis of the pathogenic etiology of atopic dermatitis [12]. FLG is a component of F-type keratohyalin granules, and its loss-of-function mutation has also been confirmed in atopic dermatitis patients as well as in ichthyosis vulgaris patients, and about 2/3 of the ichthyosis vulgaris cases were complicated with allergic diseases, such as atopic dermatitis, allergic rhinitis, and asthma [1]. Common physiological response in keratinization results in dephosphorylation and degradation of the FLG precursor, producing the FLG monomer, which agglutinates keratin in corneocytes to be irrefrangible. Further degradation of the FLG monomer contributes to moisture retention by the stratum corneum as a natural moisturizing factor. Although decreased FLG impairs the water-retention capacity of the stratum corneum, the minimum requirement of FLG for preventing skin dryness has yet to be defined. Expression levels of FLG are affected by environmental factors and skin inflammation [13]. Furthermore, the mutation of FLG has been confirmed only in some cases with atopic dermatitis. A recent study of Japanese subjects found that the prevalence of FLG mutations is 11.1% (n = 820) [14]. Thus, we should keep in mind that decreased FLG could be both a cause and a consequence of the skin conditions in atopic dermatitis.

6.4 Epidermal Barrier: Role of Tight Junctions

The epidermis should be the final sophisticated defense against pathogens (Fig. 6.2). To avoid entry of pathogens into the body and to avoid water leakage through paracellular space between the epidermal cells, cell adhesion structures called "tight junctions" exist. Tight junctions in the epidermal granular layer have been confirmed by both electron microscopy and immunofluorescence, and these tight junctions form the barrier of the paracellular space to regulate permeability [15]. On another front, Langerhans cells exist inside the epidermis and elongate their dendrites to reach the outside of tight junction to sample pathogens [16]. Even in this case, tight junctions are formed between extended dendrites of activated Langerhans cells and epidermal granular cells [16]. This finding shows the importance of epidermal tight junctions. Every tight junction consists of transmembrane proteins (e.g., claudins, occludin, and tricellulin), cytoplasmic adaptor proteins, and cytoskeletal linkers (e.g., zonula occludens (ZO) proteins, etc.) [15, 17, 18] (Fig. 6.2). Claudins, which are essential tight junction transmembrane proteins, have 27 family members [15]. Claudin-1 and claudin-4 are expressed in skin epithelial cells and have roles in paracellular barrier function and possibly regulation of cell differentiation, respectively [15]. Claudin-1 is the major component of the epidermal tight junction and is indispensable to prevent fatal dehydration, as shown by claudin-1 knockout (*Cldn1*KO) animals [15, 17, 18]. An SNP in the *claudin-1 (Cldn1)* gene and inflammation-mediated decreased expression of claudin-1 have been observed in subjects with atopic dermatitis and have been found to be involved in the etiology of atopic dermatitis [19, 20]. More recently, claudin-1 was found to regulate the adequacy of the paracellular barrier in a dose-dependent manner, and decreased claudin-1 was found to cause skin manifestations resembling those in atopic dermatitis [21].

Fatal dehydration in *Cldn1*KO mice has been a barrier to investigation of the pathogenic involvement of claudin-1 in atopic dermatitis. Thus, Tokumasu et al. generated six types of *Cldn1* knockdown (*Cldn1*KD) mice with different expression levels of *Cldn1* and found dysfunction of the epidermal barrier caused by decreased *Cldn-1* levels to less than half [21]. Decreased expression of Cldn-1 affected

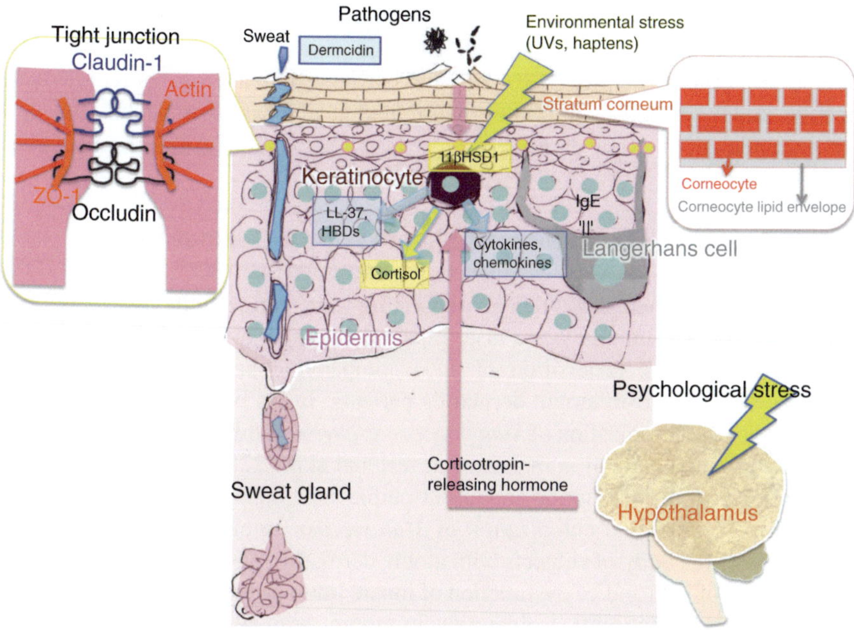

Fig. 6.2 Scheme of the defense mechanisms of the skin. Pathogens penetrate from the outside of the skin via a damaged stratum corneum. Pathogens or substances derived from pathogens pass through the tight junction, activating keratinocytes via pattern-recognition receptors. The activated keratinocytes release antimicrobial peptides (e.g., LL-37, human β-defensins [hBDs]), cytokines, and/or chemokines to recruit inflammatory cells. Keratinocytes exposed to environmental stresses will activate 11βHSD1 and produce cortisol to reduce the negative impact of environmental stimuli. Psychological stresses activate the hypothalamus in the central nervous system, causing release of corticotropin-releasing hormone (CRH) to regulate epidermal homeostasis

differentiation of keratinocytes and increased the number of K5-positive or ectopically proliferating suprabasal cells [21].

*Cldn1*KD mice develop age-related skin manifestations. *Cldn1*KD mice and moderately decreased *Cldn1* (*Cldn1*$^{\Delta/\Delta}$) mice develop wrinkled skin and dry hair at around 1 week and 2 weeks of age, respectively. This skin phenotype disappeared by 8 weeks of age. This age-related phenotypic change appears similar to the clinical course of human pediatric atopic dermatitis cases, as most human pediatric patients outgrow the disease. *Cldn1*KD mice with severely decreased *Cldn1* (*Cldn1*$^{\Delta/-}$) show more severe skin manifestations with severe desquamation and wrinkled skin at the age of 8 weeks or older [21]. These findings indicate that expression of *Cldn-1* will affect the severity of atopic dermatitis symptoms. Also, increased numbers of skin-homing innate immune cells, such as neutrophils and macrophages, in *Cldn1*KD mice indicated that epidermal barrier dysfunction requires functional augmentation of innate immunity to cope with penetration of certain pathogens from the outside [21].

Further elucidation of the precise mechanism of epidermal barrier dysfunction may lead to a better understanding of the pathogenesis and natural clinical course of atopic dermatitis. The epidermal barrier may, therefore, provide a therapeutic target and may contribute to formulation of novel therapeutic strategies for management of atopic dermatitis.

6.5 Defense Mechanism of Skin in Atopic Dermatitis

Host defense mechanisms, such as regulating skin permeability (as mentioned above) and innate immunity, are also impaired in atopic dermatitis. These abnormalities lead to the acquisition of an accompanying bacterial infection (e.g., impetigo contagiosa) in atopic dermatitis patients. It has been confirmed that the frequency of the colonization of *Staphylococcus aureus* is different between lesional and non-lesional skin and is increased in lesional skin [22]. Viral infections (e.g., Kaposi's varicelliform eruption and molluscum contagiosum) and fungal infections (e.g., tinea corporis and colonization of *Malassezia*) are also frequently found in large areas of the body of subjects with atopic dermatitis [23]. Aberrantly increased permeability of skin and/or dysfunction of innate immune responses are involved in the increased susceptibility to infection in atopic dermatitis [23] (Fig. 6.2). The innate immune system in the skin surface is formulated with genetically encoded molecules that are inherent in the human skin and skin appendages themselves [23]. Receptors that recognize the highly conserved structure in pathogens, the so-called pattern-recognition receptors (PRRs), such as Toll-like receptors (TLRs) and collectin proteins, are expressed on keratinocytes and Langerhans cells and induce the innate immune response by binding with pathogen-associated molecular patterns (PAMPs) characterized by cell wall products such as LPS, peptidoglycan, and viral double-stranded RNA derived from common pathogens [23, 24]. The innate immune response is characterized by the release of antimicrobial peptides (AMPs), chemokines, and cytokines and will immediately inhibit the infection [23, 25]. AMPs are released from keratinocytes and are also contained in sweat [23, 26] (Fig. 6.2). Continuous secretion of dermcidin from sweat glands contributes to the regulation of the proper skin surface microbiome [27].

These innate defense mechanisms are impaired by Th2-type inflammation, which is the prominent inflammation in atopic dermatitis, by decreasing the release of antibacterial peptides, such as human cathelicidin product (hCAP), cathelicidin (LL-37), and human β-defensins (hBDs) [26]. Because LL-37 is necessary for the formation of a mature stratum corneum, alterations in the release of AMPs negatively impact the innate defense mechanism via increasing the permeability of the skin [7].

In addition to responding to infection by pathogens, the innate host defense responses of keratinocyte are induced by environmental stresses, such as UV irradiation or exposure to haptens via production of cortisol associated with activation of 11β-hydroxysteroid dehydrogenase type 1 (11βHSD1) [28–32]. Cortisol derived from keratinocytes, which are exposed to environmental stimuli, minimizes damage of the skin. Decreased expression of 11βHSD1 in keratinocytes has been found in atopic dermatitis and leads to the impairment of the innate host defense response [30, 32, 33]. As for treatment strategies to target 11βHSD1, topical application of cholesterol restores the expression of 11βHSD1 in keratinocytes and reduces the severity of hapten-evoked dermatitis [33].

Conclusion

The skin barrier, which is characterized by both proper permeability of the skin and innate immunity, largely contributes to host defense mechanisms. The identified molecular-based mechanisms have been found to be impaired in atopic dermatitis. Understanding the importance of barrier function leads to the notion that care of the skin to improve the skin barrier should take precedent over anything. The question of whether there is a difference in the mechanism of barrier dysfunction between each case is a point of interest, and resolution of these issues will contribute to the development of therapeutic strategies for each case.

Conflict of Interest The authors have no conflicts of interest to declare.

References

1. Proksch E, Folster-Holst R, Jensen JM. Skin barrier function, epidermal proliferation and differentiation in eczema. J Dermatol Sci. 2006;43:159–69.
2. Seidenari S, Girusti G. Objective assessment of the skin of child affected by atopic dermatitis: a study of pH, capacitance and TEWL in eczematous and clinically uninvolved skin. Acta Derm Venereol. 1995;75(6):429–33.
3. Grimalt R, Mengeaud V, Cambazard F. The steroid-sparing effect of an emollient therapy in infants with atopic dermatitis: a randomized controlled study. Dermatology. 2007;214:61–7.
4. Murota H, Takahashi A, Nishioka M, et al. Showering reduces atopic dermatitis in elementary school students. Eur J Dermatol. 2010;20:410–1.
5. Elias PM, Wood LC, Freingold KR. Epidermal pathogenesis of inflammatory dermatoses. Am J Contact Dermat. 1999;10:119–26.
6. Elias PM. Stratum corneum as an innate immune element. Semin Immunopathol. 2007;29:3–14.
7. Elias PM. Stratum corneum defensive functions: an integrated view. J Invest Dermatol. 2005;125:183–200.
8. Walley AJ, Chanvanas S, Moffatt MF, et al. Gene polymorphism in Netherton and common atopic disease. Nat Genet. 2001;29:175–8.
9. Elias PM, Schmutt M. Abnormal skin barrier in the etiopathogenesis of atopic dermatitis. Curr Opin Allergy Clin Immunol. 2009;9:437–46.
10. Saeki H, Nakahara T, Tanaka A, Kabashima K, Sugaya M, Murota H, Ebihara T, Kataoka Y, Aihara M, Etoh T, Katoh N, Committee for Clinical Practice Guidelines for the Management of Atopic Dermatitis of Japanese Dermatological Association. Clinical practice guidelines for the management of atopic dermatitis 2016. J Dermatol. 2016;43:1117–45.
11. Hachem JP, Houben E, Crumrine D, et al. Serine protease signaling of epidermal permeability barrier homeostasis. J Invest Dermatol. 2006;126:2074–86.
12. Fleckman P, Brumbaugh S. Absence of the granular layer and keratohyalin define a morphologically distinct subset of individuals with ichthyosis vulgaris. Exp Dermatol. 2002;11:327–36.
13. Kono M, Nomura T, Ohguchi Y, Mizuno O, Suzuki S, Tsujiuchi H, Hamajima N, McLean WH, Shimizu H, Akiyama M. Comprehensive screening for a complete set of Japanese-population-specific filaggrin gene mutations. Allergy. 2014;69:537–40.

14. Egawa G, Kabashima K. Multifactorial skin barrier deficiency and atopic dermatitis: essential topics to prevent the atopic march. J Allergy Clin Immunol. 2016;138:350–8.
15. Tamura A, Tsukita S. Paracellular barrier and channel functions of TJ claudins in organizing biological systems: advances in the field of barriology revealed in knockout mice. Semin Cell Dev Biol. 2014;36:177–85.
16. Kubo A, Nagao K, Yokouchi M, Sasaki H, Amagai M. External antigen uptake by Langerhans cells with reorganization of epidermal tight junction barriers. J Exp Med. 2009;206:2937–46.
17. Furuse M, et al. Claudin-based tight junctions are crucial for the mammalian epidermal barrier: a lesson from claudin-1-deficient mice. J Cell Biol. 2002;156:1099–111.
18. Sugawara T, et al. Tight junction dysfunction in the stratum granulosum leads to aberrant stratum corneum barrier function in claudin-1-deficient mice. J Dermatol Sci. 2013;70:12–8.
19. De Benedetto A, Slifka MK, Rafaels NM, Kuo IH, Georas SN, Boguniewicz M, Hata T, Schneider LC, Hanifin JM, Gallo RL, Johnson DC, Barnes KC, Leung DY, Beck LA. Reductions in claudin-1 may enhance susceptibility to herpes simplex virus 1infections in atopic dermatitis. J Allergy Clin Immunol. 2011;128:242–6.
20. De Benedetto A, Rafaels NM, McGirt LY, Ivanov AI, Georas SN, Cheadle C, Berger AE, Zhang K, Vidyasagar S, Yoshida T, Boguniewicz M, Hata T, Schneider LC, Hanifin JM, Gallo RL, Novak N, Weidinger S, Beaty TH, Leung DY, Barnes KC, Beck LA. Tight junction defects in patients with atopic dermatitis. J Allergy Clin Immunol. 2011;127:773–86.
21. Tokumasu R, Yamaga K, Yamazaki Y, Murota H, Suzuki K, Tamura A, Bando K, Furuta Y, Katayama I, Tsukita S. Dose-dependent role of claudin-1 in vivo in orchestrating features of atopic dermatitis. Proc Natl Acad Sci U S A. 2016;113(28):E4061–8.
22. Totté JE, van der Feltz WT, Hennekam M, van Belkum A, van Zuuren EJ, Pasmans SG. Prevalence and odds of Staphylococcus aureus carriage in atopic dermatitis: a systematic review and meta-analysis. Br J Dermatol. 2016;175:687–95.
23. McGirt LY, Beck LA. Innate immune defects in atopic dermatitis. J Allergy Clin Immunol. 2006;118:202–8.
24. Medzhitov R, Janeway C Jr. Innate immunity. N Engl J Med. 2000;343:338–44.
25. Esche C, Stellato C, Beck LA. Chemokines: key players in innate and adaptive immunity. J Invest Dermatol. 2005;125:615–28.
26. Murota H, Matsui S, Ono E, Kijima A, Kikuta J, Ishii M, Katayama I. Sweat, the driving force behind normal skin: an emerging perspective on functional biology and regulatory mechanisms. J Dermatol Sci. 2015;77(1):3–10.
27. Rieg S, Saborowski V, Kern WV, Jonas D, Bruckner-Tuderman L, Hofmann SC. Expression of the sweat-derived innate defence antimicrobial peptide dermcidin is not impaired in Staphylococcus aureus colonization or recurrent skin infections. Clin Exp Dermatol. 2014;39(2):209–12.
28. Terao M, Murota H, Kimura A, Kato A, Ishikawa A, Igawa K, Miyoshi E, Katayama I. 11β-Hydroxysteroid dehydrogenase-1 is a novel regulator of skin homeostasis and a candidate target for promoting tissue repair. PLoS One. 2011;6:e25039.
29. Itoi S, Terao M, Murota H, Katayama I. 11β-Hydroxysteroid dehydrogenase 1 contributes to the pro-inflammatory response of keratinocytes. Biochem Biophys Res Commun. 2013;440:265–70.
30. Terao M, Itoi S, Matsumura S, Yang L, Murota H, Katayama I. Local glucocorticoid activation by 11β-Hydroxysteroid dehydrogenase 1 in keratinocytes: the role in Hapten-induced dermatitis. Am J Pathol. 2016;186:1499–510.
31. Itoi-Ochi S, Terao M, Murota H, Katayama I. Local corticosterone activation by 11β-hydroxysteroid dehydrogenase 1 in keratinocytes: the role in narrow-band UVB-induced dermatitis. Dermatoendocrinol. 2016;8(1):e1119958.
32. Terao M, Katayama I. Local cortisol/corticosterone activation in skin physiology and pathology. J Dermatol Sci. 2016;84(1):11–6.
33. Murota H, Itoi S, Terao M, Matsui S, Kawai H, Satou Y, Suda K, Katayama I. Topical cholesterol treatment ameliorates hapten-evoked cutaneous hypersensitivity by sustaining expression of 11β-HSD1 in epidermis. Exp Dermatol. 2014;23:68–70.

7 Immunological Perspectives: Th2 Cells/ Mast Cells/Basophils/Eosinophils

Takashi Hashimoto and Takahiro Satoh

Abstract

Atopic dermatitis (AD) is a chronic allergic skin disease with severe pruritus. The "three musketeers" of skin barrier dysfunction, allergy/immunology, and pruritus are considered to play important roles. Th2 immunity mediated by the cytokines interleukin (IL)-4, IL-13, IL-5, and IL-31 has been considered as a key immune process in the pathogenesis of AD. Other cytokines (e.g., TSLP) and chemokines (e.g., TARC/CCL17 and MDC/CCL22) also play important roles in Th2 skewing and the development of skin inflammation. Mast cells release several preformed mediators, as well as newly synthesized proteins and cytokines upon stimulation, contributing to the inflammatory processes and pruritus. Eosinophils have been implicated in tissue remodeling. Basophils may contribute to Th2 skewing but may also exert as-yet unidentified but crucial functions that need to be elucidated in future work.

Keywords

Atopic dermatitis • Basophils • Eosinophils • Mast cells • Th2 immunity

T. Hashimoto, M.D., Ph.D. (✉)
Department of Dermatology, Graduate School, Tokyo Medical and Dental University, 1-5-45, Yushima, Bunkyo-ku, 113-8519 Tokyo, Japan
e-mail: hashderm@tmd.ac.jp

T. Satoh
Department of Dermatology, National Defense Medical College, 3-2, Namiki, Tokorozawa, 359-8513 Saitama, Japan
e-mail: tasaderm@ndmc.ac.jp

I. Katayama et al. (eds.), *Evolution of Atopic Dermatitis in the 21st Century*,
https://doi.org/10.1007/978-981-10-5541-6_7

7.1 Introduction

Atopic dermatitis (AD) is a chronic allergic skin disease involving severe pruritus [1]. The pathogenesis of AD is multifactorial, and the "three musketeers" of skin barrier dysfunction, allergy/immunology, and pruritus are considered to play important roles [2]. For a long time, T-helper (Th)2 immunity has been considered as a main component in the pathogenesis of AD, since AD is characterized by the predominant expression of Th2-type cytokines with high serum immunoglobulin (Ig)E levels and blood eosinophilia [3]. Recent studies have revealed that the high prevalence of loss-of-function mutations of filaggrin in AD patients and skin barrier dysfunction also plays central roles [4]. Skin barrier dysfunctions provoke inflammation of immunity biased toward Th2, which in turn leads to further impairment of barrier function [5]. In addition, Th2 immunity provokes pruritus via the production of thymic stromal lymphopoietin (TSLP) and the itch-related cytokine interleukin (IL)-31 [6]. Scratching also leads to skin barrier disruption.

This chapter reviews the contribution of Th2 immunity and related immune cells, such as mast cells, eosinophils, and basophils, to the pathogenesis of AD.

7.2 Th2 Immunity

7.2.1 Th2 Immunity in AD

Immunological responses can be classified into three major categories: Th1, Th2, and Th17. In general, allergic diseases are explained by the Th1/Th2/Th17 concept. Th1 cells produce IL-2 and interferon (IFN)-γ. Th2 cells produce IL-4, IL-5, IL-13, and IL-31. IL-17 and IL-22 are produced by Th17 cells.

AD is clinically characterized by skin inflammation, pruritus, peripheral blood eosinophilia, and elevated serum concentrations of IgE. These features are simply explained by Th2 immunity. IL-4 and IL-13 promote Th2 cell differentiation and IgE generation. IL-5 plays a pivotal role in the development, survival, and proliferation of eosinophils [7]. IL-31 is implicated in pruritus [6] (Fig. 7.1). In acute skin lesions of AD, T cells producing Th2-type cytokines infiltrate into the dermis [8]. The contribution of Th2 immunity to AD is supported by a recent clinical study in which a Th2 cytokine receptor antagonist, dupilumab, alleviated AD symptoms [9].

Despite these findings, chronic skin lesions have been shown to be mediated by immunity biased toward Th1 [10]. Th17 cells, which play an essential role in the pathogenesis of psoriasis, may also contribute to the acute phase of AD [11, 12], although this does not appear as prominent as in psoriasis [13]. The role of Th17 immunity in the pathogenesis of AD is uncertain, but IL-17 is hypothesized to enhance the development of AD and prolong exaggeration of skin symptoms [11].

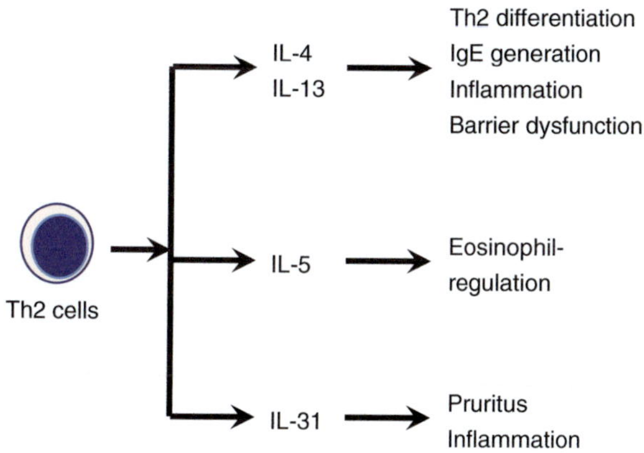

Fig. 7.1 Major Th2-related cytokines. Th2 cells secrete various cytokines. IL-4 and IL-13 promote Th2 differentiation, IgE generation, and inflammation and disrupt epidermal barrier function. IL-5 is implicated in eosinophil regulation. IL-31 is associated with pruritus and inflammation

7.2.2 TSLP

TSLP is a member of the IL-7-like cytokines and is expressed by epidermal keratinocytes, mast cells, dendritic cells (DCs), and fibroblasts [14]. TSLP is now receiving attention as an important player in the pathogenesis of AD.

Elevated levels of TSLP are observed in both acute and chronic skin lesions of AD but not in contact allergic dermatitis from nickel or lupus erythematosus lesions [14]. In addition, levels of TSLP expression in the stratum corneum correlate with the Severity Scoring of AD (SCORAD) index [15].

Allergen injection into the skin in individuals with AD causes rapid dermal TSLP expression [16], with Th2 cytokines (IL-4 and IL-13) in conjunction with pro-inflammatory cytokines (tumor necrosis factor [TNF]-α or IL-1α) inducing TSLP production from human keratinocytes [17]. TSLP generation in keratinocytes is also induced by innate immune responses mediated by Toll-like receptor 2/6 and 5 signals [18–20] and protease-activated receptor (PAR)-2 activation through the proteolytic activity of house dust mite allergen [21]. In addition, periostin released from fibroblasts stimulated by IL-4 and IL-13 induces the expression of keratinocyte TSLP [22]. Even more importantly, epidermal TSLP expression is simply stimulated by skin injury or barrier disruption [23, 24].

A crucial role of TSLP in the pathogenesis of AD is in the promotion of Th2 immune responses. Activation of naive CD4 (+) T cells with TSLP induces IL-4 gene transcription, which in turn upregulates TSLP receptor (TSLPR) expression on those cells. This positive feedback mechanism further promotes Th2 cell differentiation [25–27].

TSLP induces the activation and migration of CD11c (+) DCs. These DCs, when primed with specific antigen in the absence of IL-12, promote Th2 cell differentiation from naive CD4 (+) T cells [14, 28]. In addition, TSLP stimulates DCs to produce Th2 cell-attracting chemokines, such as CCL17/thymus and activation-regulated chemokine (TARC) and CCL22/macrophage-derived chemokine (MDC) [14]. Production of CCL17/TARC and CCL22/MDC is increased in AD patients compared with healthy donors. In addition, serum levels correlate with disease activity [29–31]. CCL17/TARC appears to be generated not only by TSLP-primed DCs but also by activated blood mononuclear cells, endothelial cells, and epidermal keratinocytes [32–34]. CCL22/MDC is secreted by macrophages and DCs [35].

A recent study indicated that pruritus is directly provoked by TSLP through TSLPR on transient receptor potential cation channel subfamily A member 1 (TRPA-1)-positive peripheral sensory nerve fibers [36]. Scratching in turn induces epidermal keratinocytes to express TSLP, forming the vicious cycle of AD [24].

7.2.3 IL-31

Activated Th2 cells produce IL-31 [6]. IL-31 is highly expressed in the lesional skin of AD, and serum levels of IL-31 correlate with the clinical severity of AD [37, 38].

IL-31 is a pruritogenic cytokine [39] but also induces skin inflammation. Cutaneous injection of IL-31 into the skin of mice evokes inflammatory cell infiltration. Cell accumulation induced by IL-31 may be partly explained by the fact that epidermal keratinocytes produce CCL17/TARC and CCL22/MDC in response to IL-31 [39].

7.2.4 IL-18 and IL-33

IL-18 and IL-33 belong to the IL-1 family of cytokines. IL-18 has been generally known as a Th1 cytokine but also contributes to Th2 immunity. IL-18 stimulates basophils, mast cells, and CD4 (+) T cells to produce IL-4 and IL-13 [40–42]. AD patients display elevated serum concentrations of IL-18, with these levels correlating with disease severity and serum IgE [43].

IL-33 promotes the maturation of mast cells and Th2 cells and enhances the production of IL-13 and other cytokines and chemokines from mast cells [44–47]. High levels of IL-33 mRNA expression are observed in the lesional skin of AD [48].

7.3 Mast Cells

Mast cells are tissue-resident inflammatory cells that possess metachromatic cytoplasmic granules. Mast cells express a variety of cell surface receptors including stem cell factor (SCF) receptor CD117 (also known as c-kit) and a high-affinity IgE receptor, Fc epsilon receptor I (FcεRI) [49, 50].

Increased numbers of dermal mast cells are observed in skin lesions of AD [51]. Mast cells show various stages of degranulation in acute skin lesions but are fully granulated in chronic skin lesions [3]. However, whether and how mast cells contribute to the pathogenesis of AD remains unclear [52].

Th2 skewing in AD may affect mast cell proliferation and activation. IL-4 enhances the IgE-induced upregulation of FcεRI on mast cells [53]. IL-5 promotes the proliferation of mast cells in conjunction with SCF [54]. In contrast, the Th1-related cytokine IFN-γ decreases mast cell numbers [50].

Mast cells activated by IgE plus antigens produce and secrete three categories of substances: (1) chemical and protein mediators (histamine, serotonin, heparin, proteases, and even major basic protein [MBP]) [55]; (2) a wide variety of cytokines (e.g., IL-3, IL-4, IL-5, IL-6, and IL-13), chemokines (e.g., CCL3/macrophage inflammatory protein [MIP]-1α, CCL4/MIP-1β, CCL5/regulated on activation, normal T cell expressed and secreted [RANTES], and CXCL10/IFNγ-induced protein-10 [IP-10]), and growth factors (e.g., SCF); and (3) lipid mediators (prostaglandins [PGs], leukotrienes [LTs], etc.).

Histamine is a representative pruritogen released by mast cells. In addition, mast cells produce a tryptase that cleaves and activates its receptor PAR-2 on nerve fibers, provoking pruritus [56].

Mast cell-derived histamine appears to play important roles in tissue remodeling [51]. Synthesis of collagen and periostin by fibroblasts is induced by histamine. Periostin, in turn, stimulates fibroblast collagen synthesis [57] and also induces keratinocyte proliferation [58].

Mast cells are capable of generating Th2-related cytokines (IL-4, IL-5, IL-13, and IL-13), thereby contributing to Th2 immunity. In skin lesions of AD, a high proportion of dermal mast cells express IL-31 [59].

PGD_2 is one of the cyclooxygenase metabolites of arachidonic acid. Mast cells are one of major producers of PGD2 in the skin. Chemoattractant receptor-homologous molecule on Th2 cells (CRTH2), a receptor for PGD_2, is expressed on Th2 cells, eosinophils, basophils, and type 2 innate lymphoid cells (ILC2) [60, 61]. CRTH2 provides stimulatory signals in those cells and exerts chemotactic activity. CRTH2 has been shown to play an essential role in mouse models of AD [62].

7.4 Eosinophils

Eosinophils are granulocytes containing two major types of granules: specific and primary. Specific granules contain cationic proteins such as eosinophil MBP, eosinophil peroxidase (EPO), eosinophil cationic protein (ECP), and eosinophil-derived neurotoxin (EDN). These cationic proteins are protective against bacteria, parasites, and/or viruses but are also toxic to tissue cells [63]. Primary granules show enriched levels of Charcot-Leyden crystal protein (galectin-10) [7, 50]. Eosinophils exert their function by releasing pro-inflammatory mediators, including these proteins, cytokines (e.g., TNF, transforming growth factor [TGF], IL-1, IL-3, IL-4, IL-5, IL-8, IL-10, and IL-13), and eicosanoids (e.g., LTC4, LTD4, and LTE4) [64, 65].

In histology, eosinophils are usually seen in the acute phase of AD but are barely observed in chronic lichenified lesions. However, significant deposition of eosinophil MBP can be detected in the dermis. Tissue eosinophilia is often associated with blood eosinophilia and correlates with the severity of AD [66].

The Th2-related cytokine IL-5 is a key cytokine for eosinophils, and elevated levels of IL-5 mRNA are detected in the skin lesions of AD [67]. IL-5 is produced mainly by stromal cells in bone marrow and by Th2 cells. In addition to IL-5, eotaxins (CCL11/eotaxin and CCL26/eotaxin-3), IL-3, and granulocyte-macrophage colony-stimulating factor (GM-CSF) also promote the development and differentiation of eosinophils from CD34 (+) hematopoietic progenitor cells [68]. Eosinophils that have developed in the bone marrow then mobilize into the blood circulation in response to IL-5 and/or eotaxin stimulation [69, 70] and migrate to inflamed tissues where Th2 immune mechanisms predominate. IL-4 and IL-13 induce P-selectin and endothelial cell vascular cell adhesion molecule 1 (VCAM-1) expression on dermal endothelial cells [71, 72]. Endothelial P-selectin promotes eosinophil rolling on endothelial cells via P-selectin glycoprotein ligand-1 (PSGL-1) [73]. In addition, since very late antigen-4 (VLA-4), a ligand for VCAM-1, is expressed on eosinophils, but not on neutrophils, the IL-4/IL-13-VLA-4 axis may represent a key step in eosinophilic inflammation [74]. IL-4 and IL-13 stimulate dermal fibroblasts to produce eotaxins [75, 76]. Eotaxins and the Th2-related protein TSLP exert chemoattractant activity for eosinophils [77].

On the other hand, IFN-γ, a Th1 cytokine, stimulates dermal fibroblasts to produce CCL5/RANTES [78] and ecalectin (galectin-9) [79], which are both eosinophil chemoattractants [80, 81]. Eosinophils express CXCR3 and exhibit chemotaxis to CXCL10/IP-10 and CXCL9/monokine induced by IFN-γ (Mig) [82]. Importantly, eosinophils themselves generate a Th1 cytokine, IL-12 [83]. Eosinophils may thus participate in the immune reactions of not only Th2-type inflammation but also Th1-type inflammation, such as chronic lesions of AD (Fig. 7.2).

The pathogenic roles of eosinophils in skin inflammation have been a focus of debate, and whether toxic granule proteins (ECP, EDN, EPO, and MBP) derived from eosinophils cause tissue damage remains contentious. One study has demonstrated that dermal eosinophilia induced by intradermal CCL5/RANTES injection did not provoke macroscopic changes in the skin of atopic patients [84]. More importantly, the monoclonal IL-5 antibody mepolizumab has been found to ameliorate only peripheral eosinophilia, not other AD symptoms [85].

A number of recent lines of evidence have suggested a possible contribution of eosinophils to tissue remodeling. TGF-β1 derived from eosinophils promotes fibroblast proliferation, collagen synthesis, and lattice contraction [86]. Eosinophils also produce metalloproteinase 9, vascular endothelial growth factor, basic fibroblast growth factor, and angiogenin [87–89]. In AD patients, intradermal allergen challenge has been found to induce infiltration of TGF-β1 (+) eosinophils, α-smooth muscle action (+) myofibroblasts, and procollagen-I (+) cells [90], which was inhibited by anti-IL-5 monoclonal antibody and TGF-β1-neutralizing antibody [90, 91].

In a murine model of prurigo reactions, the presence of dermal eosinophils correlated with scratching behavior [92]. In a model of contact toxicant reactions, skin innervation and scratching behaviors were dependent on eosinophils [93]. Eosinophils promote branching of sensory neurons in vitro [94]. In humans, MBP and EPO stimulate mast cells to release histamine through Mas-related gene (*Mrgx2*) [95]. Eosinophils may thus participate in the development of intractable itch in AD.

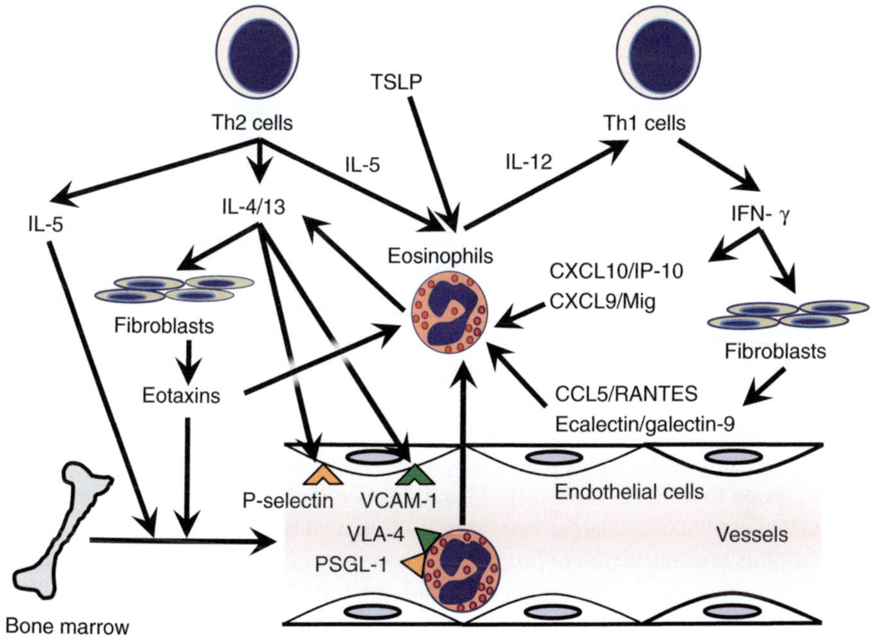

Fig. 7.2 Eosinophil migration into inflamed skin. IL 5 mobilizes the eosinophil pool from bone marrow into the peripheral circulation. The Th2 cytokines IL-4/IL-13 stimulate fibroblasts to generate eosinophil chemokine eotaxins and endothelial cells to express the cell adhesion molecules P-selectin and VCAM-1. The Th1 cytokine IFN-γ mediates CXCL10/IP-10, CXCL9/Mig, CCL5/RANTES, and ecalectin/galectin-9 production, leading to eosinophil accumulation in inflammatory lesions biased toward Th1. IP-10, IFNγ-induced protein-10; Mig, monokine induced by IFN-γ; PSGL-1, P-selectin glycoprotein ligand-1; RANTES, regulated on activation, normal T cell expressed and secreted; VCAM-1, vascular cell adhesion molecule 1; VLA-4, very late antigen-4

7.5 Basophils

Basophils constitute less than 1% of peripheral blood leukocytes and have a half-life of 1–3 days [50]. Basophils share some functional and morphological similarities with mast cells (e.g., expression of the high-affinity IgE receptor FcεRI and secretion of histamine). These similarities initially led to the idea that basophils were minor and redundant relatives or blood-circulating precursors of tissue-resident mast cells [96]. However, recent accumulated evidence has indicated non-redundant roles of basophils compared to mast cells in innate and acquired immunity. In a number of skin diseases, basophils have been demonstrated to be present in skin lesions [97].

With regard to the hematopoiesis of human basophils, a close lineage relationship with eosinophils has recently been demonstrated, as seen in the presence of immature basophils with a basophil-eosinophil hybrid phenotype and the capacity to generate eosinophil-specific MBP [98].

Both TSLP and IL-3 promote the development and maturation of basophils from bone marrow progenitor cells [99]. The Th2 cytokine IL-4 induces expression of VCAM-1. Like eosinophils, human basophils express the VCAM-1 ligand VLA-4 [74]. In addition, P- and E-selectin also contribute, at least partially, to the adhesion of human basophils to endothelium [100]. In mice, functional PSGL-1, modified by α(1,3) fucosyltransferases (FTs)-IV and (FT)-VII, and L-selectin play roles in the initial recruitment of basophils in chronic allergic inflammation [101]. CCL11/eotaxin, CCL2/monocyte chemotactic protein (MCP)-1, CCL13/MCP-4, and histamine (through the histamine H4 receptor) are thought to be chemoattractive for basophils [102–104].

IL-3 from activated T cells promotes basophil development [105]. When activated by FcεRI cross-linking, IL-3-elicited basophils degranulate and release histamine, leukotrienes (e.g., LTB4, LTD4, LTE4), PGs (e.g., PGD2 and PGE2), and cytokines (e.g., IL-4 and IL-13) [106–108]. TSLP, a key player in Th2 immunity of AD, also regulates basophil development and peripheral basophilia [99]. TSLP-elicited basophils respond to IL-3, IL-18, and IL-33 and produce IL-4 [99]. Of note, the amounts of secreted cytokines are larger than from IL-3-elicited basophils.

Basophils are considered to function as antigen-presenting cells (APCs) in mice [109]. However, human basophils have not yet been confirmed to possess APC activity [110–112].

Basophil infiltration is observed in the lesional skin of AD patients [97]. Although a few basophils are present in AD lesions, patch testing with house dust mite antigen has been found to result in significant basophil infiltration into the dermis and even epidermis within 48 h after exposure [97]. In allergen-induced late-phase reactions of AD, maximal eosinophil infiltration occurred at 6 h, whereas peak basophil accumulation was seen at 24 h, one-third of which had morphologic appearances suggestive of degranulation [113, 114].

In a murine model of IgE-dependent eosinophilic dermatitis, infiltration of eosinophils was seen to be dependent on basophils [115]. In IgE-mediated chronic allergic inflammation (IgE-CAI) [116], basophils are indispensable for the induction of eosinophils and other inflammatory cells, even though dermal basophils constituted only 2% of total infiltrative cells [92, 116]. Based on these findings, we can assume that basophils play important roles in the pathogenesis of human AD, despite constituting only a minority population among inflammatory cells. However, whether and how basophils play a pathogenetic role in AD remains to be determined and warrants a focus on elucidation in the near future.

Conclusions

Th2-type immunity represents a key inflammatory process in the pathogenesis of AD. Th1 and Th17 immunity also appear to be involved in inflammation. Mast cells and eosinophils participate in not only inflammatory processes but also in pruritus and tissue remodeling. Further research is needed to clarify the actual pathogenetic roles of basophils in AD.

References

1. Weidinger S, Novak N. Atopic dermatitis. Lancet. 2016;387(10023):1109–22.
2. Kabashima K. New concept of the pathogenesis of atopic dermatitis: interplay among the barrier, allergy, and pruritus as a trinity. J Dermatol Sci. 2013;70(1):3–11.
3. Bieber T. Atopic dermatitis. Ann Dermatol. 2010;22(2):125–37.
4. Palmer CN, Irvine AD, Terron-Kwiatkowski A, Zhao Y, Liao H, Lee SP, et al. Common loss-of-function variants of the epidermal barrier protein filaggrin are a major predisposing factor for atopic dermatitis. Nat Genet. 2006;38(4):441–6.
5. Howell MD, Kim BE, Gao P, Grant AV, Boguniewicz M, Debenedetto A, et al. Cytokine modulation of atopic dermatitis filaggrin skin expression. J Allergy Clin Immunol. 2007;120(1):150–5.
6. Sonkoly E, Muller A, Lauerma AI, Pivarcsi A, Soto H, Kemeny L, et al. IL-31: a new link between T cells and pruritus in atopic skin inflammation. J Allergy Clin Immunol. 2006;117(2):411–7.
7. Simon D, Braathen LR, Simon HU. Eosinophils and atopic dermatitis. Allergy. 2004;59(6):561–70.
8. Werfel T, Allam JP, Biedermann T, Eyerich K, Gilles S, Guttman-Yassky E, et al. Cellular and molecular immunologic mechanisms in patients with atopic dermatitis. J Allergy Clin Immunol. 2016;138(2):336–49.
9. Simpson EL, Bieber T, Guttman-Yassky E, Beck LA, Blauvelt A, Cork MJ, et al. Two phase 3 trials of dupilumab versus placebo in atopic dermatitis. N Engl J Med. 2016;375(24):2335–48.
10. Grewe M, Gyufko K, Schöpf E, Krutmann J. Lesional expression of interferon-gamma in atopic eczema. Lancet. 1994;343(8888):25–6.
11. Koga C, Kabashima K, Shiraishi N, Kobayashi M, Tokura Y. Possible pathogenic role of Th17 cells for atopic dermatitis. J Invest Dermatol. 2008;128(11):2625–30.
12. Noda S, Suárez-Fariñas M, Ungar B, Kim SJ, de Guzman Strong C, Xu H, et al. The Asian atopic dermatitis phenotype combines features of atopic dermatitis and psoriasis with increased TH17 polarization. J Allergy Clin Immunol. 2015;136(5):1254–64.
13. Guttman-Yassky E, Lowes MA, Fuentes-Duculan J, Zaba LC, Cardinale I, Nograles KE, et al. Low expression of the IL-23/Th17 pathway in atopic dermatitis compared to psoriasis. J Immunol. 2008;181(10):7420–7.
14. Soumelis V, Reche PA, Kanzler H, Yuan W, Edward G, Homey B, et al. Human epithelial cells trigger dendritic cell mediated allergic inflammation by producing TSLP. Nat Immunol. 2002;3(7):673–80.
15. Sano Y, Masuda K, Tamagawa-Mineoka R, Matsunaka H, Murakami Y, Yamashita R, et al. Thymic stromal lymphopoietin expression is increased in the horny layer of patients with atopic dermatitis. Clin Exp Immunol. 2013;171(3):330–7.
16. Corrigan CJ, Jayaratnam A, Wang Y, Liu Y, de Waal Malefyt R, Meng Q, et al. Early production of thymic stromal lymphopoietin precedes infiltration of dendritic cells expressing its receptor in allergen-induced late phase cutaneous responses in atopic subjects. Allergy. 2009;64(7):1014–22.
17. Bogiatzi SI, Fernandez I, Bichet JC, Marloie-Provost MA, Volpe E, Sastre X, et al. Cutting edge: proinflammatory and Th2 cytokines synergize to induce thymic stromal lymphopoietin production by human skin keratinocytes. J Immunol. 2007;178(6):3373–7.
18. Kinoshita H, Takai T, Le TA, Kamijo S, Wang XL, Ushio H, et al. Cytokine milieu modulates release of thymic stromal lymphopoietin from human keratinocytes stimulated with double-stranded RNA. J Allergy Clin Immunol. 2009;123(1):179–86.
19. Vu AT, Baba T, Chen X, Le TA, Kinoshita H, Xie Y, et al. Staphylococcus aureus membrane and diacylated lipopeptide induce thymic stromal lymphopoietin in keratinocytes through the Toll-like receptor 2-Toll-like receptor 6 pathway. J Allergy Clin Immunol. 2010;126(5):985–93, 993.e1–3.

20. Le TA, Takai T, Vu AT, Kinoshita H, Chen X, Ikeda S, et al. Flagellin induces the expression of thymic stromal lymphopoietin in human keratinocytes via toll-like receptor 5. Int Arch Allergy Immunol. 2011;155(1):31–7.
21. Kouzaki H, O'Grady SM, Lawrence CB, Kita H. Proteases induce production of thymic stromal lymphopoietin by airway epithelial cells through protease-activated receptor-2. J Immunol. 2009;183(2):1427–34.
22. Shiraishi H, Masuoka M, Ohta S, Suzuki S, Arima K, Taniguchi K, et al. Periostin contributes to the pathogenesis of atopic dermatitis by inducing TSLP production from keratinocytes. Allergol Int. 2012;61(4):563–72.
23. Angelova-Fischer I, Fernandez IM, Donnadieu MH, Bulfone-Paus S, Zillikens D, Fischer TW, et al. Injury to the stratum corneum induces in vivo expression of human thymic stromal lymphopoietin in the epidermis. J Invest Dermatol. 2010;130(10):2505–7.
24. Oyoshi MK, Larson RP, Ziegler SF, Geha RS. Mechanical injury polarizes skin dendritic cells to elicit a T(H)2 response by inducing cutaneous thymic stromal lymphopoietin expression. J Allergy Clin Immunol. 2010;126(5):976–84, 984.e1–5.
25. Kitajima M, Lee HC, Nakayama T, Ziegler SF. TSLP enhances the function of helper type 2 cells. Eur J Immunol. 2011;41(7):1862–71.
26. Omori M, Ziegler S. Induction of IL-4 expression in CD4(+) T cells by thymic stromal lymphopoietin. J Immunol. 2007;178(3):1396–404.
27. Rochman I, Watanabe N, Arima K, Liu YJ, Leonard WJ. Cutting edge: direct action of thymic stromal lymphopoietin on activated human CD4+ T cells. J Immunol. 2007;178(11):6720–4.
28. Ito T, Wang YH, Duramad O, Hori T, Delespesse GJ, Watanabe N, et al. TSLP-activated dendritic cells induce an inflammatory T helper type 2 cell response through OX40 ligand. J Exp Med. 2005;202(9):1213–23.
29. Kakinuma T, Nakamura K, Wakugawa M, Mitsui H, Tada Y, Saeki H, et al. Thymus and activation-regulated chemokine in atopic dermatitis: serum thymus and activation-regulated chemokine level is closely related with disease activity. J Allergy Clin Immunol. 2001;107(3):535–41.
30. Kakinuma T, Nakamura K, Wakugawa M, Mitsui H, Tada Y, Saeki H, et al. Serum macrophage-derived chemokine (MDC) levels are closely related with the disease activity of atopic dermatitis. Clin Exp Immunol. 2002;127(2):270–3.
31. Shimada Y, Takehara K, Sato S. Both Th2 and Th1 chemokines (TARC/CCL17, MDC/CCL22, and Mig/CXCL9) are elevated in sera from patients with atopic dermatitis. J Dermatol Sci. 2004;34(3):201–8.
32. Shoda T, Futamura K, Kobayashi F, Saito H, Matsumoto K, Matsuda A. Expression of thymus and activation-regulated chemokine (TARC) by human dermal cells, but not epidermal keratinocytes. J Dermatol Sci. 2014;76(2):90–5.
33. Nomura T, Terada N, Kim WJ, Nakano K, Fukuda Y, Wakita A, et al. Interleukin-13 induces thymus and activation-regulated chemokine (CCL17) in human peripheral blood mononuclear cells. Cytokine. 2002;20(2):49–55.
34. Vestergaard C, Bang K, Gesser B, Yoneyama H, Matsushima K, Larsen CG. A Th2 chemokine, TARC, produced by keratinocytes may recruit CLA+CCR4+ lymphocytes into lesional atopic dermatitis skin. J Invest Dermatol. 2000;115(4):640–6.
35. Vulcano M, Albanesi C, Stoppacciaro A, Bagnati R, D'Amico G, Struyf S, et al. Dendritic cells as a major source of macrophage-derived chemokine/CCL22 in vitro and in vivo. Eur J Immunol. 2001;31(3):812–22.
36. Wilson SR, Thé L, Batia LM, Beattie K, Katibah GE, McClain SP, et al. The epithelial cell-derived atopic dermatitis cytokine TSLP activates neurons to induce itch. Cell. 2013;155(2):285–95.
37. Raap U, Wichmann K, Bruder M, Ständer S, Wedi B, Kapp A, et al. Correlation of IL-31 serum levels with severity of atopic dermatitis. J Allergy Clin Immunol. 2008;122(2):421–3.
38. Ezzat MH, Hasan ZE, Shaheen KY. Serum measurement of interleukin-31 (IL-31) in paediatric atopic dermatitis: elevated levels correlate with severity scoring. J Eur Acad Dermatol Venereol. 2011;25(3):334–9.

39. Dillon SR, Sprecher C, Hammond A, Bilsborough J, Rosenfeld-Franklin M, Presnell SR, et al. Interleukin 31, a cytokine produced by activated T cells, induces dermatitis in mice. Nat Immunol. 2004;5(7):752–60.
40. Yoshimoto T, Tsutsui H, Tominaga K, Hoshino K, Okamura H, Akira S, et al. IL-18, although antiallergic when administered with IL-12, stimulates IL-4 and histamine release by basophils. Proc Natl Acad Sci U S A. 1999;96(24):13962–6.
41. Yoshimoto T, Mizutani H, Tsutsui H, Noben-Trauth N, Yamanaka K, Tanaka M, et al. IL-18 induction of IgE: dependence on CD4+ T cells, IL-4 and STAT6. Nat Immunol. 2000;1(2):132–7.
42. Tsutsui H, Yoshimoto T, Hayashi N, Mizutani H, Nakanishi K. Induction of allergic inflammation by interleukin-18 in experimental animal models. Immunol Rev. 2004;202:115–38.
43. Yoshizawa Y, Nomaguchi H, Izaki S, Kitamura K. Serum cytokine levels in atopic dermatitis. Clin Exp Dermatol. 2002;27(3):225–9.
44. Schmitz J, Owyang A, Oldham E, Song Y, Murphy E, McClanahan TK, et al. IL-33, an interleukin-1-like cytokine that signals via the IL-1 receptor-related protein ST2 and induces T helper type 2-associated cytokines. Immunity. 2005;23(5):479–90.
45. Iikura M, Suto H, Kajiwara N, Oboki K, Ohno T, Okayama Y, et al. IL-33 can promote survival, adhesion and cytokine production in human mast cells. Lab Investig. 2007;87(10):971–8.
46. Allakhverdi Z, Smith DE, Comeau MR, Delespesse G. Cutting edge: the ST2 ligand IL-33 potently activates and drives maturation of human mast cells. J Immunol. 2007;179(4):2051–4.
47. Liew FY, Pitman NI, McInnes IB. Disease-associated functions of IL-33: the new kid in the IL-1 family. Nat Rev Immunol. 2010;10(2):103–10.
48. Pushparaj PN, Tay HK, H'ng SC, Pitman N, Xu D, McKenzie A, et al. The cytokine interleukin-33 mediates anaphylactic shock. Proc Natl Acad Sci U S A. 2009;106(24):9773–8.
49. Kawakami T, Ando T, Kimura M, Wilson BS, Kawakami Y. Mast cells in atopic dermatitis. Curr Opin Immunol. 2009;21(6):666–78.
50. Stone KD, Prussin C, Metcalfe DD. IgE, mast cells, basophils, and eosinophils. J Allergy Clin Immunol. 2010;125(2 Suppl 2):S73–80.
51. Murota H, Bae S, Hamasaki Y, Maruyama R, Katayama I. Emedastine difumarate inhibits histamine-induced collagen synthesis in dermal fibroblasts. J Investig Allergol Clin Immunol. 2008;18(4):245–52.
52. Otsuka A, Kabashima K. Mast cells and basophils in cutaneous immune responses. Allergy. 2015;70(2):131–40.
53. Yamaguchi M, Sayama K, Yano K, Lantz CS, Noben-Trauth N, Ra C, et al. IgE enhances fc epsilon receptor I expression and IgE-dependent release of histamine and lipid mediators from human umbilical cord blood-derived mast cells: synergistic effect of IL-4 and IgE on human mast cell fc epsilon receptor I expression and mediator release. J Immunol. 1999;162(9):5455–65.
54. Ochi H, Hirani WM, Yuan Q, Friend DS, Austen KF, Boyce JA. T helper cell type 2 cytokine-mediated comitogenic responses and CCR3 expression during differentiation of human mast cells in vitro. J Exp Med. 1999;190(2):267–80.
55. Nakajima T, Matsumoto K, Suto H, Tanaka K, Ebisawa M, Tomita H, et al. Gene expression screening of human mast cells and eosinophils using high-density oligonucleotide probe arrays: abundant expression of major basic protein in mast cells. Blood. 2001;98(4):1127–34.
56. Steinhoff M, Neisius U, Ikoma A, Fartasch M, Heyer G, Skov PS, et al. Proteinase-activated receptor-2 mediates itch: a novel pathway for pruritus in human skin. J Neurosci. 2003;23(15):6176–80.
57. Yang L, Murota H, Serada S, Fujimoto M, Kudo A, Naka T, et al. Histamine contributes to tissue remodeling via periostin expression. J Invest Dermatol. 2014;134(8):2105–13.
58. Taniguchi K, Arima K, Masuoka M, Ohta S, Shiraishi H, Ontsuka K, et al. Periostin controls keratinocyte proliferation and differentiation by interacting with the paracrine IL-1α/IL-6 loop. J Invest Dermatol. 2014;134(5):1295–304.
59. Niyonsaba F, Ushio H, Hara M, Yokoi H, Tominaga M, Takamori K, et al. Antimicrobial peptides human beta-defensins and cathelicidin LL-37 induce the secretion of a pruritogenic cytokine IL-31 by human mast cells. J Immunol. 2010;184(7):3526–34.

60. Hirai H, Tanaka K, Yoshie O, Ogawa K, Kenmotsu K, Takamori Y, et al. Prostaglandin D2 selectively induces chemotaxis in T helper type 2 cells, eosinophils, and basophils via seven-transmembrane receptor CRTH2. J Exp Med. 2001;193(2):255–61.
61. Xue L, Salimi M, Panse I, Mjösberg JM, McKenzie AN, Spits H, et al. Prostaglandin D2 activates group 2 innate lymphoid cells through chemoattractant receptor-homologous molecule expressed on TH2 cells. J Allergy Clin Immunol. 2014;133(4):1184–94.
62. Satoh T, Moroi R, Aritake K, Urade Y, Kanai Y, Sumi K, et al. Prostaglandin D2 plays an essential role in chronic allergic inflammation of the skin via CRTH2 receptor. J Immunol. 2006;177(4):2621–9.
63. Walsh GM. Eosinophil granule proteins and their role in disease. Curr Opin Hematol. 2001;8(1):28–33.
64. Hogan SP, Rosenberg HF, Moqbel R, Phipps S, Foster PS, Lacy P, et al. Eosinophils: biological properties and role in health and disease. Clin Exp Allergy. 2008;38(5):709–50.
65. Blanchard C, Rothenberg ME. Biology of the eosinophil. Adv Immunol. 2009;101:81–121.
66. Kiehl P, Falkenberg K, Vogelbruch M, Kapp A. Tissue eosinophilia in acute and chronic atopic dermatitis: a morphometric approach using quantitative image analysis of immunostaining. Br J Dermatol. 2001;145(5):720–9.
67. Jeong CW, Ahn KS, Rho NK, Park YD, Lee DY, Lee JH, et al. Differential in vivo cytokine mRNA expression in lesional skin of intrinsic vs. extrinsic atopic dermatitis patients using semiquantitative RT-PCR. Clin Exp Allergy. 2003;33(12):1717–24.
68. Rosenberg HF, Phipps S, Foster PS. Eosinophil trafficking in allergy and asthma. J Allergy Clin Immunol. 2007;119(6):1303–10. quiz 1311-2
69. Collins PD, Marleau S, Griffiths-Johnson DA, Jose PJ, Williams TJ. Cooperation between interleukin-5 and the chemokine eotaxin to induce eosinophil accumulation in vivo. J Exp Med. 1995;182(4):1169–74.
70. Satoh T, Yokozeki H, Nishioka K. Pathogenic roles of eosinophils in guinea-pig contact sensitivity: regulation of dermal eosinophilia with remotely administered IL-5. Clin Exp Immunol. 2000;122(3):300–7.
71. Ying S, Meng Q, Barata LT, Robinson DS, Durham SR, Kay AB. Associations between IL-13 and IL-4 (mRNA and protein), vascular cell adhesion molecule-1 expression, and the infiltration of eosinophils, macrophages, and T cells in allergen-induced late-phase cutaneous reactions in atopic subjects. J Immunol. 1997;158(10):5050–7.
72. Miyazaki Y, Satoh T, Nishioka K, Yokozeki H. STAT-6-mediated control of P-selectin by substance P and interleukin-4 in human dermal endothelial cells. Am J Pathol. 2006;169(2):697–707.
73. Satoh T, Kaneko M, Wu MH, Yokozeki H, Nishioka K. Contribution of selectin ligands to eosinophil recruitment into the skin of patients with atopic dermatitis. Eur J Immunol. 2002;32(5):1274–81.
74. Schleimer RP, Sterbinsky SA, Kaiser J, Bickel CA, Klunk DA, Tomioka K, et al. IL-4 induces adherence of human eosinophils and basophils but not neutrophils to endothelium. Association with expression of VCAM-1. J Immunol. 1992;148(4):1086–92.
75. Mochizuki M, Bartels J, Mallet AI, Christophers E, Schröder JM. IL-4 induces eotaxin: a possible mechanism of selective eosinophil recruitment in helminth infection and atopy. J Immunol. 1998;160(1):60–8.
76. Dulkys Y, Schramm G, Kimmig D, Knöss S, Weyergraf A, Kapp A, et al. Detection of mRNA for eotaxin-2 and eotaxin-3 in human dermal fibroblasts and their distinct activation profile on human eosinophils. J Invest Dermatol. 2001;116(4):498–505.
77. Wong CK, Hu S, Cheung PF, Lam CW. Thymic stromal lymphopoietin induces chemotactic and prosurvival effects in eosinophils: implications in allergic inflammation. Am J Respir Cell Mol Biol. 2010;43(3):305–15.
78. Fukuoka M, Ogino Y, Sato H, Ohta T, Komoriya K, Nishioka K, et al. RANTES expression in psoriatic skin, and regulation of RANTES and IL-8 production in cultured epidermal keratinocytes by active vitamin D3 (tacalcitol). Br J Dermatol. 1998;138(1):63–70.
79. Asakura H, Kashio Y, Nakamura K, Seki M, Dai S, Shirato Y, et al. Selective eosinophil adhesion to fibroblast via IFN-gamma-induced galectin-9. J Immunol. 2002;169(10):5912–8.

80. Kameyoshi Y, Dörschner A, Mallet AI, Christophers E, Schröder JM. Cytokine RANTES released by thrombin-stimulated platelets is a potent attractant for human eosinophils. J Exp Med. 1992;176(2):587–92.
81. Matsumoto R, Matsumoto H, Seki M, Hata M, Asano Y, Kanegasaki S, et al. Human ecalectin, a variant of human galectin-9, is a novel eosinophil chemoattractant produced by T lymphocytes. J Biol Chem. 1998;273(27):16976–84.
82. Jinquan T, Jing C, Jacobi HH, Reimert CM, Millner A, Quan S, et al. CXCR3 expression and activation of eosinophils: role of IFN-gamma-inducible protein-10 and monokine induced by IFN-gamma. J Immunol. 2000;165(3):1548–56.
83. Grewe M, Czech W, Morita A, Werfel T, Klammer M, Kapp A, et al. Human eosinophils produce biologically active IL-12: implications for control of T cell responses. J Immunol. 1998;161(1):415–20.
84. Beck LA, Dalke S, Leiferman KM, Bickel CA, Hamilton R, Rosen H, et al. Cutaneous injection of RANTES causes eosinophil recruitment: comparison of nonallergic and allergic human subjects. J Immunol. 1997;159(6):2962–72.
85. Oldhoff JM, Darsow U, Werfel T, Katzer K, Wulf A, Laifaoui J, et al. Anti-IL-5 recombinant humanized monoclonal antibody (mepolizumab) for the treatment of atopic dermatitis. Allergy. 2005;60(5):693–6.
86. Levi-Schaffer F, Garbuzenko E, Rubin A, Reich R, Pickholz D, Gillery P, et al. Human eosinophils regulate human lung- and skin-derived fibroblast properties in vitro: a role for transforming growth factor beta (TGF-beta). Proc Natl Acad Sci U S A. 1999; 96(17):9660–5.
87. Horiuchi T, Weller PF. Expression of vascular endothelial growth factor by human eosinophils: upregulation by granulocyte macrophage colony-stimulating factor and interleukin-5. Am J Respir Cell Mol Biol. 1997;17(1):70–7.
88. Schwingshackl A, Duszyk M, Brown N, Moqbel R. Human eosinophils release matrix metalloproteinase-9 on stimulation with TNF-alpha. J Allergy Clin Immunol. 1999; 104(5):983–9.
89. Hoshino M, Takahashi M, Aoike N. Expression of vascular endothelial growth factor, basic fibroblast growth factor, and angiogenin immunoreactivity in asthmatic airways and its relationship to angiogenesis. J Allergy Clin Immunol. 2001;107(2):295–301.
90. Phipps S, Ying S, Wangoo A, Ong YE, Levi-Schaffer F, Kay AB. The relationship between allergen-induced tissue eosinophilia and markers of repair and remodeling in human atopic skin. J Immunol. 2002;169(8):4604–12.
91. Phipps S, Flood-Page P, Menzies-Gow A, Ong YE, Kay AB. Intravenous anti-IL-5 monoclonal antibody reduces eosinophils and tenascin deposition in allergen challenged human atopic skin. J Invest Dermatol. 2004;122(6):1406–12.
92. Hashimoto T, Satoh T, Yokozeki H. Protective role of STAT6 in basophil-dependent Prurigo-like allergic skin inflammation. J Immunol. 2015;194(10):4631–40.
93. Lee JJ, Protheroe CA, Luo H, Ochkur SI, Scott GD, Zellner KR, et al. Eosinophil-dependent skin innervation and itching following contact toxicant exposure in mice. J Allergy Clin Immunol. 2015;135(2):477–87.
94. Foster EL, Simpson EL, Fredrikson LJ, Lee JJ, Lee NA, Fryer AD, et al. Eosinophils increase neuron branching in human and murine skin and in vitro. PLoS One. 2011;6(7):e22029.
95. Fujisawa D, Kashiwakura J, Kita H, Kikukawa Y, Fujitani Y, Sasaki-Sakamoto T, et al. Expression of Mas-related gene X2 on mast cells is upregulated in the skin of patients with severe chronic urticaria. J Allergy Clin Immunol. 2014;134(3):622–633.e9.
96. Karasuyama H, Yamanishi Y. Basophils have emerged as a key player in immunity. Curr Opin Immunol. 2014;31:1–7.
97. Ito Y, Satoh T, Takayama K, Miyagishi C, Walls AF, Yokozeki H. Basophil recruitment and activation in inflammatory skin diseases. Allergy. 2011;66(8):1107–13.
98. Grundström J, Reimer JM, Magnusson SE, Nilsson G, Wernersson S, Hellman L. Human cord blood derived immature basophils show dual characteristics, expressing both basophil and eosinophil associated proteins. PLoS One. 2012;7(10):e48308.

99. Siracusa MC, Saenz SA, Hill DA, Kim BS, Headley MB, Doering TA, et al. TSLP promotes interleukin-3-independent basophil haematopoiesis and type 2 inflammation. Nature. 2011;477(7363):229–33.
100. Kepley CL, Andrews RP, Brown DC, Chigaev A, Sklar LA, Oliver JM, et al. Regulation of human basophil adhesion to endothelium under flow conditions: different very late antigen 4 regulation on umbilical cord blood-derived and peripheral blood basophils. J Allergy Clin Immunol. 2002;110(3):469–75.
101. Saeki K, Satoh T, Yokozeki H. α(1,3) Fucosyltransferases IV and VII are essential for the initial recruitment of basophils in chronic allergic inflammation. J Invest Dermatol. 2013;133(9):2161–9.
102. Garcia-Zepeda EA, Combadiere C, Rothenberg ME, Sarafi MN, Lavigne F, Hamid Q, et al. Human monocyte chemoattractant protein (MCP)-4 is a novel CC chemokine with activities on monocytes, eosinophils, and basophils induced in allergic and nonallergic inflammation that signals through the CC chemokine receptors (CCR)-2 and -3. J Immunol. 1996;157(12):5613–26.
103. Iikura M, Ebisawa M, Yamaguchi M, Tachimoto H, Ohta K, Yamamoto K, et al. Transendothelial migration of human basophils. J Immunol. 2004;173(8):5189–95.
104. Mommert S, Kleiner S, Gehring M, Eiz-Vesper B, Stark H, Gutzmer R, et al. Human basophil chemotaxis and activation are regulated via the histamine H4 receptor. Allergy. 2016;71(9):1264–73.
105. Hida S, Yamasaki S, Sakamoto Y, Takamoto M, Obata K, Takai T, et al. Fc receptor gamma-chain, a constitutive component of the IL-3 receptor, is required for IL-3-induced IL-4 production in basophils. Nat Immunol. 2009;10(2):214–22.
106. MacGlashan D Jr, White JM, Huang SK, Ono SJ, Schroeder JT, Lichtenstein LM. Secretion of IL-4 from human basophils. The relationship between IL-4 mRNA and protein in resting and stimulated basophils. J Immunol. 1994;152(6):3006–16.
107. Gibbs BF, Haas H, Falcone FH, Albrecht C, Vollrath IB, Noll T, et al. Purified human peripheral blood basophils release interleukin-13 and preformed interleukin-4 following immunological activation. Eur J Immunol. 1996;26(10):2493–8.
108. Ugajin T, Satoh T, Kanamori T, Aritake K, Urade Y, Yokozeki H. FcεRI, but not FcγR, signals induce prostaglandin D2 and E2 production from basophils. Am J Pathol. 2011;179(2):775–82.
109. Otsuka A, Nakajima S, Kubo M, Egawa G, Honda T, Kitoh A, et al. Basophils are required for the induction of Th2 immunity to haptens and peptide antigens. Nat Commun. 2013;4:1739.
110. Kitzmüller C, Nagl B, Deifl S, Walterskirchen C, Jahn-Schmid B, Zlabinger GJ, et al. Human blood basophils do not act as antigen-presenting cells for the major birch pollen allergen Bet v 1. Allergy. 2012;67(5):593–600.
111. Eckl-Dorna J, Ellinger A, Blatt K, Ghanim V, Steiner I, Pavelka M, et al. Basophils are not the key antigen-presenting cells in allergic patients. Allergy. 2012;67(5):601–8.
112. Sharma M, Hegde P, Aimanianda V, Beau R, Maddur MS, Sénéchal H, et al. Circulating human basophils lack the features of professional antigen presenting cells. Sci Rep. 2013;3:1188.
113. Macfarlane AJ, Kon OM, Smith SJ, Zeibecoglou K, Khan LN, Barata LT, et al. Basophils, eosinophils, and mast cells in atopic and nonatopic asthma and in late-phase allergic reactions in the lung and skin. J Allergy Clin Immunol. 2000;105(1 Pt 1):99–107.
114. Ying S, Robinson DS, Meng Q, Barata LT, McEuen AR, Buckley MG, et al. C-C chemokines in allergen-induced late-phase cutaneous responses in atopic subjects: association of eotaxin with early 6-hour eosinophils, and of eotaxin-2 and monocyte chemoattractant protein-4 with the later 24-hour tissue eosinophilia, and relationship to basophils and other C-C chemokines (monocyte chemoattractant protein-3 and RANTES). J Immunol. 1999;163(7):3976–84.
115. Cheng LE, Sullivan BM, Retana LE, Allen CD, Liang HE, Locksley RM. IgE-activated basophils regulate eosinophil tissue entry by modulating endothelial function. J Exp Med. 2015;212(4):513–24.
116. Obata K, Mukai K, Tsujimura Y, Ishiwata K, Kawano Y, Minegishi Y, et al. Basophils are essential initiators of a novel type of chronic allergic inflammation. Blood. 2007;110(3):913–20.

Etiopathology of Atopic Dermatitis: Immunological Aspects of Dendritic Cells (DCs) and Innate Lymphoid Cells (ILCs)

8

Saeko Nakajima, Tetsuya Honda, and Kenji Kabashima

Abstract

Dendritic cells (DCs) form a heterogeneous group of antigen-presenting cells that play different roles in skin immunology. Recent studies have revealed the existence of distinct DC populations in the skin, highlighting the complexity of the cutaneous DC network in the steady state and inflammatory conditions.

Recently, another new skin immune cell subset, innate lymphoid cells (ILCs), which are part of a heterogeneous family of innate immune cells, has emerged as an important contributor to inflammatory skin diseases, such as atopic dermatitis (AD) and psoriasis.

In this review, we will summarize the current understanding of the functions of cutaneous DCs and ILCs in the pathogenesis of AD and will discuss the potential implications of their functions in AD.

Keywords

Langerhans cells (LCs) • Dendritic cells (DCs) • Type 2 innate lymphoid cells (ILC2s)

8.1 Introduction

The skin is classified into two distinct regions, the epidermis and the dermis, separated by the basement membrane. The epidermis is derived from ectoderm and presents as an epithelial layer that is composed mainly of keratinocytes. Keratinocytes constitute 90–95% of the cells in the epidermis; the remaining cells include Langerhans cells

S. Nakajima • T. Honda • K. Kabashima (✉)
Department of Dermatology, Kyoto University Graduate School of Medicine, 54 Shogoin Kawara, Sakyo, Kyoto 606-8507, Japan
e-mail: fujiko@kuhp.kyoto-u.ac.jp; hontetsu@kuhp.kyoto-u.ac.jp; kaba@kuhp.kyoto-u.ac.jp

I. Katayama et al. (eds.), *Evolution of Atopic Dermatitis in the 21st Century*, https://doi.org/10.1007/978-981-10-5541-6_8

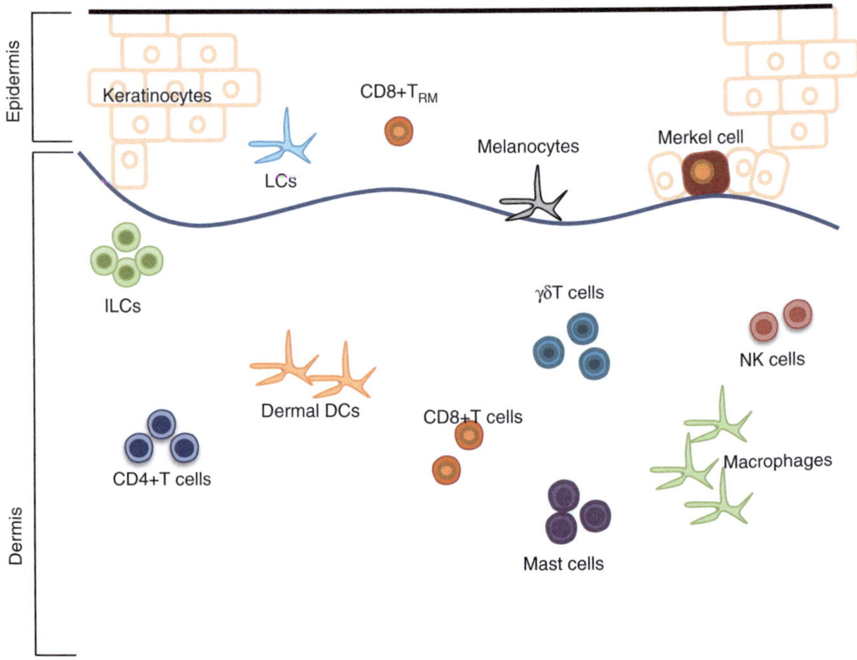

Fig. 8.1 Description of skin immune cells. *LCs* Langerhans cells, T_{RM} resident memory T cells, *dermal DCs* dermal dendritic cells, *ILCs* innate lymphoid cells, *γδT cells* gamma delta T cells, *NK cells* natural killer cells

(LCs), skin-resident memory CD8$^+$ T cells, melanocytes, and Merkel cells. In addition, murine epidermis contains approximately the same percentage of the γδ T cell subset (called dendritic epidermal T cells [DETC]), as that of LCs [1, 2]. A much more heterogeneous population of immune cells reside in the dermis, including dermal dendritic cells (dDCs), mast cells, CD4$^+$ and CD8$^+$ T cells, dermal γδ T cells, macrophages, natural killer (NK) cells, and innate lymphoid cells (ILCs) [2, 3] (Fig. 8.1).

Atopic dermatitis (AD) is a pruritic, chronic, retractable inflammatory skin disease that is induced by the complex interaction between susceptibility genes encoding skin barrier components and host immune responses [4–10]. Type 2 helper T (Th2) cells and related cytokines such as IL-4, IL-5, and IL-13 have been reported to play important roles in its pathogenesis [10–15]. Cutaneous DCs acquire protein antigens and drive the differentiation/proliferation of a distinct Th cell subset including Th2 cells and provoke antigen-specific T cell responses to external pathogens [16]. In addition to Th2 cells, several recent papers have indicated that type 2 ILCs (ILC2s) are enriched in the lesional skin of AD patients and might play a critical role in driving the Th2-type immune response in AD [17–20].

This review will define the functions of cutaneous DCs and ILCs in the pathogenesis of AD, with a focus on studies performed by Japanese researchers, and will discuss the potential implications of these functions in the context of skin immune responses in AD.

8.2 The Role of Cutaneous DCs in the Pathogenesis of AD

8.2.1 DC Subsets in the Skin

Several subsets of DCs have been identified in the skin of both mice and humans. LCs comprise a skin DC subset that resides in the epidermis. Both human and murine LCs constitutively express a lectin receptor, namely, langerin/CD207, which is capable of binding sugar moieties commonly found on a variety of microorganisms [21]. They also express the E-cadherin and epithelial cell adhesion molecules (EpCAMs), which anchor LCs to keratinocytes [22, 23], and CD205 that is implicated in antigen capture and antigen processing [24, 25]. Human LCs highly express CD1a, a member of the group 1 CD1 protein, which is capable of presenting microbial lipid antigens to T cells [26] (Table 8.1).

DCs in the dermis consist of dermal-resident DCs and migratory LCs traveling to the lymphatic vessels [27]. Recent studies have shown that murine dermal-resident DCs are further classified into two populations including langerin-positive dDCs (langerin$^+$ dDCs) and langerin-negative dDCs (langerin$^-$ dDCs) [28–30]. The langerin$^+$ dDC population represents 10–20% of the total dDC pool. In contrast to LCs, langerin$^+$ dDCs express integrin αEβ7 (also called CD103) [31], lack the adhesion molecules E-cadherin and EpCAM, and express low levels of the integrin CD11b. Langerin$^+$ dDCs express the same high levels of CD24 as LCs but do not express CX3CR1, F4/80, or signal-regulatory protein alpha (SIRPα); they also express low levels of CD11b and EpCAM [32] (Table 8.1). Langerin$^-$ dDCs represent the majority (up to 70%) of the dDC pool and express high levels of integrin

Table 8.1 Dendritic cell population in the skin of human and mice

	Localization	Cell type	Cellular markers
Human	Epidermis	LC	CD45, MHC class II, CD1a, CD207 (langerin), E-cadherin, EpCAM
		IDEC	CD1a, CD1b, CD1c, CD11c, FcεRI, CD23, HLA-DR, CD11b, CD206, CD36
	Dermis	CD1c$^+$ dDC	CD1c, CD1a$^{+/-}$, CD45, CD11b, CD11c, MHC class II
		CD14$^+$ dDC	CD1c, CD45, CD11b, CD11c, CD14, MHC class II, CD209 (DC-SIGN)
		CD141$^+$ dDC	CD1c, CD45, CD11c, CD141
		pDC	CD303 (CLEC4C), CD304 (neuropilin), CD123 (IL-3R)
		Tip-DC	CD11c, TNF-α, iNOS
Mouse	Epidermis	LC	CD45, CD11b, CD11c, CD24, MHC class II, CD205, CD207, E-cadherin, EpCAM
	Dermis	Langerin$^-$ dDC	CD45, CD11b^{hi}, CD11c, CD24, MHC class II, CD205, SIRP-1α
		Langerin$^+$ dDC	CD45, CD11b^{dim}, CD11c, CD24, CD103, MHC class II, CD207
		pDC	B220, Siglec-H, PDCA-1

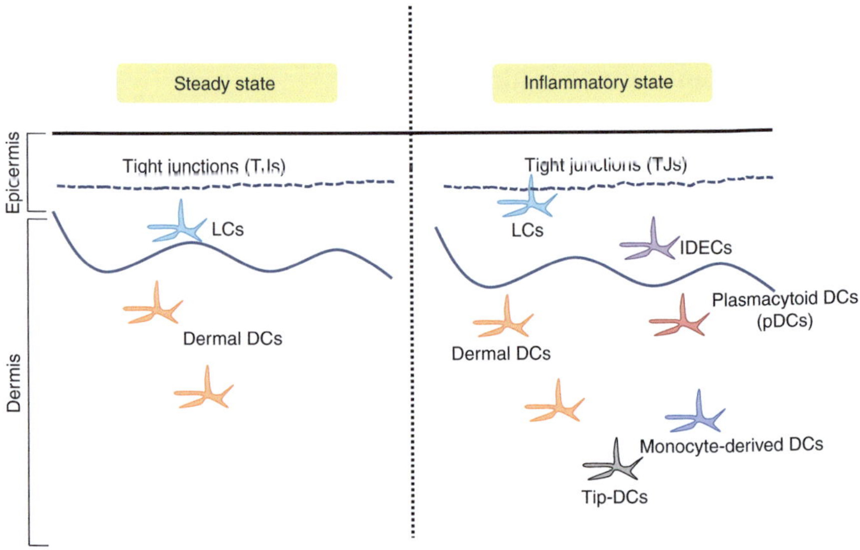

Fig. 8.2 Cutaneous dendritic cells in the steady state and in the inflammatory state. *TJs* tight junctions, *LCs* Langerhans cells, *dermal DCs* dermal dendritic cells, *IDECs* inflammatory dendritic epidermal cells, *Tip-DCs* tumor necrosis factor and inducible nitric oxide synthase-producing dendritic cells, *pDCs* plasmacytoid dendritic cells. In steady state, LCs reside in the epidermis beneath the TJ barrier. Dermal DCs reside in the dermis. In inflammatory condition, such as AD, LCs elongate their dendrite through TJs, capturing external antigens. IDECs recruit into the epidermis. Tip-DCs, pDCs, and monocyte-derived DCs also recruit into the dermis from the circulation

CD11b and several macrophage markers, such as F4/80, CX3CR1, and SIRPα [32]. In human, dDCs are classified into three subsets (i.e., CD1a + dDCs, CD14+ dDCs, and CD141+ dDCs), depending on the expression pattern of surface molecules, although their functional differences remain unclear [33] (Table 8.1).

In inflamed skin, two additional subsets of DCs can be found: a DC population derived from blood monocytes (monocyte-derived DCs) [19] and plasmacytoid DCs (pDCs) [2, 34] (Table 8.1, Fig. 8.2). Another subset of the identified DC subpopulation referred to as TNF-α and inducible NO synthase (iNOS)-producing DCs (Tip-DCs) has been reported to be critical against bacterial infections [35]. In AD patients, inflammatory dendritic epidermal cells (IDECs) appear in the epidermis (Table 8.1, Fig. 8.2).

8.2.2 Cutaneous DCs in the Pathogenesis of AD

Since AD is a Th2-type immune response to protein antigens, and cutaneous DCs can induce Th2 cell differentiation, it has been suggested that cutaneous DCs initiate AD [36]. It remains unclear, however, which cutaneous DC subset mediates epicutaneous sensitization to protein antigens.

Kubo et al. showed that protein antigens of large molecular size are localized above the size-selective barrier, the tight junction (TJ), and that activated LCs extend their dendrites through the TJ to take up antigens [37]. Therefore, it can be hypothesized that LCs, not dermal DCs, initiate epicutaneous sensitization with protein antigens in the development of AD.

Nakajima et al. and Ouchi et al. showed that, in a murine AD model, which is induced by epicutaneous sensitization with protein antigen, depletion of LCs led to significantly attenuated induction of IgE/IgG1 upon epicutaneous sensitization with protein antigens [38, 39]. Moreover, Nakajima et al. showed that thymic stromal lymphopoietin (TSLP) receptor (TSLPR) expression on LCs is enhanced upon protein antigen exposure to the skin and that mice lacking TSLPR on LCs exhibited significantly attenuated Th2 cell differentiation in the AD model [38].

TSLP is a cytokine that is produced mainly by non-hematopoietic cells such as fibroblasts and epithelial cells, including epidermal keratinocytes. It has been reported that TSLP plays an important role in the induction of Th2 responses through the activation of DCs via the expression of OX40L [40]. TSLP stimulation also causes LCs to express OX40L [38]. In addition, cutaneous DCs can elicit a Th2 response in a mechanical injury model, in which TSLP is produced by keratinocytes [41]. These results indicate that TSLP produced by keratinocytes acts on LCs, which induces Th2-type immune responses in the murine AD model [38] (Fig. 8.3). In keeping with this, it has been reported that TSLP is highly expressed in the lesional

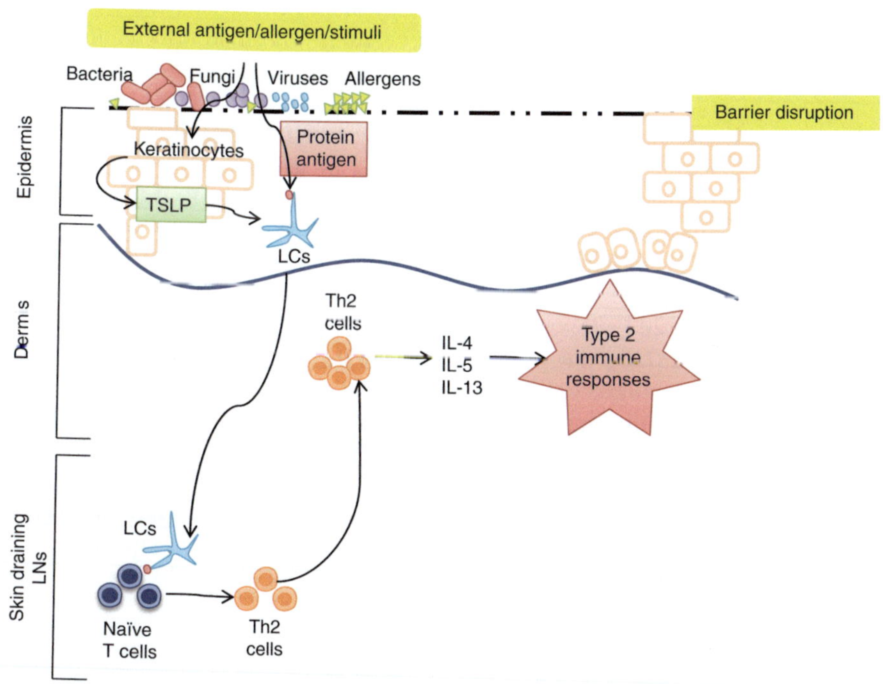

Fig. 8.3 Role of LCs in the pathogenesis of AD. Upon stimulation, keratinocytes produce TSLP. TSLP will activate LCs and induce LCs to uptake external antigens, migrate to the skin-draining lymph nodes, and induce Th2 cell differentiation

skin of AD patients and that it activates human LCs in vitro [42–44], suggesting that LCs induce Th2-type immune response in human AD as well.

In the epidermis of human AD patients, both LCs and IDECs have been detected. Both LCs and IDECs express FcεRI on the surface and have been assumed to enable specific allergen uptake through IgE-dependent antigen capture [45, 46]. Yoshida et al., however, revealed that LCs, not IDECs, extend their dendrites through the TJ with a polarized distribution of langerin but not FcεRI in human AD skin [47]. These results again suggest that LCs mediate Th2-type immune responses in a langerin-dependent manner in the pathogenesis of AD.

8.3 The Role of ILCs in the Pathogenesis of AD

8.3.1 ILCs in the Skin

ILCs are part of a family of innate immune cells that are derived from a common lymphoid progenitor, and their development is partially or completely dependent on the common γ-chain (γc or CD132), IL-7, Notch, and the transcription factor inhibitor of DNA binding 2 [48]. ILCs are predominantly tissue-resident cells that lack antigen-specific receptors, such as T and B cell receptors. Instead, ILCs rapidly respond to various environmental stimuli with cytokine production [49].

The ILC family can be subdivided into three groups based on their requirement for activating cytokines, expression of transcription factors, and production of effector cytokines (Fig. 8.4). Group 1 ILC comprises NK cells and ILC1s; both of them are activated by IL-12 depending on transcription factor T-bet and produce interferon (IFN)-γ. Groups 2 ILC contains ILC2s that are activated by epithelial cell-derived cytokines/chemokines, such as IL-25, IL-33, and TSLP. ILC2s express GATA3 and produce Th2-type cytokines, e.g., IL-4, IL-5, and IL-13 upon activation. Group 3 ILC comprises lymphoid tissue inducer (LTi) cells and ILC3s. ILC3s can be further subdivided based on their expression of natural cytotoxicity receptors. They are activated by IL-1β and IL-23, are dependent on RORγt, and produce IL-17A and/or IL-22 [50]. Intriguingly, all of the ILC-activating cytokines can be produced by skin immune cells, such as keratinocytes, LCs, and dDCs.

All three ILC subsets have been identified in healthy human adult skin, where ILC3s are the most abundant and ILC2s make up 25% of the total ILC pool [20, 51–54]. In addition to NK cells, ILC2s were the first ILCs to be identified in both healthy and AD skin [52]. Although ILCs are present in both epidermis and dermis, the majority are found in the dermis, where ILC2s constitute 5–10% of $CD45^+$ cells [55].

8.3.2 ILC2s in the Pathogenesis of AD

ILC2s were originally identified in the gut and gut-associated lymphoid tissues and were found to contribute to immunity against parasitic helminth in the absence of an adaptive immune system [56–59]. Subsequent studies showed that ILC2s play key

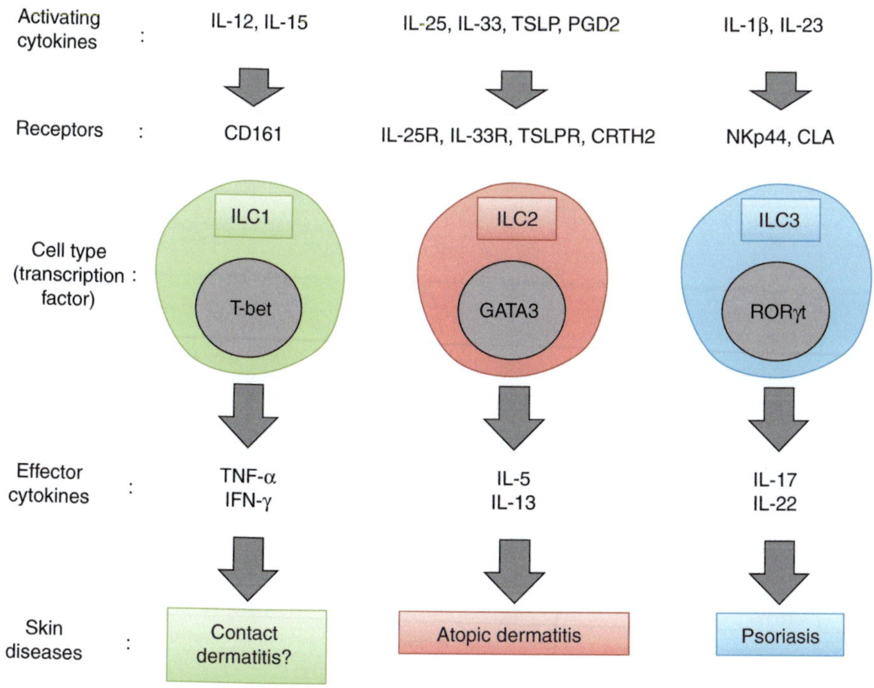

Fig. 8.4 Regulation and function of each subset of innate lymphoid cells (ILCs) in the human skin. Human skin ILC1s express CD161 and can be activated by IL-12 and IL-15 to produce its effector cytokines TNF-α and IFN-γ. Human skin ILC2s can be activated by epithelial cell-derived cytokines/eicosanoid (e.g., IL-25, IL-33, TSLP, and PGD2) and produce its effector cytokines IL-5 and IL-13; they have thus been implicated in AD. Human skin ILC3s produce IL-17 and IL-22 in response to IL-1β and IL-23 and have been implicated in psoriasis

roles in airway hyperreactivity [60] and epithelial tissue repair in the lung [61]. These studies demonstrated that ILC2s were predominantly regulated by the epithelial cell-derived cytokines IL-25 and IL-33 [62] (Fig. 8.5).

When ILC2s were first identified in the skin, they were also found to be enriched in the lesional skin of AD patients [20, 52]. Type 2 cytokines, including IL-5 and IL-13, have long been suspected to play a key role in the pathogenesis of AD [63–65]. It was also revealed that ILC2s that produce IL-5 and IL-13 were found to be both necessary and sufficient for the development of AD-like disease in a low-dose vitamin D3-induced murine AD model [52, 55].

Mast cell numbers are elevated in chronic AD and likely drive IgE-mediated pathology in the disease [66]. Mast cells can also be directly activated by toxins derived from the skin-resident bacteria, *Staphylococcus aureus*, which is commonly found in the lesional skin of AD patients [67, 68]. Mast cell hyperplasia during inflammation is mediated by IL-3 and IL-9 [69, 70]. IL-9 can also augment the inflammatory cytokine response by mast cells following IgE-mediated activation [55]. ILC2s are a key source of IL-9 in vivo [71], suggesting that ILC2s potentially affect the severity of AD by regulating the number and function of mast cells in the

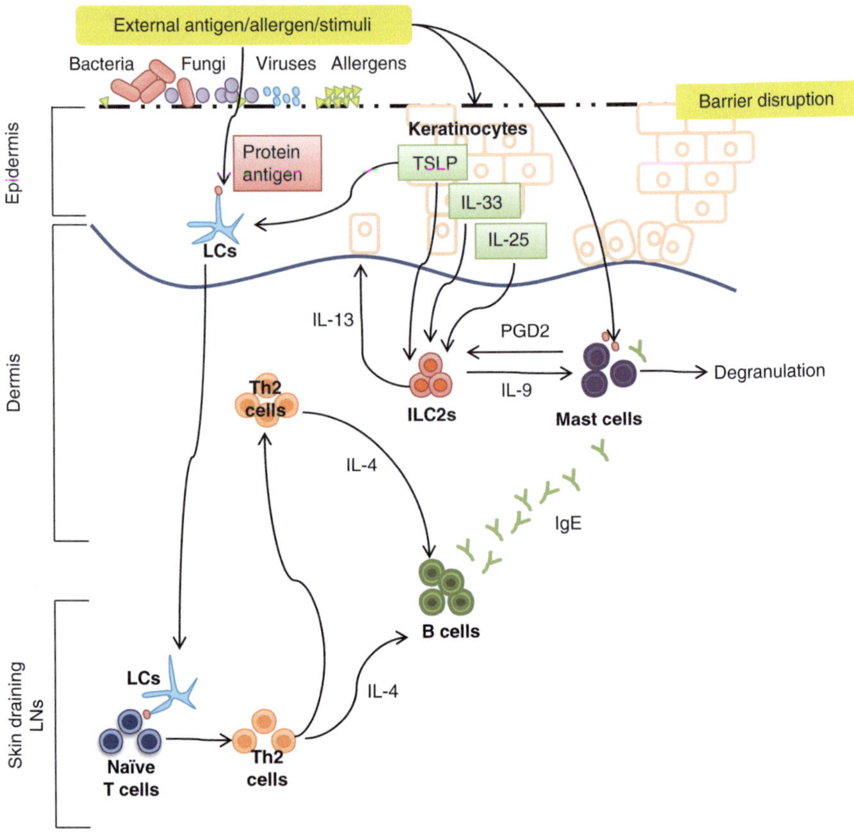

Fig. 8.5 Potential roles of ILC2s in AD. ILC2s are activated by epithelial cell-derived cytokines IL-33, IL-25, and TSLP, all of which are associated with barrier disruption and are upregulated in AD. ILC2 cell-derived IL-9 may increase mast cell numbers in the skin and enhance their responses to IgE-mediated activation in AD. Activated mast cell-derived PGD2 promotes ILC2 migration in the skin

lesional skin (Fig. 8.5). It has also been shown that prostaglandin D2 (PGD2) promotes the migration of skin ILC2s and induces type 2 cytokine production from skin ILC2s. Moreover, the supernatant of IgE/anti-IgE-activated mast cells induces migration and cytokine production by human skin ILC2s [72]. Since mast cells produce PGD2 by means of activation through FcεRI, they might play a role in migration and cytokine production by ILC2s through the effects of PGD2.

As mentioned earlier, TSLP is a crucial cytokine that causes cutaneous DCs to induce Th2 cells. ILC2s express the receptor for TSLP, and TSLP signaling in ILC2s promotes cytokine production [73]. Activation of cutaneous ILC2s was found to be dependent on TSLP signaling, suggesting that ILC2s were critical for disease pathogenesis [52] (Fig. 8.5). In addition to TSLP, Imai et al. showed that transgenic overexpression of IL-33 under a keratin 14 promoter is sufficient to induce spontaneous AD-like dermatitis in association with the accumulation of

ILC2s [74]. This human and mouse evidence indicates that ILC2s are important players in the pathogenesis of AD, where their activity likely depends on the severity of AD, coinfections, and dysfunction of the skin barrier.

Conclusion

With their constitutional plasticity, LCs and ILC2s in the skin play crucial roles in initiating and modulating type 2 immune responses in AD. As many papers have demonstrated, both Th2 cells and ILC2s seem to play crucial roles in the pathogenesis of AD. The magnitude of their effect and/or their interplay, however, remains to be further elucidated.

Recent advances in our knowledge of the skin immune network and pathology in the pathogenesis of AD have opened avenues for the development of therapies that trigger skin DCs and/or ILC2s with specialized properties to control immunity.

Acknowledgments This work was supported in part by Grants-in-Aid for Scientific Research from the Ministry of Education, Culture, Sports, Science, and Technology and the Ministry of Health, Labor, and Welfare of Japan.

References

1. Kaplan DH, Igyarto BZ, Gaspari AA. Early immune events in the induction of allergic contact dermatitis. Nat Rev Immunol. 2012;12(2):114–24. doi:10.1038/nri3150.
2. Nestle FO, Di Meglio P, Qin JZ, Nickoloff BJ. Skin immune sentinels in health and disease. Nat Rev Immunol. 2009;9(10):679–91. doi:10.1038/nri2622.
3. Otsuka A, Kabashima K. Mast cells and basophils in cutaneous immune responses. Allergy. 2015;70(2):131–40. doi:10.1111/all.12526.
4. Brunner PM, Silverberg JI, Guttman-Yassky E, Paller AS, Kabashima K, Amagai M, et al. Increasing comorbidities suggest that atopic dermatitis is a systemic disorder. J Invest Dermatol. 2016. doi:10.1016/j.jid.2016.08.022.
5. Dainichi T, Hanakawa S, Kabashima K. Classification of inflammatory skin diseases: a proposal based on the disorders of the three-layered defense systems, barrier, innate immunity and acquired immunity. J Dermatol Sci. 2014;76(2):81–9. doi:10.1016/j.jdermsci.2014.08.010.
6. Egawa G, Kabashima K. Multifactorial skin barrier deficiency and atopic dermatitis: essential topics to prevent the atopic march. J Allergy Clin Immunol. 2016;138(2):350–8.e1. doi:10.1016/j.jaci.2016.06.002.
7. Kabashima K. New concept of the pathogenesis of atopic dermatitis: interplay among the barrier, allergy, and pruritus as a trinity. J Dermatol Sci. 2013;70(1):3–11. doi:10.1016/j.jdermsci.2013.02.001.
8. Moniaga CS, Kabashima K. Filaggrin in atopic dermatitis: flaky tail mice as a novel model for developing drug targets in atopic dermatitis. Inflamm Allergy Drug Targets. 2011;10(6):477–85.
9. Saeki H, Nakahara T, Tanaka A, Kabashima K, Sugaya M, Murota H, et al. Clinical practice guidelines for the management of atopic dermatitis 2016. J Dermatol. 2016;43(10):1117–45. doi:10.1111/1346-8138.13392.
10. Werfel T. The role of leukocytes, keratinocytes, and allergen-specific IgE in the development of atopic dermatitis. J Invest Dermatol. 2009;129(8):1878–91. doi:10.1038/jid.2009.71.
11. Amano W, Nakajima S, Kunugi H, Numata Y, Kitoh A, Egawa G, et al. The Janus kinase inhibitor JTE-052 improves skin barrier function through suppressing signal transducer and activator of transcription 3 signaling. J Allergy Clin Immunol. 2015;136(3):667–677. e7. doi:10.1016/j.jaci.2015.03.051.

12. Ewald DA, Noda S, Oliva M, Litman T, Nakajima S, Li X et al. Major differences between human atopic dermatitis and murine models, as determined by using global transcriptomic profiling. J Allergy Clin Immunol. 2016. doi:10.1016/j.jaci.2016.08.029.
13. Nemoto O, Furue M, Nakagawa H, Shiramoto M, Hanada R, Matsuki S, et al. The first trial of CIM331, a humanized antihuman interleukin-31 receptor A antibody, in healthy volunteers and patients with atopic dermatitis to evaluate safety, tolerability and pharmacokinetics of a single dose in a randomized, double-blind, placebo-controlled study. Br J Dermatol. 2016;174(2):296–304. doi:10.1111/bjd.14207.
14. Noda S, Suarez-Farinas M, Ungar B, Kim SJ, de Guzman SC, Xu H, et al. The Asian atopic dermatitis phenotype combines features of atopic dermatitis and psoriasis with increased TH17 polarization. J Allergy Clin Immunol. 2015;136(5):1254–64. doi:10.1016/j.jaci.2015.08.015.
15. Nomura T, Kabashima K, Miyachi Y. The panoply of alphabetaT cells in the skin. J Dermatol Sci. 2014;76(1):3–9. doi:10.1016/j.jdermsci.2014.07.010.
16. Banchereau J, Briere F, Caux C, Davoust J, Lebecque S, Liu YJ, et al. Immunobiology of dendritic cells. Annu Rev Immunol. 2000;18:767–811. doi:10.1146/annurev.immunol.18.1.767.
17. Kim BS, Wojno ED, Artis D. Innate lymphoid cells and allergic inflammation. Curr Opin Immunol. 2013;25(6):738–44. doi:10.1016/j.coi.2013.07.013.
18. Kim BS, Wang K, Siracusa MC, Saenz SA, Brestoff JR, Monticelli LA, et al. Basophils promote innate lymphoid cell responses in inflamed skin. J Immunol. 2014;193(7):3717–25. doi:10.4049/jimmunol.1401307.
19. Leon B, Ardavin C. Monocyte-derived dendritic cells in innate and adaptive immunity. Immunol Cell Biol. 2008;86(4):320–4. doi:10.1038/icb.2008.14.
20. Salimi M, Barlow JL, Saunders SP, Xue L, Gutowska-Owsiak D, Wang X, et al. A role for IL-25 and IL-33-driven type-2 innate lymphoid cells in atopic dermatitis. J Exp Med. 2013;210(13):2939–50. doi:10.1084/jem.20130351.
21. Valladeau J, Saeland S. Cutaneous dendritic cells. Semin Immunol. 2005;17(4):273–83. doi:10.1016/j.smim.2005.05.009.
22. Borkowski TA, Letterio JJ, Farr AG, Udey MC. A role for endogenous transforming growth factor beta 1 in Langerhans cell biology: the skin of transforming growth factor beta 1 null mice is devoid of epidermal Langerhans cells. J Exp Med. 1996;184(6):2417–22.
23. Tang A, Amagai M, Granger LG, Stanley JR, Udey MC. Adhesion of epidermal Langerhans cells to keratinocytes mediated by E-cadherin. Nature. 1993;361(6407):82–5. doi:10.1038/361082a0.
24. Inaba K, Swiggard WJ, Inaba M, Meltzer J, Mirza A, Sasagawa T, et al. Tissue distribution of the DEC-205 protein that is detected by the monoclonal antibody NLDC-145. I. Expression on dendritic cells and other subsets of mouse leukocytes. Cell Immunol. 1995;163(1):148–56.
25. Jiang W, Swiggard WJ, Heufler C, Peng M, Mirza A, Steinman RM, et al. The receptor DEC-205 expressed by dendritic cells and thymic epithelial cells is involved in antigen processing. Nature. 1995;375(6527):151–5. doi:10.1038/375151a0.
26. Hunger RE, Sieling PA, Ochoa MT, Sugaya M, Burdick AE, Rea TH, et al. Langerhans cells utilize CD1a and langerin to efficiently present nonpeptide antigens to T cells. J Clin Invest. 2004;113(5):701–8. doi:10.1172/JCI19655.
27. Merad M, Ginhoux F, Collin M. Origin, homeostasis and function of Langerhans cells and other langerin-expressing dendritic cells. Nat Rev Immunol. 2008;8(12):935–47. doi:10.1038/nri2455.
28. Bursch LS, Wang L, Igyarto B, Kissenpfennig A, Malissen B, Kaplan DH, et al. Identification of a novel population of Langerin+ dendritic cells. J Exp Med. 2007;204(13):3147–56. doi:10.1084/jem.20071966.
29. Ginhoux F, Collin MP, Bogunovic M, Abel M, Leboeuf M, Helft J, et al. Blood-derived dermal langerin+ dendritic cells survey the skin in the steady state. J Exp Med. 2007;204(13):3133–46. doi:10.1084/jem.20071733.
30. Poulin LF, Henri S, de Bovis B, Devilard E, Kissenpfennig A, Malissen B. The dermis contains langerin+ dendritic cells that develop and function independently of epidermal Langerhans cells. J Exp Med. 2007;204(13):3119–31. doi:10.1084/jem.20071724.

31. Cepek KL, Shaw SK, Parker CM, Russell GJ, Morrow JS, Rimm DL, et al. Adhesion between epithelial cells and T lymphocytes mediated by E-cadherin and the alpha E beta 7 integrin. Nature. 1994;372(6502):190–3. doi:10.1038/372190a0.
32. Ginhoux F, Liu K, Helft J, Bogunovic M, Greter M, Hashimoto D, et al. The origin and development of nonlymphoid tissue CD103+ DCs. J Exp Med. 2009;206(13):3115–30. doi:10.1084/jem.20091756.
33. Patel VI, Metcalf JP. Identification and characterization of human dendritic cell subsets in the steady state: a review of our current knowledge. J Invest Med. 2016;64(4):833–47. doi:10.1136/jim-2016-000072.
34. Liu YJ. IPC: professional type 1 interferon-producing cells and plasmacytoid dendritic cell precursors. Annu Rev Immunol. 2005;23:275–306. doi:10.1146/annurev.immunol.23.021704.115633.
35. Serbina NV, Salazar-Mather TP, Biron CA, Kuziel WA, Pamer EG. TNF/iNOS-producing dendritic cells mediate innate immune defense against bacterial infection. Immunity. 2003; 19(1):59–70.
36. Novak N, Peng W, Yu C. Network of myeloid and plasmacytoid dendritic cells in atopic dermatitis. Adv Exp Med Biol. 2007;601:97–104.
37. Kubo A, Nagao K, Yokouchi M, Sasaki H, Amagai M. External antigen uptake by Langerhans cells with reorganization of epidermal tight junction barriers. J Exp Med. 2009;206(13):2937–46. doi:10.1084/jem.20091527.
38. Nakajima S, Igyarto BZ, Honda T, Egawa G, Otsuka A, Hara-Chikuma M, et al. Langerhans cells are critical in epicutaneous sensitization with protein antigen via thymic stromal lymphopoietin receptor signaling. J Allergy Clin Immunol. 2012;129(4):1048–55.e6. doi:10.1016/j.jaci.2012.01.063.
39. Ouchi T, Kubo A, Yokouchi M, Adachi T, Kobayashi T, Kitashima DY, et al. Langerhans cell antigen capture through tight junctions confers preemptive immunity in experimental staphylococcal scalded skin syndrome. J Exp Med. 2011;208(13):2607–13. doi:10.1084/jem.20111718.
40. Ito T, Wang YH, Duramad O, Hori T, Delespesse GJ, Watanabe N, et al. TSLP-activated dendritic cells induce an inflammatory T helper type 2 cell response through OX40 ligand. J Exp Med. 2005;202(9):1213–23. doi:10.1084/jem.20051135.
41. Oyoshi MK, Larson RP, Ziegler SF, Geha RS. Mechanical injury polarizes skin dendritic cells to elicit a T(H)2 response by inducing cutaneous thymic stromal lymphopoietin expression. J Allergy Clin Immunol. 2010;126(5):976–84, 84.e1–5. doi:10.1016/j.jaci.2010.08.041.
42. Ebner S, Nguyen VA, Forstner M, Wang YH, Wolfram D, Liu YJ, et al. Thymic stromal lymphopoietin converts human epidermal Langerhans cells into antigen-presenting cells that induce proallergic T cells. J Allergy Clin Immunol. 2007;119(4):982–90. doi:10.1016/j.jaci.2007.01.003.
43. Liu YJ. Thymic stromal lymphopoietin: master switch for allergic inflammation. J Exp Med. 2006;203(2):269–73. doi:10.1084/jem.20051745.
44. Soumelis V, Reche PA, Kanzler H, Yuan W, Edward G, Homey B, et al. Human epithelial cells trigger dendritic cell mediated allergic inflammation by producing TSLP. Nat Immunol. 2002;3(7):673–80. doi:10.1038/ni805.
45. Bieber T. Atopic dermatitis. N Engl J Med. 2008;358(14):1483–94. doi:10.1056/NEJMra074081.
46. Wollenberg A, Rawer HC, Schauber J. Innate immunity in atopic dermatitis. Clin Rev Allergy Immunol. 2011;41(3):272–81. doi:10.1007/s12016-010-8227-x.
47. Yoshida K, Kubo A, Fujita H, Yokouchi M, Ishii K, Kawasaki H, et al. Distinct behavior of human Langerhans cells and inflammatory dendritic epidermal cells at tight junctions in patients with atopic dermatitis. J Allergy Clin Immunol. 2014;134(4):856–64. doi:10.1016/j.jaci.2014.08.001.
48. Mjosberg J, Eidsmo L. Update on innate lymphoid cells in atopic and non-atopic inflammation in the airways and skin. Clin Exp Allergy. 2014;44(8):1033–43. doi:10.1111/cea.12353.
49. Fan X, Rudensky AY. Hallmarks of tissue-resident lymphocytes. Cell. 2016;164(6):1198–211. doi:10.1016/j.cell.2016.02.048.

50. Sonnenberg GF, Mjosberg J, Spits H, Artis D. SnapShot: innate lymphoid cells. Immunity. 2013;39(3):622-e1. doi:10.1016/j.immuni.2013.08.021.
51. Dyring-Andersen B, Geisler C, Agerbeck C, Lauritsen JP, Gudjonsdottir SD, Skov L, et al. Increased number and frequency of group 3 innate lymphoid cells in nonlesional psoriatic skin. Br J Dermatol. 2014;170(3):609–16. doi:10.1111/bjd.12658.
52. Kim BS, Siracusa MC, Saenz SA, Noti M, Monticelli LA, Sonnenberg GF, et al. TSLP elicits IL-33-independent innate lymphoid cell responses to promote skin inflammation. Sci Transl Med. 2013;5(170):170ra16. doi:10.1126/scitranslmed.3005374.
53. Teunissen MB, Munneke JM, Bernink JH, Spuls PI, Res PC, Te Velde A, et al. Composition of innate lymphoid cell subsets in the human skin: enrichment of NCR(+) ILC3 in lesional skin and blood of psoriasis patients. J Invest Dermatol. 2014;134(9):2351–60. doi:10.1038/jid.2014.146.
54. Villanova F, Flutter B, Tosi I, Grys K, Sreeneebus H, Perera GK, et al. Characterization of innate lymphoid cells in human skin and blood demonstrates increase of NKp44+ ILC3 in psoriasis. J Invest Dermatol. 2014;134(4):984–91. doi:10.1038/jid.2013.477.
55. Roediger B, Kyle R, Yip KH, Sumaria N, Guy TV, Kim BS, et al. Cutaneous immunosurveillance and regulation of inflammation by group 2 innate lymphoid cells. Nat Immunol. 2013;14(6):564–73. doi:10.1038/ni.2584.
56. Fallon PG, Ballantyne SJ, Mangan NE, Barlow JL, Dasvarma A, Hewett DR, et al. Identification of an interleukin (IL)-25-dependent cell population that provides IL-4, IL-5, and IL-13 at the onset of helminth expulsion. J Exp Med. 2006;203(4):1105–16. doi:10.1084/jem.20051615.
57. Moro K, Yamada T, Tanabe M, Takeuchi T, Ikawa T, Kawamoto H, et al. Innate production of T(H)2 cytokines by adipose tissue-associated c-Kit(+)Sca-1(+) lymphoid cells. Nature. 2010;463(7280):540–4. doi:10.1038/nature08636.
58. Neill DR, Wong SH, Bellosi A, Flynn RJ, Daly M, Langford TK, et al. Nuocytes represent a new innate effector leukocyte that mediates type-2 immunity. Nature. 2010;464(7293):1367–70. doi:10.1038/nature08900.
59. Price AE, Liang HE, Sullivan BM, Reinhardt RL, Eisley CJ, Erle DJ, et al. Systemically dispersed innate IL-13-expressing cells in type 2 immunity. Proc Natl Acad Sci U S A. 2010;107(25):11489–94. doi:10.1073/pnas.1003988107.
60. Chang YJ, Kim HY, Albacker LA, Baumgarth N, McKenzie AN, Smith DE, et al. Innate lymphoid cells mediate influenza-induced airway hyper-reactivity independently of adaptive immunity. Nat Immunol. 2011;12(7):631–8. doi:10.1038/ni.2045.
61. Monticelli LA, Sonnenberg GF, Abt MC, Alenghat T, Ziegler CG, Doering TA, et al. Innate lymphoid cells promote lung-tissue homeostasis after infection with influenza virus. Nat Immunol. 2011;12(11):1045–54. doi:10.1031/ni.2131.
62. Monticelli LA, Sonnenberg GF, Artis D. Innate lymphoid cells: critical regulators of allergic inflammation and tissue repair in the lung. Curr Opin Immunol. 2012;24(3):284–9. doi:10.1016/j.coi.2012.03.012.
63. Akdis M, Akdis CA, Weigl L, Disch R, Blaser K. Skin-homing, CLA+ memory T cells are activated in atopic dermatitis and regulate IgE by an IL-13-dominated cytokine pattern: IgG4 counter-regulation by CLA- memory T cells. J Immunol. 1997;159(9):4611–9.
64. Bos JD, Wierenga EA, Sillevis Smitt JH, van der Heijden FL, Kapsenberg ML. Immune dysregulation in atopic eczema. Arch Dermatol. 1992;128(11):1509–12.
65. Plaut M. Antigen-specific lymphokine secretory patterns in atopic disease. J Immunol. 1990;144(12):4497–500.
66. Liu FT, Goodarzi H, Chen HY. IgE, mast cells, and eosinophils in atopic dermatitis. Clin Rev Allergy Immunol. 2011;41(3):298–310. doi:10.1007/s12016-011-8252-4.
67. Kong HH, Oh J, Deming C, Conlan S, Grice EA, Beatson MA, et al. Temporal shifts in the skin microbiome associated with disease flares and treatment in children with atopic dermatitis. Genome Res. 2012;22(5):850–9. doi:10.1101/gr.131029.111.
68. Nakamura Y, Oscherwitz J, Cease KB, Chan SM, Munoz-Planillo R, Hasegawa M, et al. Staphylococcus delta-toxin induces allergic skin disease by activating mast cells. Nature. 2013;503(7476):397–401. doi:10.1038/nature12655.

69. Lantz CS, Boesiger J, Song CH, Mach N, Kobayashi T, Mulligan RC, et al. Role for interleukin-3 in mast-cell and basophil development and in immunity to parasites. Nature. 1998;392(6671):90–3. doi:10.1038/32190.
70. Townsend JM, Fallon GP, Matthews JD, Smith P, Jolin EH, McKenzie NA. IL-9-deficient mice establish fundamental roles for IL-9 in pulmonary mastocytosis and goblet cell hyperplasia but not T cell development. Immunity. 2000;13(4):573–83.
71. Wilhelm C, Hirota K, Stieglitz B, Van Snick J, Tolaini M, Lahl K, et al. An IL-9 fate reporter demonstrates the induction of an innate IL-9 response in lung inflammation. Nat Immunol. 2011;12(11):1071–7. doi:10.1038/ni.2133.
72. Xue L, Salimi M, Panse I, Mjosberg JM, McKenzie AN, Spits H, et al. Prostaglandin D2 activates group 2 innate lymphoid cells through chemoattractant receptor-homologous molecule expressed on TH2 cells. J Allergy Clin Immunol. 2014;133(4):1184–94. doi:10.1016/j.jaci.2013.10.056.
73. Mjosberg J, Bernink J, Golebski K, Karrich JJ, Peters CP, Blom B, et al. The transcription factor GATA3 is essential for the function of human type 2 innate lymphoid cells. Immunity. 2012;37(4):649–59. doi:10.1016/j.immuni.2012.08.015.
74. Imai Y, Yasuda K, Sakaguchi Y, Haneda T, Mizutani H, Yoshimoto T, et al. Skin-specific expression of IL-33 activates group 2 innate lymphoid cells and elicits atopic dermatitis-like inflammation in mice. Proc Natl Acad Sci U S A. 2013;110(34):13921–6. doi:10.1073/pnas.1307321110.

Cytokine Network

9

Kenji Izuhara, Satoshi Nunomura, Shoichiro Ohta, Masahiro Ogawa, and Yasuhiro Nanri

Abstract

Immune dysregulation, barrier defects, and increased skin infections combine to lead to the onset of atopic dermatitis (AD). It was previously thought that type 2 inflammation was dominant in the acute phase of AD, and then in the chronic phase, it became type 1 inflammation. However, it is now widely accepted that both type 2 inflammation and inflammation induced by T_H22 cells are dominant in both the acute and chronic phases of AD. In type 2 inflammation, IL-4, IL-13, and IL-5, which are signature type 2 cytokines, are highly expressed and are involved in forming the characteristic features of AD. Epithelial cell-derived cytokines—thymic stromal lymphopoietin, IL-33, and IL-25—initiate type 2 inflammation by controlling various cells, including group 2 innate lymphoid cells. Moreover, IL-31, a newly identified type 2 cytokine, induces itch by acting on sensory neurons. IL-22, a signature cytokine derived from T_H22 cells, is significantly expressed in AD skin and is believed to contribute to the pathogenesis of AD as well as type 2 cytokines by acting on keratinocytes. Based on both basic and clinical findings, several antibodies targeting cytokines have been developed as therapeutic agents against AD, among which dupilumab, targeting the IL-4 receptor α chain shared with IL-4R and IL-13R, has become the first molecularly targeted drug for the treatment of AD.

Keywords

Cytokine • Type 2 inflammation • T_H22 cell • Epithelial cell-derived cytokine • Dupilumab

---

K. Izuhara (✉) • S. Nunomura • S. Ohta • M. Ogawa • Y. Nanri
Division of Medical Biochemistry, Department of Biomolecular Sciences,
Saga Medical School, 5-1-1 Nabeshima, Saga 849-8501, Japan
e-mail: kizuhara@cc.saga-u.ac.jp

I. Katayama et al. (eds.), *Evolution of Atopic Dermatitis in the 21st Century*,
https://doi.org/10.1007/978-981-10-5541-6_9

9.1 Introduction

Atopic dermatitis (AD) is the most common chronic inflammatory skin disease and is characterized by eczematous lesions and pruritus. A combination of barrier defects, immune dysregulation, and increased skin infections contributes to the pathogenesis of AD [1]; these factors do not act independently but interact with each other. It is of note that immune dysregulation leads to barrier defects or susceptibility to infections. In this chapter, we describe how the cytokine network working within the immune system is dysregulated in the pathogenesis of AD and what agents targeting cytokines are developed for therapeutic drugs for treatment of AD.

9.2 Type 2 Signature Cytokines

Historically, the T_H1/T_H2 paradigm has been proposed as an immune mechanism, and allergic inflammation including AD has been explained as the dominance of the T_H2 status [2]. Although the details of T_H2 immunity, now called type 2 immunity, have been further clarified and the involvement of immune systems other than type 1 and type 2 immunity has been demonstrated, classic type 2 immunity has explained a great deal about the underlying mechanism of allergic inflammation. Based on the findings, some agents, including dupilumab, have emerged as therapeutic drugs for AD. Here, we demonstrate the significance and roles of type 2 signature cytokines—IL-4, IL-5, and IL-13—in allergic skin inflammation (Fig. 9.1).

9.2.1 IL-4/IL-13

IL-4 and IL-13 are related type 2 signature cytokines. T_H2 cells produce both IL-4 and IL-13, as do mast cells, eosinophils, and basophils [3]. Recently, it has turned out that group 2 innate lymphoid cells (ILCs) are important sources of IL-13 [4–6] and to a lesser extent of IL-4 [7, 8]. IL-4 binds to either type 1 IL-4 receptor (IL-4R), composed of the IL-4R subunit α (IL-4Rα) and the cytokine receptor common subunit γ, or type 2 IL-4R, composed of IL-4Rα and the IL-13R subunit α-1 chain [9]. Type 2 IL-4R also acts as IL-13R. Hematopoietic/immune cells mainly express type 1 IL-4R, whereas type 2 IL-4R/IL-13R is ubiquitously expressed on non-hematopoietic cells or tissue-resident cells. Due to the different distributions of IL-4R/IL-13R and the concentrations of IL-4/IL-13, IL-4 exerts its functions, such as expansion of T_H2 cells and IgE synthesis in B cells, mainly on hematopoietic/immune cells, whereas IL-13 does so on non-hematopoietic cells or tissue-resident cells.

Analyses of gene-manipulated mice have shown the importance of IL-4 or IL-13 in the pathogenesis of AD; ectopic expression of IL-4 [10, 11] or IL-13 [12] in the skin caused xerosis and pruritic inflammatory skin accompanied with elevated type 2 immune responses, which reproduced all key features of human AD. Both IL-4 and IL-13 are pleiotropic cytokines contributing to the pathogenesis

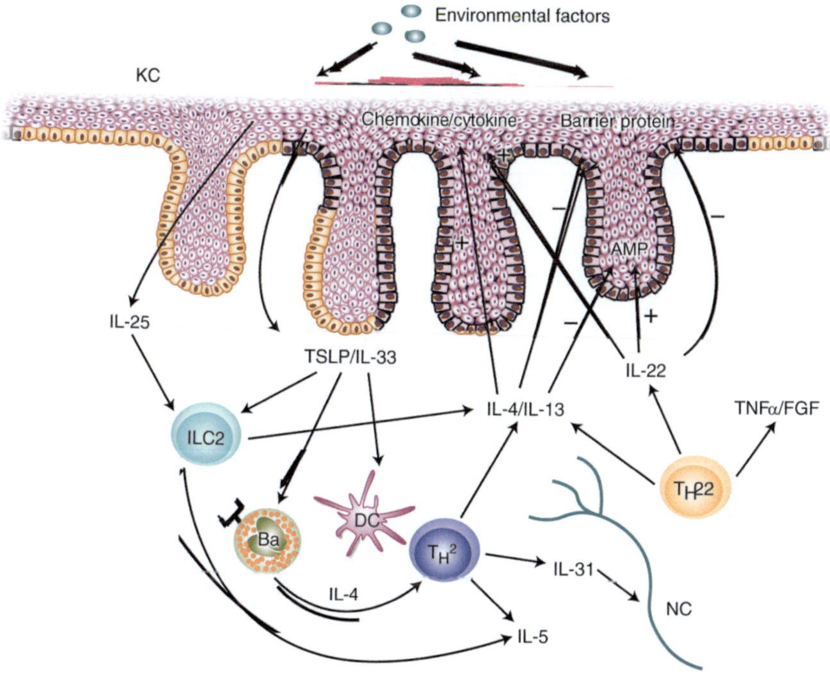

Fig. 9.1 Dysregulated cytokine network in the pathogenesis of AD. Various environmental factors act on keratinocytes (KC) inducing epithelial cell-derived cytokines—TSLP, IL-33, and IL-25. These cytokines initiate type 2 inflammation by controlling group 2 ILCs (ILC2), DCs, and basophils (Ba). These cells activate T_H2 cells or produce IL-5 and IL-13. T_H2 cells secrete type 2 cytokines—IL-4, IL-5, IL-13, and IL-31— whereas T_H22 cells secrete IL-22, IL-13, TNFα, and FGF. IL-4/IL-13 and IL-22 have common effects on keratinocytes: upregulation of chemokine and cytokine production and downregulation of barrier proteins. However, these cytokines have opposite effects regarding AMP production; IL-4/IL-13 downregulates it, whereas IL-22 enhances it. Moreover, IL-31 activates neuronal cells (NC) inducing itch

of AD by acting on tissue-resident cells such as keratinocytes or fibroblasts as well as on immune cells. The actions of IL-4 and IL-13 in the pathogenesis of AD are summarized as follows: (1) chemokine production, (2) barrier defect in epidermis, (3) susceptibility to infections, and (4) fibrosis, particularly in the case of IL-13. Either IL-4 or IL-13 by itself or together with other cytokines such as TNFα and IFN-γ can induce several chemokines for recruiting inflammatory cells such as thymus and activation-regulated chemokine (TARC)/CCL17, eotaxin-2/CCL24, and eotaxin-3/CCL26, which are highly expressed in the AD skin [13–16]. Either IL-4 or IL-13 downregulates expression of the components in the epidermal differentiation complex, such as filaggrin, loricrin, and involucrin [17, 18], leading to the barrier defect of the epidermis. Moreover, IL-4 and IL-13 inhibit production of antimicrobial peptides (AMPs), human β defensin (HBD)-2, and HBD-3 [19], consistent with the finding that AD patients showed low expression of cathelicidin (LL-37) and HBD-2 [20], which at least partially explains the susceptibility to infections in AD patients. Mice overexpressing ectopically IL-13 in the skin showed significant fibrosis [12], which is a typical feature of chronic AD patients. We found that periostin, a component of fibrosis in AD, is a downstream molecule of IL-4 or IL-13 and plays a key role in the pathogenesis of AD [21]. Periostin produced in IL-4- or IL-13-stimulated fibroblasts is critical for the appearance of AD-like phenotypes—type 2 inflammation, hyperplasia or dysregulated differentiation of keratinocytes, and fibrosis—in mice painted with house dust mites (HDM). Direct effects of periostin on keratinocytes via integrins can at least partially explain its actions.

9.2.2 IL-5

IL-5 is critical for eosinophil development, survival, and proliferation [22]. T_H2 cells are the main IL-5-producing cells; mast cells, eosinophils, and basophils as well as epithelial cells and smooth muscles also produce IL-5. Group 2 ILCs are another important source of IL-5 as well as IL-13 [4–6]. IL-5 binds to the heterodimeric receptor composed of the IL-5R subunit α (IL-5Rα) and the cytokine receptor common subunit β shared with IL-3 and granulocyte-macrophage colony-stimulating factor.

Ectopic expression of IL-5 in mouse skin caused infiltration of eosinophils in the epidermis [23], which recaptured the phenotypic changes in AD patients. Interestingly, a number of sensory neurons also significantly increased in the epidermis of these mice, suggesting the importance of IL-5 in neuron branching in AD. Moreover, IL-5 production in peripheral blood mononuclear cells stimulated by HDM extract in AD infants was correlated with the severity of AD [24]. However, anti-IL-5 antibody (Ab, mepolizumab) did not show efficacy for AD patients as described later [25], although it showed good efficacy for asthma patients [26, 27], suggesting that the roles of eosinophils are different in the pathogenesis of AD and asthma.

9.3 Epithelial Cell-Derived Cytokines

Epithelial cells constitute a first physical, chemical, and immunological barrier that may be classified as a part of the innate defense system [28]. Dendritic cells (DCs), group 2 ILCs, and basophils are the immune cells that initiate type 2 immune responses, and these cells act very collaboratively. Epithelial cells secrete various factors—cytokines, chemokines, other proteins, and chemicals—to control these immune cells. Among them, thymic stromal lymphopoietin (TSLP), IL-33, and IL-25 are the most important factors in the pathogenesis of AD.

9.3.1 TSLP

TSLP is an IL-7-like cytokine highly expressed in AD skin. TSLP binds to the heterodimeric receptor composed of the TSLP receptor and the IL-7R subunit α

(IL-7Rα). TSLP is mainly produced in keratinocytes and other epithelial cells [29, 30]. Various extrinsic and intrinsic factors induce TSLP production; environmental factors such as TLR ligands (pathogen-associated molecular patterns, or PAMPs), danger-associated molecular patterns, virus, allergens, helminthes, and chemicals can trigger TSLP production [31]. Moreover, pro-inflammatory cytokines (TNFα and IL-1α) and type 2 cytokines (IL-4 and IL-13) synergistically enhance TSLP production [32, 33]. We found that periostin, a downstream molecule of IL-4/IL-13 signals, induced TSLP production in keratinocytes by directly binding to integrins on their cell surface [21]. It was reported that basophils directly activated by protease allergens could produce TSLP as well as IL-4, suggesting that basophils are another source of TSLP in addition to keratinocytes/epithelial cells [34]. Moreover, it has been shown that mast cells are indispensable for TSLP production in the mouse model of allergic rhinitis [35].

TSLP is a pleiotropic cytokine exerting its effects on many types of cells—DCs, T cells, B cells, mast cells, eosinophils, macrophages, basophils, and group 2 ILCs. TSLP induces polarization of myeloid DCs (CD11c$^+$ cells) that drive differentiation of naïve T cells into T_H2 cells, suggesting that TSLP plays an important role for linking innate immunity and acquired immunity [29, 36]. Expression of OX40 ligand (OX40L) and inhibition of IL-12 production are critical for these effects [37]. In concordance with this finding, administration of neutralizing Abs against OX40L inhibited type 2 inflammation in mice [38]. TSLP acts as a growth factor for T cells; in particular, it has been shown that TSLP directly acts on T_H2 cells, causing their expansion [39]. TSLP acts on innate immune cells such as mast cells, basophils, and NKT cells, inducing production of pro-inflammatory and type 2 cytokines in these cells involved in the initiation of an innate phase in allergic inflammation [29, 36]. It has also been shown that TSLP activates group 2 ILCs in the skin, rather than group 2 ILCs in the lungs [40]. Moreover, it has been demonstrated that TSLP directly acts on a subset of sensory neurons expressing transient receptor potential vanilloid 1 (TRPV1), a calcium-permeable ion channel, to trigger robust itch behaviors [41]. The significance of TSLP in the pathogenesis of AD has been also confirmed using model mice; selective expression of TSLP in the skin caused spontaneous AD-like phenotypes [42], whereas genetic deficiency of TSLP or administration of neutralizing Abs against TSLP inhibited allergen-induced skin inflammation [43].

9.3.2 IL-33

IL-33 is a member of the IL-1 family and is mainly expressed by epithelial cells, fibroblasts, and endothelial cells [44]. IL-33 binds to the heterodimeric receptor composed of ST2, also known as IL-1RL1, and the IL-1R accessory protein (IL-1RAcP). IL-33 localizes to the nucleus, and cellular necrosis leads to the release of IL-33 followed by activation of IL-33 by cleavage with inflammatory proteases [44]. This suggests that IL-33 acts as an alarmin, sensing danger signals in the body, as well as high mobility group box 1 (HMGB1) and IL-1α.

Like TSLP, IL-33 is also a pleiotropic cytokine exerting its effects on many types of cells—T_H2 cells, mast cells, basophils, eosinophils, macrophages, DCs, and group 2 ILCs. IL-33 causes expansion, activation, and recruitment of T_H2 cells [45, 46]. It induces production of pro-inflammatory and type 2 cytokines in mast cells [47, 48] and basophils [49]. It potently activates eosinophils and enhances their adhesion and survival [50, 51]. In macrophages, IL-33 amplifies polarization of M2 macrophages [52]. It also activates DCs by upregulating expression of MHC class II molecules and co-stimulatory molecules [53]. Moreover, it should be noted that group 2 ILCs are main targets for IL-33 and that they are expanded by administering IL-33 [4–6].

Expression of both IL-33 and its receptor components, ST2 and IL-1RAcP, was upregulated in the lesional skin of AD patients, and expression of IL-33 and ST2 was further enhanced after HDM or staphylococcal enterotoxin B (SEB) exposure [54]. Specifically expressed IL-33 in the skin caused pruritic inflammatory skin similar to the features in AD patients accompanied with expansion of group 2 ILCs [55], suggesting the potential of IL-33 to cause the phenotypes of AD.

9.3.3 IL-25

IL-25, also known as IL-17E, is a member of the IL-17 family. IL-25 binds to the heterodimeric receptor composed of the IL-17 receptor B (IL-17RB), also known as IL-25R, and IL-17RA. IL-25-positive keratinocytes increased in AD skin [56]. DCs and activated eosinophils and basophils produce IL-25 [56, 57]. IL-25 enhances proliferation and T_H2 polarization as well as production of type 2 cytokines in T_H2 memory cells. Expression of IL-25 and IL-17RB was upregulated in AD patients, suggesting the possibility that this cytokine is involved in the pathogenesis of AD. Moreover, IL-25 targets group 2 ILCs as well as IL-33 expanding these cells and inducing secretion of IL-5 and IL-13 from these cells [4–6].

9.4 IL-31

IL-31, a newly discovered type 2 cytokine, is a member of the IL-6 cytokine family. IL-31 binds to the heterodimeric receptor composed of the IL-31 receptor subunit α (IL-31RA) and the oncostatin M receptor (OSMR). IL-31 is mainly produced in T_H2 cells, which shows that IL-31 belongs to type 2 cytokines [58], and other cells—mast cells, macrophages, DCs, keratinocytes, and fibroblasts—also express IL-31 [59].

The skin in AD patients showed high expression of both IL-31 and the superantigen SEB produced by *S. aureus* which stimulates *IL31* expression in peripheral blood mononuclear cells of AD patients [60]. Expression of IL-31 is correlated with that of IL-4 or IL-13 [61], and serum IL-31 is correlated with the severity of AD in both adults and children [62, 63]. The significance of IL-31 in the pathogenesis of AD has been confirmed using model mice; either ubiquitous or lymphocyte-specific expression of IL-31 or intradermal administration of IL-31 caused pruritic skin inflammation with alopecia, hyperkeratosis, acanthosis, and mast cell infiltration [58]. Interestingly, serum IgE/IgG1 was not altered in these mice, indicating that it is unlikely that IL-31 exerts its actions in these mice depending on the presence of immune cells.

Keratinocytes express IL-31RA, so these cells are likely one of IL-31's targets. Based on the findings that intradermal administration of IL-31 into mice caused epidermal thickening, particularly proliferation of basal cells [58, 64], epidermal cell proliferation is one action of IL-31 underlying the pathogenesis of AD. Another important target of IL-31 is neurons. Intradermal injection of IL-31 caused intense itch, suggesting the possibility that IL-31 directly acts on neurons triggering itch. Both human and mouse dorsal root ganglia neurons expressed IL-31RA [65]. These neurons largely co-expressed TRPV1, a calcium-permeable ion channel, involved in itch sensation (Kittaka and Tominaga [66]). Genetic deficiency of TRPV1 or transient receptor channel potential ankyrin subtype 1 (TRPA1), another calcium-permeable ion channel, significantly reduced IL-31-induced itch, suggesting a link between type 2 inflammation-dependent itch and the actions of IL-31 on TRPV1-expressing sensory neurons. Moreover, the gene profile by IL-31 in dorsal root ganglia suggested that IL-31 causes nerve elongation and branching in these neurons [67].

9.5 IL-22

IL-22 is a signature cytokine of T_H22 and is a member of the IL-20 cytokine family, which also includes IL-19, IL-20, IL-24, and IL-26. IL-22 binds to the heterodimeric receptor composed of the IL-10 receptor subunit β (IL-10R2) and the IL-22 receptor subunit α-1 chain (IL-22RA1). IL-22 is mainly produced by T_H22 cells and T_H17 cells [68, 69]. T_H22 cells are a T cell subset distinct from T_H1 cells, T_H2 cells, and T_H17 cells; T_H22 cells are differentiated from naïve T cells by TNF and IL-6. These cells express CCR6, CCR4, CCR10, and aryl hydrocarbon receptor, and they produce IL-22, IL-13, TNFα, and FGF. Although it has been shown that many inflammatory cytokines—TNFα, IL-6, IL-12, IL-18, and IL-23—can induce IL-22 [69], it is thought that SEB and staphylococcal α-toxin produced by *S. aureus*, whose infections are frequently complications for AD patients, are important triggers to IL-22 production in AD patients [70].

It has been shown that IL-22 is highly expressed in AD skin [71]. They compared T cell subsets in AD and in psoriasis patients, demonstrating that AD skin showed dominance of type 2 inflammation and inflammation induced by T_H22 cells, whereas psoriasis skin showed type 1/type 17 dominance. The frequency of T_C22 cells and the clinical severity of AD patients as estimated by SCORAD scores showed a positive correlation. This type 2/type 22 axis in the pathogenesis of AD has been supported by other findings that the numbers of IL-22-positive cells were correlated with the eosinophil numbers [72] and that both type 2 cytokine- and IL-22-related genes were upregulated in both acute and chronic AD lesions [73].

The functions of IL-22 in the pathogenesis of AD have been summarized as (1) enhanced proliferation and inhibition of differentiation in keratinocytes [74–78]; (2) decreased expression of the epidermal differentiation complexes such as filaggrin, loricrin, and involucrin [74, 79]; (3) enhanced inflammatory cytokines and chemokines [76]; and (4) increased AMP production such as HBD-2 and HBD-3 [74, 78, 80]. IL-22's action on AMP is inconsistent with the feature of AD skin that AMP expression is decreased, which may be one reason why AD patients are susceptible to infections. This can be explained by the dominant effects of type 2 cytokines that inhibit AMP expression. There is no formal proof showing the importance of IL-22 in the pathogenesis of AD using model mice. Gene deficiency or administration of neutralizing Abs against IL-22 has been shown to decrease psoriasis-like phenotypes in mice [81–83].

9.6 Other Cytokines

9.6.1 IFN-γ

IFN-γ is a signature cytokine of type 1 immunity. IFN-γ binds to the tetrameric receptor composed of two molecules of IFN-γ receptor 1 (IFN-γ-R1) and IFN-γ receptor 2 (IFN-γ-R2). In the past, it was widely accepted that type 2 inflammation is dominant in the acute phase of AD, and then in the chronic phase, it is switched into type 1 inflammation in which IFN-γ is highly expressed [84]. However, as mentioned earlier, it is now widely accepted that the type 1/type 17 axis is dominant in the pathogenesis of psoriasis, whereas AD showed the dominance in the type 2/type 22 axis, even in the chronic phase [71–73].

9.6.2 IL-17

IL-17 is a signature cytokine of type 17 immunity. IL-17 binds to the heterodimeric receptor composed of the IL-17 receptor A (IL-17RA) and the IL-17 receptor C (IL-17RC). There are some reports showing that expression of IL-17 is upregulated in AD skin [85, 86]. However, as mentioned earlier, the contradict concept is now widely accepted; the type 1/type 17 axis exists in the pathogenesis of psoriasis, not AD, and IL-17 expression decreases, particularly in the chronic phase [71].

9.6.3 IL-19

IL-19 is a member of the IL-20 cytokine family, as is IL-22. IL-19 binds to the heterodimeric receptor composed of the IL-20 receptor subunits α and β (IL-20RA and IL-20RB). IL-19 is induced by IL-17 and IL-4/IL-13 and enhances IL-17's actions on keratinocytes [87, 88]. IL-19 is highly expressed in pediatric AD patients rather than in adult AD patients [89]. Moreover, Asian AD patients showed higher IL-19 expression than European-American AD patients [90]. Based on this finding, it was suggested the Asian AD phenotype is a blend of the European-American AD phenotype and the psoriatic phenotype in which high expression of IL-19 is included. However, the details of the roles of IL-19 in the pathogenesis of AD remain unclear.

9.7 Cytokine-Targeted Drugs

Based on the basic and clinical studies of the contents of the cytokine network, several antibodies targeting cytokines have been developed as therapeutic agents against AD. Clinical trials have recently been completed involving dupilumab, targeting the IL-4 receptor α chain shared with IL-4R and IL-13R. Here we have summarized the agents targeting cytokines for treatment of AD (Table 9.1) and have explained the characteristics, particularly the efficacy, of several agents reported in the literature.

9.7.1 Dupilumab (Anti-IL-4Rα Ab)

Dupilumab is a fully human monoclonal Ab against IL-4Rα shared with type 1 IL-4R and type 2 IL-4R/IL-13R, so that it can inhibit both IL-4 and IL-13 signals. In phase I studies (M4A and M4B), moderate-to-severe AD patients received 75–300 mg of dupilumab once a week for 4 weeks [91]. The patients receiving dupilumab got better in a 50% improvement in the Eczema Area and Severity Index referred to as EASI-50 as well as the pruritus numerical rating scale (NRS) and TARC, but not IgE. The gene expression profiles were dramatically changed by dupilumab treatment; epidermal proliferation markers—*K16* and *MK167*—and type 2-related chemokines, *CCL17*, *CCL18*, *CCL22*, and *CCL26*, were

Table 9.1 Present status of drugs targeting cytokines for AD

Target	Biological agent	Level of development
IL-4Rα	Dupilumab (Regeneron/Sanofi)	Phase III
IL-4Rα	Pitrakinra (Aerovance)	Phase II
IL-13	Tralokinumab (MedImmune/AstraZeneca)	Phase II
IL-13	Lebrikizumab (Roche)	Phase II
IL-5	Mepolizumab (GlaxoSmithKline)	Withdrawn
TSLP	AMG-157 (Amgen)	Phase I
TSLPR	MK-8226 (Merck)	Withdrawn
IL-31R	Nemolizumab (CIM331; Chugai Pharmaceutical)	Phase II
IL-31	BMS-981164 (Bristol-Myers Squibb)	Phase I
IL-22	Fezakinumab (ILV-094, Rockefeller University)	Phase II
IL-1R1	Anakinra/Kineret (National Institute of Allergy and Infectious Diseases)	Phase I
IL-12/23p40	Ustekinumab (Stelara, Rockefeller University)	Phase II
IL-17	Secukinumab (Icahn School of Medicine at Mount Sinai)	Phase II

downregulated, whereas barrier-related genes were upregulated [92]. In the phase IIa study, monotherapy with 300 mg of dupilumab was administered to moderate-to-severe AD patients for 12 weeks (M12), showing improvements of clinical end points—EASI-50, EASI-75, Investigator's Global Assessment (IGA), the percent change in EASI, and pruritus NRS—and biomarkers such as TARC and IgE [91]. The combined therapy of dupilumab (300 mg) and topical glucocorticoids for 4 weeks (C4) showed improvements in clinical end points—EASI-50, EASI-75, pruritus NRS, IGA, and body surface area (BSA) affected—and biomarkers (TARC and IgE) and decrease of topical glucocorticoid use compared to topical glucocorticoids alone. Moreover, the phase IIb study (100–300 mg of dupilumab once per 2 or 4 weeks for 16 weeks) showed good efficacy again in improved clinical outcomes—EASI scores, SCORAD scores, patient-reported outcomes (PROs) of pruritus, the pruritus NRS, and the Dermatology Life Quality Index (DLQI)—and decreased TARC [93]. Finally, the phase III study (SOLO 1 and SOLO 2) was performed, in which 300 mg of dupilumab was administered once per 2 or 4 weeks for 16 weeks to moderate-to-severe AD patients inadequately controlled by topical treatment [94]. The IGA score, the primary end point, and EASI-75, a key secondary end point, were significantly improved. Other parameters—EASI scores, pruritus NRS, SCORAD, the Hospital Anxiety and Depression Scale (HADS), the Patient-Oriented Eczema Measure (POEM), and DLQI—were also improved. During all the studies, no serious adverse events occurred. Thus, dupilumab has become the first molecularly targeted drug for the treatment of AD to complete clinical trials.

9.7.2 Mepolizumab (Anti-IL-5 Ab)

Mepolizumab is a human monoclonal Ab against IL-5. Moderate-to-severe AD patients received two 750 mg of mepolizumab 1 week apart [25]. Peripheral blood eosinophils were significantly decreased by treatment of mepolizumab; however, the Physician Global Assessment (PGA) of improvement, SCORAD, pruritus scoring, and TARC did not show statistically significant improvements.

9.7.3 Anti-TSLP/TSLPR Ab (AMG 157/MK-8226)

Two kinds of Abs targeting TSLP/TSLPR have been applied to clinical trials. One is AMG 157 targeting TSLP, and the other is MK-8226 targeting TSLPR. The phase I study for AMG 157 was completed, but the details are unclear. The phase I study for MK-8226 was terminated due to business reasons.

9.7.4 Anti-IL-31R Ab (Nemolizumab: CIM331)

CIM331 is a human monoclonal Ab against IL-31RA, and the results of the phase I study have been reported [95]. A single dose of CIM331 up to 3.0 mg/kg was administered into healthy volunteers and AD patients. No serious adverse events occurred. In AD patients, CIM331 reduced the pruritus visual analogue scale (VAS) score and decreased the amounts of topical corticosteroids used.

Conclusions

The paradigm of how cytokines are involved in the pathogenesis of AD has significantly shifted; in the past, the sequential activation of type 2 and type 1 inflammation was proposed. However, now the type 2/T_H22 paradigm is widely accepted. Moreover, several trials for molecularly targeted drugs against AD have been performed; at this writing, dupilumab has shown efficient effects on AD patients. Thus, basic and clinical studies in the contents of the cytokine network in AD have sharply expanded; in accordance, translational research to develop therapeutic agents for AD has also flourished. It is hoped that several molecularly targeted drugs for AD will become available and that we can select optimal treatments for our AD patients in the near future.

Acknowledgments We thank Dr. Dovie R. Wylie for her critical review of this manuscript.

References

1. Czarnowicki T, Krueger JG, Guttman-Yassky E. Skin barrier and immune dysregulation in atopic dermatitis: an evolving story with important clinical implications. J Allergy Clin Immunol Pract. 2014;2:371–379.; quiz 80-1. doi:10.1016/j.jaip.2014.03.006.
2. Leung DY. Atopic dermatitis: the skin as a window into the pathogenesis of chronic allergic diseases. J Allergy Clin Immunol. 1995;96:302–18. quiz 19
3. Izuhara K, Arima K, Kanaji S, Ohta S, Kanaji T. IL-13: a promising therapeutic target for bronchial asthma. Curr Med Chem. 2006;13:2291–8.
4. Moro K, Yamada T, Tanabe M, Takeuchi T, Ikawa T, Kawamoto H, et al. Innate production of T_H2 cytokines by adipose tissue-associated c-Kit^+Sca-1^+ lymphoid cells. Nature. 2010;463:540–544. doi:nature08636 [pii]. doi:10.1038/nature08636.
5. Neill DR, Wong SH, Bellosi A, Flynn RJ, Daly M, Langford TK, et al. Nuocytes represent a new innate effector leukocyte that mediates type-2 immunity. Nature. 2010;464:1367–1370. nature08900 [pii]. doi:10.1038/nature08900.
6. Price AE, Liang HE, Sullivan BM, Reinhardt RL, Eisley CJ, Erle DJ, et al. Systemically dispersed innate IL-13-expressing cells in type 2 immunity. Proc Natl Acad Sci U S A. 2010;107:11489–11494. 1003988107 [pii]. doi:10.1073/pnas.1003988107.
7. Doherty TA, Khorram N, Lund S, Mehta AK, Croft M, Broide DH. Lung type 2 innate lymphoid cells express cysteinyl leukotriene receptor 1, which regulates TH2 cytokine production. J Allergy Clin Immunol. 2013;132:205–13. doi:10.1016/j.jaci.2013.03.048.
8. Mjosberg J, Bernink J, Golebski K, Karrich JJ, Peters CP, Blom B, et al. The transcription factor GATA3 is essential for the function of human type 2 innate lymphoid cells. Immunity. 2012;37:649–59. doi:10.1016/j.immuni.2012.08.015.
9. Izuhara K, Ohta S, Shiraishi H, Suzuki S. Interleukin 4, interleukin 13, and interleukin 9. In: Izuhara K, Holgate ST, Wills-Karp M, editors. Inflammation and allergy drug design. London: Wiley-Blackwell; 2011. p. 175–85.
10. Chan LS, Robinson N, Xu L. Expression of interleukin-4 in the epidermis of transgenic mice results in a pruritic inflammatory skin disease: an experimental animal model to study atopic dermatitis. J Invest Dermatol. 2001;117:977–83. doi:10.1046/j.0022-202x.2001.01484. x. jid1484 [pii]

11. Chen L, Martinez O, Overbergh L, Mathieu C, Prabhakar BS, Chan LS. Early up-regulation of Th2 cytokines and late surge of Th1 cytokines in an atopic dermatitis model. Clin Exp Immunol. 2004;138:375–87. doi:10.1111/j.1365-2249.2004.02649.x. CEI2649 [pii]
12. Zheng T, Oh MH, Oh SY, Schroeder JT, Glick AB, Zhu Z. Transgenic expression of interleukin-13 in the skin induces a pruritic dermatitis and skin remodeling. J Invest Dermatol. 2009;129:742–51.
13. Kagami S, Kakinuma T, Saeki H, Tsunemi Y, Fujita H, Nakamura K, et al. Significant elevation of serum levels of eotaxin-3/CCL26, but not of eotaxin-2/CCL24, in patients with atopic dermatitis: serum eotaxin-3/CCL26 levels reflect the disease activity of atopic dermatitis. Clin Exp Immunol. 2003;134:309–13.
14. Kagami S, Saeki H, Komine M, Kakinuma T, Tsunemi Y, Nakamura K, et al. Interleukin-4 and interleukin-13 enhance CCL26 production in a human keratinocyte cell line, HaCaT cells. Clin Exp Immunol. 2005;141:459–66. doi:10.1111/j.1365-2249.2005.02875.x.
15. Kakinuma T, Nakamura K, Wakugawa M, Mitsui H, Tada Y, Saeki H, et al. Thymus and activation-regulated chemokine in atopic dermatitis: serum thymus and activation-regulated chemokine level is closely related with disease activity. J Allergy Clin Immunol. 2001;107:535–541. doi:S0091-6749(01)90455-5 [pii]. doi:10.1067/mai.2001.113237.
16. Kakinuma T, Nakamura K, Wakugawa M, Yano S, Saeki H, Torii H, et al. IL-4, but not IL-13, modulates TARC (thymus and activation-regulated chemokine)/CCL17 and IP-10 (interferon-induced protein of 10kDA)/CXCL10 release by TNFα and IFN-γ in HaCaT cell line. Cytokine. 2002;20:1–6.
17. Howell MD, Kim BE, Gao P, Grant AV, Boguniewicz M, Debenedetto A, et al. Cytokine modulation of atopic dermatitis filaggrin skin expression. J Allergy Clin Immunol. 2007;120:150–5.
18. Kim BE, Leung DY, Boguniewicz M, Howell MD. Loricrin and involucrin expression is down-regulated by Th2 cytokines through STAT-6. Clin Immunol. 2008;126:332–7. doi:10.1016/j.clim.2007.11.006.
19. Nomura I, Goleva E, Howell MD, Hamid QA, Ong PY, Hall CF, et al. Cytokine milieu of atopic dermatitis, as compared to psoriasis, skin prevents induction of innate immune response genes. J Immunol. 2003;171:3262–9.
20. Ong PY, Ohtake T, Brandt C, Strickland I, Boguniewicz M, Ganz T, et al. Endogenous antimicrobial peptides and skin infections in atopic dermatitis. N Engl J Med. 2002;347:1151–60. doi:10.1056/NEJMoa021481.
21. Masuoka M, Shiraishi H, Ohta S, Suzuki S, Arima K, Aoki S, et al. Periostin promotes chronic allergic inflammation in response to Th2 cytokines. J Clin Invest. 2012;122:2590–2600. 58978 [pii]. doi:10.1172/JCI58978.
22. Llop-Guevara A, Marcinko J, Fattoub R, Jordana M. Interleukin 3, interleukin 5, and granulocyte-macrophage colony-stimulating factor. In: Izuhara K, Holgate ST, Wills-Karp M, editors. Inflammation and allergy drug design. London: Wiley-Blackwell; 2011. p. 187–96.
23. Foster EL, Simpson EL, Fredrikson LJ, Lee JJ, Lee NA, Fryer AD, et al. Eosinophils increase neuron branching in human and murine skin and in vitro. PLoS One. 2011;6:e22029. doi:10.1371/journal.pone.0022029.
24. Kimura M, Tsuruta S, Yoshida T. Correlation of house dust mite-specific lymphocyte proliferation with IL-5 production, eosinophilia, and the severity of symptoms in infants with atopic dermatitis. J Allergy Clin Immunol. 1998;101:84–9. doi:10.1016/s0091-6749(98)70197-6
25. Oldhoff JM, Darsow U, Werfel T, Katzer K, Wulf A, Laifaoui J, et al. Anti-IL-5 recombinant humanized monoclonal antibody (mepolizumab) for the treatment of atopic dermatitis. Allergy. 2005;60:693–6. doi:10.1111/j.1398-9995.2005.00791.x. ALL791 [pii]
26. Bel EH, Wenzel SE, Thompson PJ, Prazma CM, Keene ON, Yancey SW, et al. Oral glucocorticoid-sparing effect of mepolizumab in eosinophilic asthma. N Engl J Med. 2014;371:1189–97. doi:10.1056/NEJMoa1403291.
27. Ortega HG, Liu MC, Pavord ID, Brusselle GG, FitzGerald JM, Chetta A, et al. Mepolizumab treatment in patients with severe eosinophilic asthma. N Engl J Med. 2014;371:1198–207. doi:10.1056/NEJMoa1403290.

28. Hammad H, Lambrecht BN. Barrier epithelial cells and the control of type 2 immunity. Immunity. 2015;43:29–40. doi:10.1016/j.immuni.2015.07.007.
29. He R, Geha RS. Thymic stromal lymphopoietin. Ann N Y Acad Sci. 2010;1183:13–24. doi:10.1111/j.1749-6632.2009.05128.x.
30. Soumelis V, Reche PA, Kanzler H, Yuan W, Edward G, Homey B, et al. Human epithelial cells trigger dendritic cell mediated allergic inflammation by producing TSLP. Nat Immunol. 2002;3:673–80.
31. Mu Z, Zhao Y, Liu X, Chang C, Zhang J. Molecular biology of atopic dermatitis. Clin Rev Allergy Immunol. 2014;47:193–218. doi:10.1007/s12016-014-8415-1.
32. Bogiatzi SI, Fernandez I, Bichet JC, Marloie-Provost MA, Volpe E, Sastre X, et al. Proinflammatory and Th2 cytokines synergize to induce thymic stromal lymphopoietin production by human skin keratinocytes. J Immunol. 2007;178:3373–7.
33. Kinoshita H, Takai T, Le TA, Kamijo S, Wang XL, Ushio H, et al. Cytokine milieu modulates release of thymic stromal lymphopoietin from human keratinocytes stimulated with double-stranded RNA. J Allergy Clin Immunol. 2009;123:179–86.
34. Sokol CL, Barton GM, Farr AG, Medzhitov R. A mechanism for the initiation of allergen-induced T helper type 2 responses. Nat Immunol. 2008;9:310–8. doi:10.1038/ni1558.
35. Miyata M, Hatsushika K, Ando T, Shimokawa N, Ohnuma Y, Katoh R, et al. Mast cell regulation of epithelial TSLP expression plays an important role in the development of allergic rhinitis. Eur J Immunol. 2008;38:1487–92. doi:10.1002/eji.200737809.
36. Arima K, Liu Y-J. Thymic stromal lymphopoietin. In: Izuhara K, Holgate ST, Wills-Karp M, editors. Inflammation and allergy. London: Wiley-Blackwell; 2011. p. 205–14.
37. Ito T, Wang YH, Duramad O, Hori T, Delespesse GJ, Watanabe N, et al. TSLP-activated dendritic cells induce an inflammatory T helper type 2 cell response through OX40 ligand. J Exp Med. 2005;202:1213–23. doi:10.1084/jem.20051135.
38. Seshasayee D, Lee WP, Zhou M, Shu J, Suto E, Zhang J, et al. In vivo blockade of OX40 ligand inhibits thymic stromal lymphopoietin driven atopic inflammation. J Clin Invest. 2007;117:3868–78. doi:10.1172/JCI33559.
39. Omori M, Ziegler S. Induction of IL-4 expression in CD4+ T cells by thymic stromal lymphopoietin. J Immunol. 2007;178:1396–404.
40. Kim BS, Siracusa MC, Saenz SA, Noti M, Monticelli LA, Sonnenberg GF, et al. TSLP elicits IL-33-independent innate lymphoid cell responses to promote skin inflammation. Sci Transl Med. 2013;5:170ra16. doi:10.1126/scitranslmed.3005374.
41. Wilson SR, The L, Batia LM, Beattie K, Katibah GE, McClain SP, et al. The epithelial cell-derived atopic dermatitis cytokine TSLP activates neurons to induce itch. Cell. 2013;155:285–95. doi:10.1016/j.cell.2013.08.057.
42. Yoo J, Omori M, Gyarmati D, Zhou B, Aye T, Brewer A, et al. Spontaneous atopic dermatitis in mice expressing an inducible thymic stromal lymphopoietin transgene specifically in the skin. J Exp Med. 2005;202:541–9.
43. He R, Oyoshi MK, Garibyan L, Kumar L, Ziegler SF, Geha RS. TSLP acts on infiltrating effector T cells to drive allergic skin inflammation. Proc Natl Acad Sci U S A. 2008;105:11875–80.
44. Liew FY, Pitman NI, McInnes IB. Disease-associated functions of IL-33: the new kid in the IL-1 family. Nat Rev Immunol. 2010;10:103–10. doi:10.1038/nri2692.
45. Komai-Koma M, Xu D, Li Y, McKenzie AN, McInnes IB, Liew FY. IL-33 is a chemoattractant for human Th2 cells. Eur J Immunol. 2007;37:2779–86. doi:10.1002/eji.200737547.
46. Schmitz J, Owyang A, Oldham E, Song Y, Murphy E, McClanahan TK, et al. IL-33, an interleukin-1-like cytokine that signals via the IL-1 receptor-related protein ST2 and induces T helper type 2-associated cytokines. Immunity. 2005;23:479–90. doi:10.1016/j.immuni.2005.09.015.
47. Ali S, Huber M, Kollewe C, Bischoff SC, Falk W, Martin MU. IL-1 receptor accessory protein is essential for IL-33-induced activation of T lymphocytes and mast cells. Proc Natl Acad Sci U S A. 2007;104:18660–5. doi:10.1073/pnas.0705939104.
48. Allakhverdi Z, Smith DE, Comeau MR, Delespesse G. The ST2 ligand IL-33 potently activates and drives maturation of human mast cells. J Immunol. 2007;179:2051–4.

49. Suzukawa M, Iikura M, Koketsu R, Nagase H, Tamura C, Komiya A, et al. An IL-1 cytokine member, IL-33, induces human basophil activation via its ST2 receptor. J Immunol. 2008a;181:5981–9.
50. Cherry WB, Yoon J, Bartemes KR, Iijima K, Kita H. A novel IL-1 family cytokine, IL-33, potently activates human eosinophils. J Allergy Clin Immunol. 2008;121:1484–90. doi:10.1016/j.jaci.2008.04.005.
51. Suzukawa M, Koketsu R, Iikura M, Nakae S, Matsumoto K, Nagase H, et al. Interleukin-33 enhances adhesion, CD11b expression and survival in human eosinophils. Lab Investig. 2008b;88:1245–53. doi:10.1038/labinvest.2008.82.
52. Kurowska-Stolarska M, Stolarski B, Kewin P, Murphy G, Corrigan CJ, Ying S, et al. IL-33 amplifies the polarization of alternatively activated macrophages that contribute to airway inflammation. J Immunol. 2009;183:6469–77. doi:10.4049/jimmunol.0901575.
53. Rank MA, Kobayashi T, Kozaki H, Bartemes KR, Squillace DL, Kita H. IL-33-activated dendritic cells induce an atypical TH2-type response. J Allergy Clin Immunol. 2009;123:1047–54. doi:10.1016/j.jaci.2009.02.026.
54. Savinko T, Matikainen S, Saarialho-Kere U, Lehto M, Wang G, Lehtimaki S, et al. IL-33 and ST2 in atopic dermatitis: expression profiles and modulation by triggering factors. J Invest Dermatol. 2012;132:1392–400. doi:10.1038/jid.2011.446.
55. Imai Y, Yasuda K, Sakaguchi Y, Haneda T, Mizutani H, Yoshimoto T, et al. Skin-specific expression of IL-33 activates group 2 innate lymphoid cells and elicits atopic dermatitis-like inflammation in mice. Proc Natl Acad Sci U S A. 2013;110:13921–6. doi:10.1073/pnas.1307321110.
56. Hvid M, Vestergaard C, Kemp K, Christensen GB, Deleuran B, Deleuran M. IL-25 in atopic dermatitis: a possible link between inflammation and skin barrier dysfunction? J Invest Dermatol. 2011;131:150–7. doi:10.1038/jid.2010.277.
57. Wang YH, Angkasekwinai P, Lu N, Voo KS, Arima K, Hanabuchi S, et al. IL-25 augments type 2 immune responses by enhancing the expansion and functions of TSLP-DC-activated Th2 memory cells. J Exp Med. 2007;204:1837–47. doi:10.1084/jem.20070406. jem.20070406 [pii]
58. Dillon SR, Sprecher C, Hammond A, Bilsborough J, Rosenfeld-Franklin M, Presnell SR, et al. Interleukin 31, a cytokine produced by activated T cells, induces dermatitis in mice. Nat Immunol. 2004;5:752–60. doi:10.1038/ni1084.
59. Cornelissen C, Luscher-Firzlaff J, Baron JM, Luscher B. Signaling by IL-31 and functional consequences. Eur J Cell Biol. 2012;91:552–66. doi:10.1016/j.ejcb.2011.07.006.
60. Sonkoly E, Muller A, Lauerma AI, Pivarcsi A, Soto H, Kemeny L, et al. IL-31: a new link between T cells and pruritus in atopic skin inflammation. J Allergy Clin Immunol. 2006;117:411–7. doi:10.1016/j.jaci.2005.10.033.
61. Neis MM, Peters B, Dreuw A, Wenzel J, Bieber T, Mauch C, et al. Enhanced expression levels of IL-31 correlate with IL-4 and IL-13 in atopic and allergic contact dermatitis. J Allergy Clin Immunol. 2006;118:930–7. doi:10.1016/j.jaci.2006.07.015.
62. Raap U, Weissmantel S, Gehring M, Eisenberg AM, Kapp A, Folster-Holst R. IL-31 significantly correlates with disease activity and Th2 cytokine levels in children with atopic dermatitis. Pediatr Allergy Immunol. 2012;23:285–8. doi:10.1111/j.1399-3038.2011.01241.x.
63. Raap U, Wichmann K, Bruder M, Stander S, Wedi B, Kapp A, et al. Correlation of IL-31 serum levels with severity of atopic dermatitis. J Allergy Clin Immunol. 2008;122:421–3. doi:10.1016/j.jaci.2008.05.047.
64. Singh B, Jegga AG, Shanmukhappa KS, Edukulla R, Khurana GH, Medvedovic M, et al. IL-31-driven skin remodeling involves epidermal cell proliferation and thickening that lead to impaired skin-barrier function. PLoS One. 2016;11:e0161877. doi:10.1371/journal.pone.0161877.
65. Cevikbas F, Wang X, Akiyama T, Kempkes C, Savinko T, Antal A, et al. A sensory neuron-expressed IL-31 receptor mediates T helper cell-dependent itch: involvement of TRPV1 and TRPA1. J Allergy Clin Immunol. 2014;133:448–60. doi:10.1016/j.jaci.2013.10.048.
66. Kittaka H, Tominaga M. The molecular and cellular mechanisms of itch and the involvement of TRP channels in the peripheral sensory nerve system and skin. Allergol Int. 2017;66:22–30. doi:10.1016/j.alit.2016.10.003

67. Feld M, Garcia R, Buddenkotte J, Katayama S, Lewis K, Muirhead G, et al. The pruritus- and TH2-associated cytokine IL-31 promotes growth of sensory nerves. J Allergy Clin Immunol. 2016;138:500–8.e24. doi:10.1016/j.jaci.2016.02.020.
68. Eyerich K, Eyerich S. Th22 cells in allergic disease. Allergo J Int. 2015;24:1–7. doi:10.1007/s40629-015-0039-3.
69. Mirshafiey A, Simhag A, El Rouby NM, Azizi G. T-helper 22 cells as a new player in chronic inflammatory skin disorders. Int J Dermatol. 2015;54:880–8. doi:10.1111/ijd.12883.
70. Niebuhr M, Scharonow H, Gathmann M, Mamerow D, Werfel T. Staphylococcal exotoxins are strong inducers of IL-22: A potential role in atopic dermatitis. J Allergy Clin Immunol. 2010;126:1176–83.e4. doi:10.1016/j.jaci.2010.07.041.
71. Nograles KE, Zaba LC, Shemer A, Fuentes-Duculan J, Cardinale I, Kikuchi T, et al. IL-22-producing "T22" T cells account for upregulated IL-22 in atopic dermatitis despite reduced IL-17-producing TH17 T cells. J Allergy Clin Immunol. 2009;123:1244–52.e2. doi:10.1016/j.jaci.2009.03.041.
72. Simon D, Aeberhard C, Erdemoglu Y, Simon HU. Th17 cells and tissue remodeling in atopic and contact dermatitis. Allergy. 2014;69:125–31. doi:10.1111/all.12351.
73. Gittler JK, Shemer A, Suarez-Farinas M, Fuentes-Duculan J, Gulewicz KJ, Wang CQ, et al. Progressive activation of T_H2/T_H22 cytokines and selective epidermal proteins characterizes acute and chronic atopic dermatitis. J Allergy Clin Immunol. 2012;130:1344–54. doi:10.1016/j.jaci.2012.07.012.
74. Boniface K, Bernard FX, Garcia M, Gurney AL, Lecron JC, Morel F. IL-22 inhibits epidermal differentiation and induces proinflammatory gene expression and migration of human keratinocytes. J Immunol. 2005;174:3695–702.
75. Nograles KE, Zaba LC, Guttman-Yassky E, Fuentes-Duculan J, Suarez-Farinas M, Cardinale I, et al. Th17 cytokines interleukin (IL)-17 and IL-22 modulate distinct inflammatory and keratinocyte-response pathways. Br J Dermatol. 2008;159:1092–102. doi:10.1111/j.1365-2133.2008.08769.x.
76. Sa SM, Valdez PA, Wu J, Jung K, Zhong F, Hall L, et al. The effects of IL-20 subfamily cytokines on reconstituted human epidermis suggest potential roles in cutaneous innate defense and pathogenic adaptive immunity in psoriasis. J Immunol. 2007;178:2229–40.
77. Wolk K, Haugen HS, Xu W, Witte E, Waggie K, Anderson M, et al. IL-22 and IL-20 are key mediators of the epidermal alterations in psoriasis while IL-17 and IFN-γ are not. J Mol Med. 2009;87:523–36. doi:10.1007/s00109-009-0457-0.
78. Wolk K, Witte E, Wallace E, Docke WD, Kunz S, Asadullah K, et al. IL-22 regulates the expression of genes responsible for antimicrobial defense, cellular differentiation, and mobility in keratinocytes: a potential role in psoriasis. Eur J Immunol. 2006;36:1309–23. doi:10.1002/eji.200535503.
79. Gutowska-Owsiak D, Schaupp AL, Salimi M, Taylor S, Ogg GS. Interleukin-22 downregulates filaggrin expression and affects expression of profilaggrin processing enzymes. Br J Dermatol. 2011;165:492–8. doi:10.1111/j.1365-2133.2011.10400.x.
80. Guilloteau K, Paris I, Pedretti N, Boniface K, Juchaux F, Huguier V et al. Skin inflammation induced by the synergistic action of IL-17A, IL-22, oncostatin M, IL-1α, and TNFα recapitulates some features of psoriasis. J Immunol. 2010. doi:10.4049/jimmunol.0902464.
81. Ma HL, Liang S, Li J, Napierata L, Brown T, Benoit S, et al. IL-22 is required for Th17 cell-mediated pathology in a mouse model of psoriasis-like skin inflammation. J Clin Invest. 2008;118:597–607. doi:10.1172/jci33263.
82. Pantelyushin S, Haak S, Ingold B, Kulig P, Heppner FL, Navarini AA, et al. $Ror\gamma t^+$ innate lymphocytes and γδ T cells initiate psoriasiform plaque formation in mice. J Clin Invest. 2012;122:2252–6. doi:10.1172/jci61862.
83. Van Belle AB, de Heusch M, Lemaire MM, Hendrickx E, Warnier G, Dunussi-Joannopoulos K, et al. IL-22 is required for imiquimod-induced psoriasiform skin inflammation in mice. J Immunol. 2012;188:462–9. doi:10.4049/jimmunol.1102224.
84. Grewe M, Bruijnzeel-Koomen CA, Schopf E, Thepen T, Langeveld-Wildschut AG, Ruzicka T, et al. A role for Th1 and Th2 cells in the immunopathogenesis of atopic dermatitis. Immunol Today. 1998;19:359–61.

85. Koga C, Kabashima K, Shiraishi N, Kobayashi M, Tokura Y. Possible pathogenic role of Th17 cells for atopic dermatitis. J Invest Dermatol. 2008;128:2625–30.
86. Toda M, Leung DY, Molet S, Boguniewicz M, Taha R, Christodoulopoulos P, et al. Polarized in vivo expression of IL-11 and IL-17 between acute and chronic skin lesions. J Allergy Clin Immunol. 2003;111:875–81.
87. Huang F, Wachi S, Thai P, Loukoianov A, Tan KH, Forteza RM, et al. Potentiation of IL-19 expression in airway epithelia by IL-17A and IL-4/IL-13: important implications in asthma. J Allergy Clin Immunol. 2008;121:1415–21.e1–3. doi:10.1016/j.jaci.2008.04.016.
88. Witte E, Kokolakis G, Witte K, Philipp S, Doecke WD, Babel N, et al. IL-19 is a component of the pathogenetic IL-23/IL-17 cascade in psoriasis. J Invest Dermatol. 2014;134:2757–67. doi:10.1038/jid.2014.308.
89. Esaki H, Brunner PM, Renert-Yuval Y, Czarnowicki T, Huynh T, Tran G, et al. Early-onset pediatric atopic dermatitis is TH2 but also TH17 polarized in skin. J Allergy Clin Immunol. 2016;138:1639–51. doi:10.1016/j.jaci.2016.07.013.
90. Noda S, Suarez-Farinas M, Ungar B, Kim SJ, de Guzman SC, Xu H, et al. The Asian atopic dermatitis phenotype combines features of atopic dermatitis and psoriasis with increased TH17 polarization. J Allergy Clin Immunol. 2015;136:1254–64. doi:10.1016/j.jaci.2015.08.015.
91. Beck LA, Thaci D, Hamilton JD, Graham NM, Bieber T, Rocklin R, et al. Dupilumab treatment in adults with moderate-to-severe atopic dermatitis. N Engl J Med. 2014;371:130–9. doi:10.1056/NEJMoa1314768.
92. Hamilton JD, Suarez-Farinas M, Dhingra N, Cardinale I, Li X, Kostic A, et al. Dupilumab improves the molecular signature in skin of patients with moderate-to-severe atopic dermatitis. J Allergy Clin Immunol. 2014;134:1293–300. doi:10.1016/j.jaci.2014.10.013.
93. Thaci D, Simpson EL, Beck LA, Bieber T, Blauvelt A, Papp K, et al. Efficacy and safety of dupilumab in adults with moderate-to-severe atopic dermatitis inadequately controlled by topical treatments: a randomised, placebo-controlled, dose-ranging phase 2b trial. Lancet. 2016;387:40–52. doi:10.1016/s0140-6736(15)00388-8.
94. Simpson EL, Bieber T, Guttman-Yassky E, Beck LA, Blauvelt A, Cork MJ, et al. Two phase 3 trials of Dupilumab versus placebo in atopic dermatitis. N Engl J Med. 2016;375:2335–48. doi:10.1056/NEJMoa1610020.
95. Nemoto O, Furue M, Nakagawa H, Shiramoto M, Hanada R, Matsuki S, et al. The first trial of CIM331, a humanized antihuman interleukin-31 receptor a antibody, in healthy volunteers and patients with atopic dermatitis to evaluate safety, tolerability and pharmacokinetics of a single dose in a randomized, double-blind, placebo-controlled study. Br J Dermatol. 2016;174: 296–304. doi:10.1111/bjd.14207.

Factors that Exacerbate Itching in Patients with Atopic Dermatitis

10

Hiroyuki Murota and Ichiro Katayama

Abstract

Patients with atopic dermatitis (AD) exhibit different clinical symptoms, progression, and treatment responses during childhood and adulthood. In adults, itching of the skin is followed by the formation of well-circumscribed plaques or polymorphous dermatoses at the site of itching and is often accompanied by dryness. AD patients show hypersensitivity to various external stimuli that can exacerbate itching, such as heat and perspiration, which leads to scratching and further aggravation of skin lesions. This hypersensitivity exhibited by AD patients may arise from abnormal elongation of sensory nerves into the epidermis as well as sensitization of peripheral or central nerves. Itching can worsen when excess sweat is left on the skin or when insufficient sweating results in heat retention. Endogenous factors such as cytokines and chemical messengers can also induce itch by stimulating nerve fibers in the skin. Itching can be caused not only by stimulation of the skin surface but also by visual and auditory stimulation, with psychologically induced "contagious itch" being stronger in AD patients than in healthy individuals. Furthermore, itch often increases in the evening when sympathetic nerve activity decreases. This chapter discusses factors that exacerbate itching in AD and guidance for the proper management of the disease.

Keywords

Atopic dermatitis • Itch • Exacerbate • Dry skin • Temperature • Sweat • Psychological factors

H. Murota (✉) • I. Katayama
Dermatology, Department of Integrated Medicine, Graduate School of Medicine, Osaka University, 2-2, Yamadaoka, Suita-shi, Osaka 565-0871, Japan
e-mail: h-murota@derma.med.osaka-u.ac.jp

I. Katayama et al. (eds.), *Evolution of Atopic Dermatitis in the 21st Century*,
https://doi.org/10.1007/978-981-10-5541-6_10

10.1 Clinical Characteristics of Itching in Patients with Atopic Dermatitis (AD)

Patients with AD exhibit different clinical features depending on their age and duration of disease. The primary characteristics of AD at different developmental stages have been described by Sulzberger, who was responsible for naming AD [1]. In childhood, AD presents as eczematous changes and serous papules (Fig. 10.1) that produce intense itching, which may lead to excoriation and the formation of new papules induced by scratching. In adulthood, the clinical manifestations of AD are more varied. Over 100 years ago, Brocq and Jacquet [2] described AD as a chronic "disseminated neurodermatitis" characterized by mental nervousness, persistent itching before the visible appearance of skin abnormalities, emergence of circumscribed plaques at the location of itching, distributed skin lesions similar to neurodermatoses, skin dryness, skin pigmentation, and hypertrophied skin papillae. Around the same time, "Besnier's prurigo" [3] was described as a type of "diathetic prurigo" characterized by itching followed by nonspecific skin lesions in infants and "paroxystic and chronic polymorphous and pruriginous dermatoses, Hebra's prurigo type," in young adults. Such historical descriptions of the clinical course of dermatitis and its response to treatment are still valuable to modern clinical practice [1–4]. Today, AD is characterized by itching before the appearance of dermatitis, and AD-associated itching is known to be aggravated by a variety of factors such as heat, perspiration, psychological stress, specific foods and alcohol, wool fibers, and the common cold [5] (Fig. 10.2); therefore, the active avoidance of these factors is necessary for reducing itching.

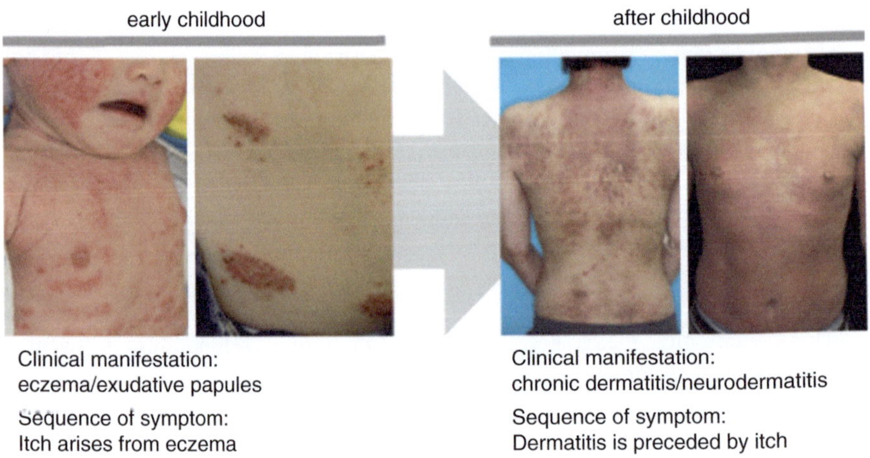

Fig. 10.1 The clinical features of AD vary depending on patient age and duration of disease. In infancy and childhood, AD is characterized by eczematous changes accompanied by strong itching. In adulthood, AD manifests as chronic dermatitis (also called disseminated neurodermatitis) with skin lesions appearing at the sites where itching first occurred (Reprinted from ref. [82] with permission of Japanese Society of Allergology)

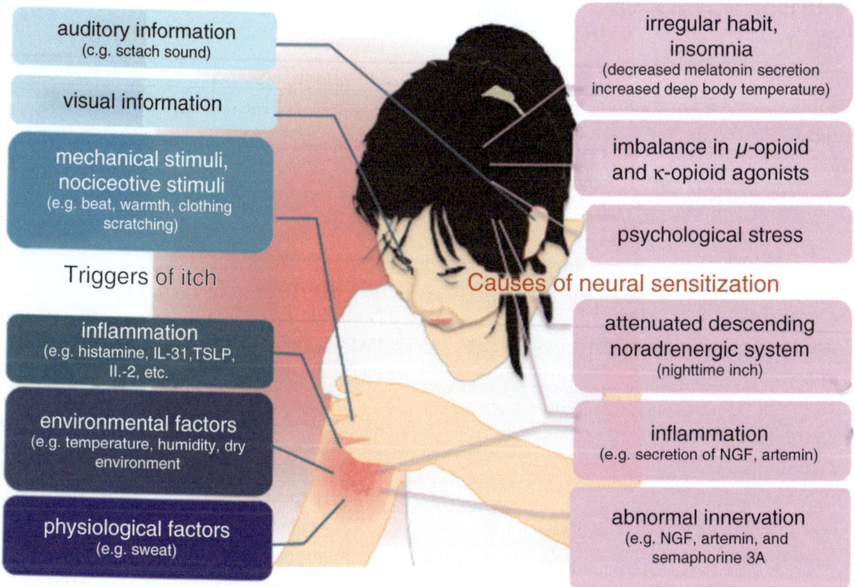

Fig. 10.2 Illustration of triggers of itch and causes of skin hypersensitivity (Reprinted from ref. [82] with permission of Japanese Society of Allergology)

Furthermore, because children and adults with AD show different symptoms and responses to treatment, additional research is required to elucidate the distinct mechanisms underlying AD-related itching at each developmental stage.

10.2 Neural Transmission and Processing of AD-Related Itching

Electrical impulses traveling through peripheral nerve fibers transmit itching-related signals to the brain, which produces a bodily reaction. Recent studies using animal models of AD indicate that astrogliosis in the dorsal horn of the spinal cord contributes to chronic itching and that the itching sensation is processed in the central nervous system [6]. Although the transmission and processing of AD-related itching in humans requires further clarification, the general process of the neural transmission of itch is summarized here.

Thermal and mechanical stimuli activate receptors on free nerve endings in the skin, which leads to the opening of ion channels and the transmission of electrical current to the spinal cord. Several different itching-related ligands and receptors have been described in the literature (Table 10.1). In particular, itch ligands (i.e., pruritogens) can induce an itching sensation by activating the histaminergic transient receptor potential cation channel subfamily V member 1

Table 10.1 Major itch-related ligands and receptors

Ligand	Receptor	Ref.
Histamine	Histamine receptors	[61]
Kallikreins, tryptase, endogenous/exogenous proteases	Protease-activated receptor 2	[62, 63]
Bradykinin	Bradykinin receptors	[64]
Serotonin (5-HT)	5-HT receptor	[65]
Endothelin-1	Endothelin receptors	[66, 67]
Interleukin (IL)-31	IL-31 receptor	[30]
Thymic stromal lymphopoietin (TSLP)	TSLP receptor	[29]
Substance P	Neurokinin-1 receptor	[68, 69]
Platelet-activating factor (PAF)	PAF receptor	[70]
Leukotriene B4 (LTB4)	LTB4 receptor	[71]
Electrophiles, oxidants, pro-inflammatory agents	TRPA1	[72, 73]
12-HPETE	TRPV1	[74]
Artemin	GDNF family receptor α3	[27]
IL-2	IL-2 receptor	[75]
Gastrin-releasing peptide (GRP)	GRP receptor	[76, 77]
β-endorphin	μ-opioid receptor	[78, 79]
Acetylcholine	Acetylcholine receptor	[80]
Calcitonin gene-related peptide (CGRP)	CGRP receptor	[81]

(Reprinted from ref. [82] with permission of Japanese Society of Allergology)

(TRPV1) and the non-histaminergic transient receptor potential cation channel member A1 (TRPA1) [7–10], and inhibition of TRPV1 or TRPA1 reduces itching in AD-like animal models [11, 12]. Thus, TRPV1 and TRPA1 have recently received much attention as possible targets for drug development [13]. After itching-related electrical impulses are sent to the spinal cord, they are modulated by interneurons in the spinal cord [14–16] that release inhibitory neurotransmitters such as gamma-aminobutyric acid, glycine, and dynorphins, which reduce the intensity of itch-related signals [15, 16]. Therefore, the control of inhibitory interneurons is another strong candidate approach for treating chronic itching. After processing in the spinal cord, itch-related signals are sent through ascending tracts to the amygdala via the thalamus or medulla oblongata, where they are analyzed and converted into information about their location, strength, and quality [17, 18]. Although the brain circuitry underlying itching is not completely understood, activation of sympathetic neurons in the medulla or midbrain induces the release of noradrenaline, which suppresses itch-related signals through the α(2)-adrenoceptor [19, 20] [19, 21]. Hence, itching is attenuated under conditions of significant sympathetic nervous system activity, such as during the daytime or when individuals concentrate on stimuli other than the itch. However, the central processing of itch-related signals differs between AD patients and healthy individuals [22]. Thus, a greater understanding of the antipruritic nervous system will help advance approaches to treating AD-related itching.

10.3 Inflammation, Dry Skin, and Itching

In skin conditions such as eczema and dryness, molecules that cause itching (i.e., pruritogens), including cytokines and chemical messengers, are released from the affected area and act on nerve endings in the skin [23, 24] (Table 10.1). The itching caused by pruritogens triggers scratching of the affected area [24], which aggravates the dermatitis, resulting in a vicious "itch-scratch cycle." Dryness and inflammation, such as that which occurs in AD, induce elongation of sensory nerves in the epidermis under the stratum corneum, which causes skin hyperesthesia [25]. This aberrant nerve elongation in AD involves nerve growth factor, artemin, interleukin (IL)-31, and semaphorin 3A [26–28]. Histamines derived from the degranulation of mast cells and substance P released from nerve endings can act directly or indirectly on elongated nerves, causing itching. The inflammatory mediators thymic stromal lymphopoietin and IL-31, which are derived from epidermal keratinocytes and infiltrated lymphocytes, respectively, cause itching through direct actions on nerve fibers [29, 30]. Furthermore, elevated levels of autotaxins (e.g., lysophospholipase) due to cholestasis induce itching in hepatic disorders [31], and blood autotaxin concentration is correlated with itch intensity in AD patients [32].

10.4 Temperature and Itching

Healthy individuals can experience relief from histamine-evoked itching by exposure to extreme temperatures [22, 33, 34], such as taking a very hot shower or using ice to cool the itchy area. However, although AD-related itching can be suppressed by painful cold stimulation, it is worsened by painful heat stimulation [22, 33, 35]. Moreover, AD patients often report that their itchiness increases in warmer conditions [5, 36]. Thus, AD may involve abnormal hyperesthesia, causing patients to feel thermal stimulation as an itching sensation. Unfortunately, this heat-provoked itching responds poorly to treatment [36], and although it is thought to result from the sensitization of peripheral or central nerves, its underlying mechanism is still uncertain.

Peripheral nerve fibers are distributed across the dermis and are affected by factors secreted by surrounding fibroblasts. To identify molecules that contribute to skin nerve fiber hypersensitization, we comprehensively analyzed the expression of genes in dermal fibroblasts that were stimulated by allergic inflammation- and itch-related factors. We found that substance P induced the expression of artemin, a neurotrophic factor that is important for the development of sympathetic innervation, in dermal fibroblasts [27]. Whereas no artemin expression was detected in normal human skin, we found its accumulation in dermal lesions associated with AD and nummular eczema [27]. Furthermore, we observed that mice treated with artemin on their back exhibited increased sensory innervation of the skin and abnormal behavior such as rubbing their skin across their entire body when exposed to a warm temperature (38 °C), which was not observed in artemin receptor knockout mice. This finding suggests that the abnormal local accumulation of artemin in the skin causes systemic thermally provoked itching, although the underlying mechanism is unclear. However, we found that capsazepine, a selective antagonist of TRPV1, did not suppress the artemin-induced abnormal behavior, indicating that the systemic response occurs independently of TRPV1 [27].

In our clinical practice, we have encountered AD patients who developed itching immediately after taking a hot bath or removing their clothes, which we assume arises from a rapid change in the temperature of the skin surface. This phenomenon has been confirmed by experimental studies. For instance, Pfab and colleagues observed increased itching when histamine-treated skin was exposed to rapidly alternating cool and warm temperatures (between 25 and 32 °C) [37]. Therefore, even within temperature ranges typically encountered in daily life, rapid changes in temperature can intensify itch. Therefore, patients with AD should be careful to avoid extreme temperatures in their daily life, such as hot bathwater or cold air conditioning. Japanese guidelines for AD recommend that the temperature of bathwater should be set between 38 and 40 °C [38].

10.5 Perspiration and Itching

Mammals are homeothermic organisms that maintain a stable body temperature through thermal control mechanisms such as perspiration, expiration, and heat transfer [39]. In humans, perspiration through eccrine sweat glands distributed throughout the body is an important physiological function that regulates body temperature [39].

Sweat contains several molecules that are beneficial for the skin, such as natural moisture-retaining factors (e.g., urea, sodium lactate), bactericidal peptides (e.g., dermcidin, cathelicidin, β-defensin), and secretory IgA to defend against infection [40]. Sweat also inhibits cysteine and serine protease activity, helps prevent inflammatory responses to allergens, and aids in the formation of mature stratum corneum [41–44]. Although sweat can reduce the intensity of experimentally induced itching in healthy individuals [45], many patients with AD report that sweating aggravates itching [46]. In one study, basophils derived from AD patients showed positive reactions in a histamine release test to semipurified antigens extracted from the sweat of healthy subjects, suggesting the existence of a "sweat allergy" [47]. However, another study failed to detect positive reactions in a longer-term sweat patch test [48]. Thus, sweat may provoke an acute, but not a delayed, allergic reaction. Interestingly, an antigen derived from *Malassezia globosa*, a fungus indigenous to the skin, was identified in the sweat of AD patients and may be involved in this "sweat allergy" [49]. In addition, reduced levels of antimicrobial components in sweat are associated with a weaker ability to defend against infection in AD patients [40].

Symptoms of AD can be aggravated by leaving excess sweat on the skin. One cause of this aggravation is that excess sweat increases the pH level of the skin surface [40]. Under normal conditions, the pH of sweat remains low because sodium bicarbonate (HCO_3^-) and alkali ions in sweat are reduced via reabsorption by sweat ducts [39]. However, excess sweat on the skin leads to a failure of HCO_3^- reabsorption, which increases the pH of the skin and thereby promotes detachment of the horny cell layer and increases susceptibility to inflammation [40]. In addition to increasing pH, various molecules contained in sweat (e.g., *Malassezia*-derived antigens) can cause itching. Moreover, the beneficial effects of sweat, such as proteinase inhibition, may be lost when excess sweat is left on the skin. Hence, AD patients are advised to wash or wipe off excess sweat with a wet towel in cases of itching accompanying perspiration.

AD patients show less ability to perspire, either due to abnormalities in the production of sweat or the obstruction of its release to the skin surface [40]. One possible mechanism by which the release of sweat is obstructed is the formation of horny plugs in sweat pores [50], although it is not clear whether this might be due to inflammation-related keratosis or dryness resulting from reduced sweating. Also, Shiohara and colleagues detected the presence of dermcidin, an antimicrobial peptide produced by sweat glands, surrounding sweat ducts in lesioned area of AD patients [51], suggesting the leakage of sweat outside of sweat ducts, which might reduce the amount of sweat discharged to the skin surface and increase heat retention. Perspiration tests using acetylcholine or temperature loading have confirmed that sweat secretion is reduced in AD patients [51–54], which is related to dysautonomia and a tendency toward an anxiogenic personality [53]. Furthermore, we recently discovered that histamine suppresses perspiration by affecting sweat glands [55], suggesting that allergic inflammation is a cause of reduced sweating in AD patients.

Because sweat aggravates AD, patients may be told to avoid sweating, although there is no evidence that this improves skin symptoms [56]. Rather, as proper treatment of skin symptoms in AD also restores perspiration function, increased sweating to facilitate heat transfer should be considered an important goal in the management of AD.

10.6 Daily Rhythms and Itching

AD patients often complain that their itching increases at night. One potential explanation is that body temperature declines overnight and fluctuates during sleep. The drops in body temperature are accompanied by dilation of peripheral vessels, which elevates skin temperature and may increase itching [57]. Another possible explanation is that transepidermal water loss increases at night, making the skin susceptible to itching. Nighttime is also associated with decreased cortisol and increased IL-2 production, which are related to inflammation [57]. Furthermore, staying up late reduces melatonin production by the pineal gland, which inhibits the normal decline in body temperature, and circadian dysregulation can cause an imbalance in agonists of μ-opioid and κ-opioid receptors, which may increase the severity of itching [57]. Therefore, AD patients are advised to practice good sleep habits and maintain regular sleep schedules.

10.7 Psychological Factors and Itching

Itching can arise not only from stimulation of the skin but also from visual or auditory information. For example, a person may have an urge to scratch himself or herself upon seeing an image suggestive of itching, such as being bitten by a mosquito, or hearing the sound of another person scratching their skin [58, 59]. This phenomenon, known as "contagious itch" [60], is stronger in AD patients than in healthy individuals [60]. The onset and worsening of itching can also be caused by psychological factors and related conditions such as insomnia.

Conclusion

The management of AD is continuing to improve through advances in our understanding of factors that exacerbate itching, their mechanisms, and their countermeasures. Because AD can be aggravated by commonplace features of our environment within a normal physiological range, it can be difficult to provide sound guidance for minimizing the symptoms of AD. As some questions remain unresolved, we hope that evidence accumulating from recent and future studies can be applied to improve the health and quality of life of patients with AD.

Conflict of Interest The authors have nothing to declare.

References

1. Hill LW, Sulzberger MB. Evolution of atopic dermatitis. Arch Dermatol Syphilol. 1935;32(3):451–63.
2. Brocq L, Jacquet L. Notes pour servir a l'histories des néurodermatitis: du lichen circumscriptus des anciens auteurs, ou lichen simplex chronique de M. le Dr. E Vidal. Ann Dermatol Syphiligr. 1891;97:193–208.
3. Besnier E. Premiére note et observations preliminaires pour servir d'introduction à l étude diathésique. Ann Dermatol Syphiligr. 1892;23:634–48.
4. Hanifin JM. Pharmacophysiology of atopic dermatitis. Clin Rev Allergy. 1986;4(1):43–65.
5. Wahlgren CF. Itch and atopic dermatitis: clinical and experimental studies. Acta Derm Venereol Suppl (Stockh). 1991;165:1–53.
6. Shiratori-Hayashi M, Koga K, Tozaki-Saitoh H, Kohro Y, Toyonaga H, Yamaguchi C, et al. STAT3-dependent reactive astrogliosis in the spinal dorsal horn underlies chronic itch. Nat Med. 2015;21(8):927–31.
7. Akiyama T, Carstens E. Spinal coding of itch and pain. In: Carstens E, Akiyama T, editors. Itch: mechanisms and Treatment. Boca Raton (FL): CRC Press/Taylor & Francis; 2014.
8. Stander S, Moormann C, Schumacher M, Buddenkotte J, Artuc M, Shpacovitch V, et al. Expression of vanilloid receptor subtype 1 in cutaneous sensory nerve fibers, mast cells, and epithelial cells of appendage structures. Exp Dermatol. 2004;13(3):129–39.
9. Wilson SR, Gerhold KA, Bifolck-Fisher A, Liu Q, Patel KN, Dong X, et al. TRPA1 is required for histamine-independent, mas-related G protein-coupled receptor-mediated itch. Nat Neurosci. 2011;14(5):595–602.
10. Lee JH, Park CK, Chen G, Han Q, Xie RG, Liu T, et al. A monoclonal antibody that targets a NaV1.7 channel voltage sensor for pain and itch relief. Cell. 2014;157(6):1393–404.

11. Yun JW, Seo JA, Jeong YS, Bae IH, Jang WH, Lee J, et al. TRPV1 antagonist can suppress the atopic dermatitis-like symptoms by accelerating skin barrier recovery. J Dermatol Sci. 2011;62(1):8–15.
12. Oh MH, Oh SY, Lu J, Lou H, Myers AC, Zhu Z, et al. TRPA1-dependent pruritus in IL-13-induced chronic atopic dermatitis. J Immunol. 2013;191(11):5371–82.
13. Wilson SR, Bautista DM. Role of transient receptor potential channels in acute and chronic itch. In: Carstens E, Akiyama T, editors. Itch: mechanisms and treatment. Boca Raton (FL): CRC Press/Taylor & Francis; 2014.
14. Ross SE, Mardinly AR, McCord AE, Zurawski J, Cohen S, Jung C, et al. Loss of inhibitory interneurons in the dorsal spinal cord and elevated itch in Bhlhb5 mutant mice. Neuron. 2010;65(6):886–98.
15. Akiyama T, Carstens E. Neural processing of itch. Neuroscience. 2013;250:697–714.
16. Pereira PJ, Lerner EA. Interneurons scratch an itch. Neuron. 2014;82(3):503–5.
17. Mochizuki H, Tanaka S, Morita T, Wasaka T, Sadato N, Kakigi R. The cerebral representation of scratching-induced pleasantness. J Neurophysiol. 2014;111(3):488–98.
18. Paus R, Schmelz M, Biro T, Steinhoff M. Frontiers in pruritus research: scratching the brain for more effective itch therapy. J Clin Invest. 2006;116(5):1174–86.
19. Gotoh Y, Omori Y, Andoh T, Kuraishi Y. Tonic inhibition of allergic itch signaling by the descending noradrenergic system in mice. J Pharmacol Sci. 2011;115(3):417–20.
20. Kuraishi Y. Noradrenergic modulation of itch transmission in the spinal cord. Handb Exp Pharmacol. 2015;226:207–17.
21. Gotoh Y, Andoh T, Kuraishi Y. Noradrenergic regulation of itch transmission in the spinal cord mediated by alpha-adrenoceptors. Neuropharmacology. 2011;61(4):825–31.
22. Ishiuji Y, Coghill RC, Patel TS, Oshiro Y, Kraft RA, Yosipovitch G. Distinct patterns of brain activity evoked by histamine-induced itch reveal an association with itch intensity and disease severity in atopic dermatitis. Br J Dermatol. 2009;161(5):1072–80.
23. Yosipovitch G. Dry skin and impairment of barrier function associated with itch - new insights. Int J Cosmet Sci. 2004;26(1):1–7.
24. Ikoma A, Steinhoff M, Stander S, Yosipovitch G, Schmelz M. The neurobiology of itch. Nat Rev Neurosci. 2006;7(7):535–47.
25. Kamo A, Tominaga M, Taneda K, Ogawa H, Takamori K. Neurotropin inhibits the increase in intraepidermal nerve density in the acetone-treated dry-skin mouse model. Clin Exp Dermatol. 2013;38(6):665–8.
26. Tominaga M, Takamori K. Itch and nerve fibers with special reference to atopic dermatitis: therapeutic implications. J Dermatol. 2014;41(3):205–12.
27. Murota H, Izumi M, Abd El-Latif MI, Nishioka M, Terao M, Tani M, et al. Artemin causes hypersensitivity to warm sensation, mimicking warmth-provoked pruritus in atopic dermatitis. J Allergy Clin Immunol. 2012;130(3):671–82. e674
28. Feld M, Garcia R, Buddenkotte J, Katayama S, Lewis K, Muirhead G, et al. The pruritus- and TH2-associated cytokine IL-31 promotes growth of sensory nerves. J Allergy Clin Immunol. 2016;138(2):500–8. e524
29. Wilson SR, The L, Batia LM, Beattie K, Katibah GE, McClain SP, et al. The epithelial cell-derived atopic dermatitis cytokine TSLP activates neurons to induce itch. Cell. 2013;155(2):285–95.
30. Sonkoly E, Muller A, Lauerma AI, Pivarcsi A, Soto H, Kemeny L, et al. IL-31: a new link between T cells and pruritus in atopic skin inflammation. J Allergy Clin Immunol. 2006;117(2):411–7.
31. Kremer AE, Martens JJ, Kulik W, Rueff F, Kuiper EM, van Buuren HR, et al. Lysophosphatidic acid is a potential mediator of cholestatic pruritus. Gastroenterology. 2010;139(3):1008–1018 e1001.
32. Nakao M, Sugaya M, Suga H, Kawaguchi M, Morimura S, Kai H, et al. Serum autotaxin levels correlate with pruritus in patients with atopic dermatitis. J Invest Dermatol. 2014;134(6):1745–7.

33. Fruhstorfer H, Hermanns M, Latzke L. The effects of thermal stimulation on clinical and experimental itch. Pain. 1986;24(2):259–69.
34. Yosipovitch G, Fast K, Bernhard JD. Noxious heat and scratching decrease histamine-induced itch and skin blood flow. J Invest Dermatol. 2005;125(6):1268–72.
35. Ikoma A, Fartasch M, Heyer G, Miyachi Y, Handwerker H, Schmelz M. Painful stimuli evoke itch in patients with chronic pruritus: central sensitization for itch. Neurology. 2004;62(2).212–7.
36. Murota H, Katayama I. Evolving understanding on the aetiology of thermally provoked itch. Eur J Pain. 2016;20(1):47–50.
37. Pfab F, Valet M, Sprenger T, Toelle TR, Athanasiadis GI, Behrendt H, et al. Short-term alternating temperature enhances histamine-induced itch: a biphasic stimulus model. J Invest Dermatol. 2006;126(12):2673–8.
38. Katayama I, Kohno Y, Akiyama K, Aihara M, Kondo N, Saeki H, et al. Japanese guideline for atopic dermatitis 2014. Allergol Int. 2014;63(3):377–98.
39. Kuno Y. Human perspiration. Springfield: Illinois; 1956.
40. Murota H, Matsui S, Ono E, Kijima A, Kikuta J, Ishii M, et al. Sweat, the driving force behind normal skin: an emerging perspective on functional biology and regulatory mechanisms. J Dermatol Sci. 2015;77(1):3–10.
41. Yokozeki H, Hibino T, Sato K. Partial purification and characterization of cysteine proteinases in eccrine sweat. Am J Phys. 1987;252(6 Pt 2):R1119–29.
42. Yokozeki H, Hibino T, Takemura T, Sato K. Cysteine proteinase inhibitor in eccrine sweat is derived from sweat gland. Am J Phys. 1991;260(2 Pt 2):R314–20.
43. Hibino T, Izaki S, Izaki M. Detection of serine proteinase inhibitors in human cornified cells. Biochem Biophys Res Commun. 1981;101(3):948–55.
44. Kato T, Takai T, Mitsuishi K, Okumura K, Ogawa H. Cystatin a inhibits IL-8 production by keratinocytes stimulated with der p 1 and der f 1: biochemical skin barrier against mite cysteine proteases. J Allergy Clin Immunol. 2005;116(1):169–76.
45. Nattkemper LA, Lee HG, Valdes-Rodriguez R, Mollanazar NK, Sanders KM, Yosipovitch G. Cholinergic induction of perspiration attenuates nonhistaminergic pruritus in the skin of patients with atopic dermatitis and healthy controls. Br J Dermatol. 2015;173(1):282–4.
46. Williams JR, Burr ML, Williams HC. Factors influencing atopic dermatitis-a questionnaire survey of schoolchildren's perceptions. Br J Dermatol. 2004;150(6):1154–61.
47. Tanaka A, Tanaka T, Suzuki H, Ishii K, Kameyoshi Y, Hide M. Semi-purification of the immunoglobulin E-sweat antigen acting on mast cells and basophils in atopic dermatitis. Exp Dermatol. 2006;15(4):283–90.
48. Adachi J, Endo K, Fukuzumi T, Kojima M, Aoki T. Negative patch test reactions to sweat in atopic dermatitis. Acta Derm Venereol. 1996;76(5):410–1.
49. Hiragun T, Ishii K, Hiragun M, Suzuki H, Kan T, Mihara S, et al. Fungal protein MGL_1304 in sweat is an allergen for atopic dermatitis patients. J Allergy Clin Immunol. 2013;132(3):608–15. e604
50. Papa C, Kligman A. Mechanism of eccrine anhidrosis. J Invest Dermatol. 1966;47:1–9.
51. Shiohara T, Doi T, Hayakawa J. Defective sweating responses in atopic dermatitis. Curr Probl Dermatol. 2011;41:68–79.
52. Eishi K, Lee JB, Bae SJ, Takenaka M, Katayama I. Impaired sweating function in adult atopic dermatitis: results of the quantitative sudomotor axon reflex test. Br J Dermatol. 2002;147(4):683–8.
53. Kijima A, Murota H, Matsui S, Takahashi A, Kimura A, Kitaba S, et al. Abnormal axon reflex-mediated sweating correlates with high state of anxiety in atopic dermatitis. Allergol Int. 2012;61(3):469–73.
54. Takahashi A, Murota H, Matsui S, Kijima A, Kitaba S, Lee JB, et al. Decreased sudomotor function is involved in the formation of atopic eczema in the cubital fossa. Allergol Int. 2013;62(4):473–8.
55. Matsui S, Murota H, Takahashi A, Yang L, Lee JB, Omiya K, et al. Dynamic analysis of histamine-mediated attenuation of acetylcholine-induced sweating via GSK3beta activation. J Invest Dermatol. 2014;134(2):326–34.

56. Saeki H, Nakahara T, Tanaka A, Kabashima K, Sugaya M, Murota H, et al. Clinical practice guidelines for the management of atopic dermatitis 2016. J Dermatol. 2016;43:1117–45.
57. Lavery MJ, Stull C, Kinney MO, Yosipovitch G. Nocturnal pruritus: the battle for a peaceful night's sleep. Int J Mol Sci. 2016;17(3):425.
58. Parsad D, Saini R. The sound of scratching: an unusual cause of neurotic excoriations. Dermatology. 1997;195(1):74.
59. Schut C, Grossman S, Gieler U, Kupfer J, Yosipovitch G. Contagious itch: what we know and what we would like to know. Front Hum Neurosci. 2015;9:57.
60. Papoiu AD, Wang H, Coghill RC, Chan YH, Yosipovitch G. Contagious itch in humans: a study of visual 'transmission' of itch in atopic dermatitis and healthy subjects. Br J Dermatol. 2011;164(6):1299–303.
61. Wahlgren CF, Hagermark O, Bergstrom R. Patients' perception of itch induced by histamine, compound 48/80 and wool fibres in atopic dermatitis. Acta Derm Venereol. 1991;71(6):488–94.
62. Steinhoff M, Neisius U, Ikoma A, Fartasch M, Heyer G, Skov PS, et al. Proteinase-activated receptor-2 mediates itch: a novel pathway for pruritus in human skin. J Neurosci. 2003;23(15):6176–80.
63. Kempkes C, Buddenkotte J, Cevikbas F, Buhl T, Steinhoff M. Role of PAR-2 in neuroimmune communication and itch. In: Carstens E, Akiyama T, editors. Itch: mechanisms and treatment. Boca Raton (FL): CRC Press/Taylor & Francis; 2014.
64. Hosogi M, Schmelz M, Miyachi Y, Ikoma A. Bradykinin is a potent pruritogen in atopic dermatitis: a switch from pain to itch. Pain. 2006;126(1–3):16–23.
65. Bautista DM, Wilson SR, Hoon MA. Why we scratch an itch: the molecules, cells and circuits of itch. Nat Neurosci. 2014;17(2):175–82.
66. Tsybikov NN, Petrisheva IV, Kuznik BI, Magen E. Plasma endothelin-1 levels during exacerbation of atopic dermatitis. Allergy Asthma Proc. 2015;36(4):320–4.
67. McQueen DS, Noble MA, Bond SM. Endothelin-1 activates ETA receptors to cause reflex scratching in BALB/c mice. Br J Pharmacol. 2007;151(2):278–84.
68. Hon KL, Lam MC, Wong KY, Leung TF, Ng PC. Pathophysiology of nocturnal scratching in childhood atopic dermatitis: the role of brain-derived neurotrophic factor and substance P. Br J Dermatol. 2007;157(5):922–5.
69. Heyer G, Hornstein OP, Handwerker HO. Reactions to intradermally injected substance P and topically applied mustard oil in atopic dermatitis patients. Acta Derm Venereol. 1991;71(4):291–5.
70. Abeck D, Andersson T, Grosshans E, Jablonska S, Kragballe K, Vahlquist A, et al. Topical application of a platelet-activating factor (PAF) antagonist in atopic dermatitis. Acta Derm Venereol. 1997;77(6):449–51.
71. Andoh T, Haza S, Saito A, Kuraishi Y. Involvement of leukotriene B4 in spontaneous itch-related behaviour in NC mice with atopic dermatitis-like skin lesions. Exp Dermatol. 2011;20(11):894–8.
72. Wilson SR, Nelson AM, Batia L, Morita T, Estandian D, Owens DM, et al. The ion channel TRPA1 is required for chronic itch. J Neurosci. 2013;33(22):9283–94.
73. Zygmunt PM, Hogestatt ED. Trpa1. Handb Exp Pharmacol. 2014;222:583–630.
74. Kim DK, Kim HJ, Kim H, Koh JY, Kim KM, Noh MS, et al. Involvement of serotonin receptors 5-HT1 and 5-HT2 in 12(S)-HPETE-induced scratching in mice. Eur J Pharmacol. 2008;579(1–3):390–4.
75. Mollanazar NK, Smith PK, Yosipovitch G. Mediators of Chronic Pruritus in Atopic Dermatitis: Getting the Itch Out? Clin Rev Allergy Immunol. 2016;51:263–92.
76. Tirado-Sanchez A, Bonifaz A, Ponce-Olivera RM. Serum gastrin-releasing peptide levels correlate with disease severity and pruritus in patients with atopic dermatitis. Br J Dermatol. 2015;173(1):298–300.
77. Kagami S, Sugaya M, Suga H, Morimura S, Kai H, Ohmatsu H, et al. Serum gastrin-releasing peptide levels correlate with pruritus in patients with atopic dermatitis. J Invest Dermatol. 2013;133(6):1673–5.
78. Georgala S, Schulpis KH, Papaconstantinou ED, Stratigos J. Raised beta-endorphin serum levels in children with atopic dermatitis and pruritus. J Dermatol Sci. 1994;8(2):125–8.

79. Stander S, Gunzer M, Metze D, Luger T, Steinhoff M. Localization of mu-opioid receptor 1A on sensory nerve fibers in human skin. Regul Pept. 2002;110(1):75–83.
80. Heyer G, Vogelgsang M, Hornstein OP. Acetylcholine is an inducer of itching in patients with atopic eczema. J Dermatol. 1997;24(10):621–5.
81. Salomon J, Baran E. The role of selected neuropeptides in pathogenesis of atopic dermatitis. J Eur Acad Dermatol Venereol. 2008;22(2):223–8.
82. Murota H, Katayama I. Exacerbating factors of itch in atopic dermatitis. Allergol Int. 2016;66:8–13. doi:10.1016/j.alit.2016.10.005.

The Role of Sweat in the Pathogenesis of Atopic Dermatitis

11

Tetsuo Shiohara, Yurie Shimoda-Komatsu, Yoshiko Mizukawa, Yuki Hayashida, and Yumi Aoyama

Abstract

Although atopic dry skin is believed to be caused by defects in skin genes that are important for maintaining skin barrier function, the role of sweat has been apparently underestimated despite its great capacity to increase skin hydration. It has become clear that sweating responses can be divided into two types depending on their functions. Under baseline conditions, sweat glands/ducts located at the dermal folds secrete basal levels of sweat in an unrecognized fashion, which is referred to as "insensible" sweating and could serve to maintain skin hydration. In contrast, another type of sweating is called "sensible" sweating that is induced by physical exercise and hot/humid environment and could function as a major thermoregulator: this type of sweating is largely delivered from sweat glands/ducts at the dermal ridges. Atopic dermatitis (AD) would initially arise from a localized defect in "insensible" sweating responses from sweat glands/ducts at the folds: this defect could start with leakage of sweat from the glands/ducts, thereby not only providing an inflammatory milieu but also resulting in dry skin. As a next step, compensatory hyperhidrosis would occur preferentially in the sweat glands/ducts at the ridges, which may exacerbate the inflammatory responses. In the final stage, patients eventually manifest the phenotype with systemic hypohidrosis. This three-stage model for the pathogenesis of AD has significant implications both in terms of future research and therapies. Therapies directed at correcting the defects at early times, while ameliorating inflammatory responses, may prove efficacious for preventing further progression of the disease.

T. Shiohara, M.D., Ph.D. (✉) • Y. Shimoda-Komatsu • Y. Mizukawa
Department of Dermatology, Kyorin University School of Medicine, 6-20-2 Shinkawa, Mitaka, Tokyo 181-8611, Japan
e-mail: tpshio@ks.kyorin-u.ac.jp

Y. Hayashida • Y. Aoyama
Department of Dermatology, Kawasaki Medical School, Kurashiki, Japan

Department of Dermatology, Kawasaki General Medical Center, Okayama, Japan

I. Katayama et al. (eds.), *Evolution of Atopic Dermatitis in the 21st Century*,
https://doi.org/10.1007/978-981-10-5541-6_11

Keywords
Atopic dermatitis • Impression mold technique • Insensible sweating • Moisturizer
Skin hydration • Sweat glands • Topography

11.1 Introduction

Although studies on the effects of climate change on inflammatory skin diseases are still lacking, current knowledge provided by epidemiological and experimental studies suggests the possibility that the prevalence of inflammatory skin diseases, such as atopic dermatitis (AD), could be profoundly influenced by climate change [1, 2]: climate factors such as low humidity could increase the prevalence of inflammatory skin diseases by negatively affecting skin barrier function. Consistent with this view, our recent study clearly demonstrates that the magnitude of contact sensitivity in mice is greatly downregulated through an increase in water content of stratum corneum only by exposing them to high humidity [3]. While previous studies explained the biophysical implications of decreasing ambient humidity on skin barrier function, none examined the possibility that many of the impaired skin barrier function that have been reported to occur in AD may be secondary to the decrease in sweating responses under low humidity conditions. In addition, given recent reports demonstrating that low humidity in atmosphere plays an important role with regard to itching [4, 5], the primary impact of climate change, such as the trend for a dry environment, on inflammatory skin diseases may be mediated through the effects on sweating responses. Thus, if the permeability barrier and antimicrobial barrier dysfunction represents the primary event in the development of AD, defective sweating responses are a logical place to look for changes that predispose individuals to the disease: most of previous studies were mainly focusing on the direct effects of climate change on the disease, apparently disregarding the effect of defective sweating responses on the development of the disease. Therefore, the purpose of this review was to briefly review recent advances in our understanding of the role of sweat in the development of AD and of the therapeutic approaches.

11.2 The Physiology of Sweating

Sweating is one of the major mechanisms by which body temperature can be kept constant in hot environments and during physical exercise. An individual can secrete up to 10 L/day of sweat under appropriate conditions [6–8], thereby cooling down body temperature as necessary. Sweat is mainly produced by ~4 millions of eccrine glands unevenly distributed widely on both hairy and glabrous skin, and eccrine glands are composed of secretory coil and a linear duct [6–8]. In humans, sweating responses are the most important means of dissipating excess heat generated by physical exercise, fever, or hot environment. In contrast, most other mammals (except for horses) have no thermoregulatory sweating system, but several mammals only exhibit sweating responses in the glabrous skin of the palm and sole, which is referred to as emotional sweating. In humans, sweat pores of eccrine glands in glabrous skin open at the dermal ridges (Fig. 11.1a), while those in the hairy skin open at the skin folds (Fig. 11.1b) [8]. In diverse physiological settings, however, sweat pores also open at the ridges in the hairy skin (Fig. 11.1c) and at the folds in the glabrous skin, respectively. The eccrine glands are innervated by postganglionic sympathetic C-type nonmyelinated fibers and periglandular neurotransmitters [6]: sweat secretion in sweat glands is regulated by the sympathetic nervous system at different levels of neuronal centers [7].

Eccrine sweat glands can respond to both core (internal) temperature and peripheral (skin) temperatures, with the former being much more efficient for both sweat induction and sweating rate [7]. Cholinergic sweat secretion is the major route and also accounts for >70% of sweating capacity in isolated human sweat glands analyzed in vitro [7]. With cholinergic stimulation, there is increased secretion of sweat. Thus, a pilocarpine sweat test is widely used for evaluating the ability to produce or deliver sweat to the surface of the skin in the presence of appropriate stimuli [9]. In addition to thermoregulation, an additional function of eccrine sweat glands is to maintain skin surface hydration by secreting moisturizing factors, such as lactate, urea, and potassium [10]. Recent studies have further demonstrated that sweat glands secrete water including several antimicrobial peptides, including dermcidin (DCD) that can contribute to the first line of defense against invading pathogens by building a constant barrier that overlies the epithelial skin [11]. Additional studies have also demonstrated that sweat contains proteolytic enzymes, IL-1α, IL-1β, IL-6, IL-8, IL-31, TNF-α, and epidermal growth factors [12–15].

Dysfunction of one or more of the processes in normal regulatory mechanisms of sweat production and secretion could be reflected in the development of anhidrosis or hypohidrosis [9]. It could result from diverse causes: they include absence or atrophy of the sweat glands, a direct damage to the glands by trauma or inflammation of the skin, and portal occlusion or dysfunction of sympathetic nerves in neuropathics [8, 9, 16].

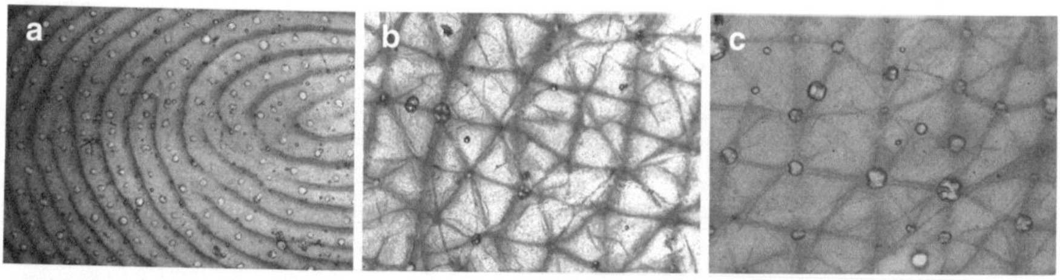

Fig. 11.1 Differential localization of sweat pores of eccrine glands in relation to skin folds and ridges. (**a**) In glabrous skin, such as fingertips, sweat pores open at the ridges under baseline conditions. (**b**) In hairy skin, such as forearm, those open at the folds under baseline conditions. (**c**) Upon thermal stimulus, those in the hairy skin also open at the ridges. Sweat droplets are visualized as small holes corresponding to each sweat pore in the impression mold technique (IMT), as described later

11.3 Measurement of Sweat Output

Research on the regulation of sweating responses under various physiologic and pathologic conditions has been hampered by the paucity of reproducible and quantitative evaluation methods, although a variety of methods for sweat testing have been devised [17]. In this regard, we have recently established impression mold technique (IMT) modified from the previously reported plastic impression method (Fig. 11.2) [17–20]: it allows an accurate quantification of individual sweat glands/ducts actively delivering sweat to the skin surface and the volume of sweat they produce over time [18–20]. In the IMT, emerging sweat droplets can be visualized as small holes corresponding to the individual sweat pores. This method is useful for determining the relation between the sweat pores and the surface topography of the skin (Fig. 11.1).

The degree of sweating can be also determined by measuring the skin surface hydration (SSH) at different time points after starting stimulus: measurements of the SSH can be performed before and after stimulus. This method seems to be superior to the IMT in terms of the easiness of obtaining the time course of sweating responses, while the IMT is superior to the SSH in terms of quantitative evaluation of sweating occurring in a well-defined location. To investigate whether sweating responses would be different depending on the localization of sweat pores relative to skin folds or ridges, the IMT is the only informative measure.

Sweating responses can be induced by different means: they include intradermal injection of cholinergic agents, physical exercise, exposure to increased temperature, and immersion of legs in warm water. According to our unpublished studies, immersion of legs in warm water was found to induce most efficient sweating responses in the glands/ducts located either at the folds or ridges, when sweating responses were evaluated by the IMT. In the IMT, sweating responses can be evaluated by both the number of sweat droplets per square centimeter, either at the folds or ridges, and the volume of sweat per square centimeter obtained by measuring the mean diameter of the outline of each droplet (Fig. 11.2).

11.4 Insensible and Sensible Sweating

There are two types of sweating [21]. The first is referred to as "insensible" sweating: in this type of sweating, an individual can secrete sweat under quiescent baseline conditions before stimulus, and water evaporates through the epidermis in an unrecognized fashion. Sweat droplets mainly detected at the folds under quiescent or " basal" baseline conditions can be regarded as basal levels of sweating or "insensible" sweating (Fig. 11.3a). Because there is a significant positive correlation between the SSH status and sweat droplet numbers detected at the folds, but not those at the ridges, under baseline conditions, sweat excreted from the sweat glands/ducts at the folds would serve to maintain skin hydration under quiescent baseline conditions. For most people and physicians, however, no or little attention has been focused on this type of sweating, despite its critical role for maintaining skin

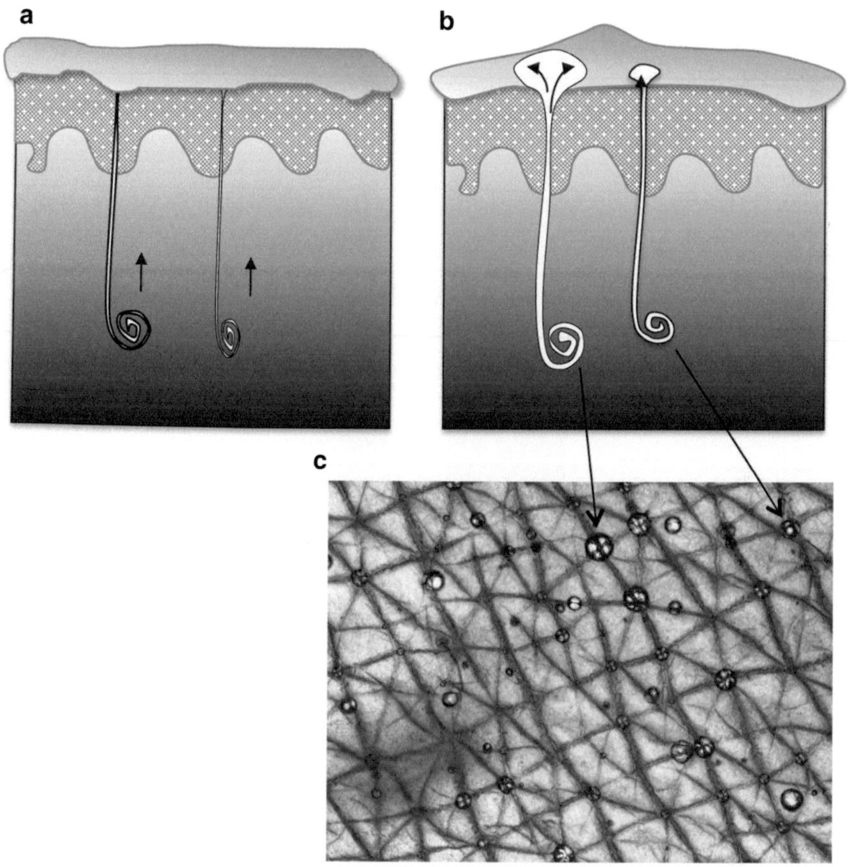

Fig. 11.2 IMT for the assessment of sweating responses. (**a**) The silicone material is mixed with a water solution and spread onto the skin. (**b**) As the silicone hardened, it retained the impression of the sweat droplets as they emerged from the sweat ducts and pushed up into the mold. Impression molds hardened in 3–4 min, and they were then removed. (**c**) The resulting sweat droplets were counted using a dissecting microscope and quantified by number and size per area over a 1 cm^2 region. Air bubbles, which were smaller than sweat droplets, can be differentiated from sweat droplets with relative ease

hydration. Perspiration by "insensible" sweating can be estimated to be <600–800 mL through the skin [21, 22].

In contrast, sweating induced by physical exercise or exposure to hot and humid environment is called "sensible" sweating [21, 22]. This type of sweating has received increasing attention over the last 10 through 20 years because it is well known that this type of sweating could function as a major thermoregulator. According to our recent unpublished observations, this type of sweating is mainly mediated by sweat produced by sweat glands/ducts at the ridges (Fig. 11.3b). Sweating responses in sweat glands/ducts at the ridges might also serve as a backup to impaired function of those at the folds, because in AD,

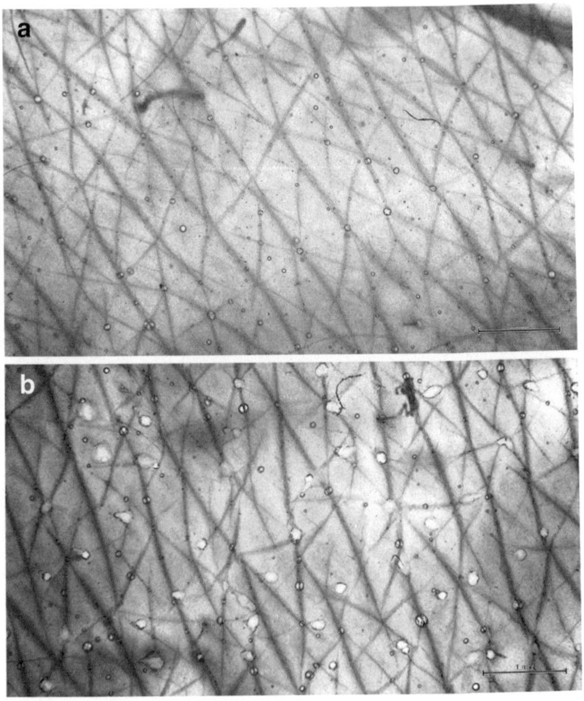

Fig. 11.3 Sweating responses in the thigh of a healthy subject evaluated by IMT before (**a**) and 30 min after thermal stimulus. (**a**) "Insensible" sweating can be detected at the folds. (**b**) "Sensible" sweating can be preferentially induced at the ridges, which is associated with the increase in size

compensatory hyperhidrosis was exclusively detected in those at the ridges, as described later [20]. Thus, measurement of sweat output depending on the surface topography of the skin, either the folds or ridges, is useful for elucidating how sweating defects could contribute to the pathogenesis of inflammatory skin diseases.

11.5 Sweating Defects in AD

There have been conflicting data regarding whether sweating responses are impaired, normal, or enhanced in patients with AD. Sulzberger et al. initially reported that there is sweat retention similar to that seen in miliaria in AD skin [23]. Lobitz and Campbell reported normal sweating responses to intradermal injection with acetylcholine and epinephrine in AD patients [24]. Other investigators soon joined the controversy. Rovensky [25] and Warndorff [26] independently reported that AD patients displayed increased sweating responses to cholinergic stimulation, while others demonstrated normal sweating responses [27]. Varying results were obtained depending on whether cholinergic or adrenergic stimulation was used. In this regard, Kiistala reported that sweating responses to either cholinergic or adrenergic stimulation were significantly decreased in AD skin and that sweating disturbances were more obvious in dry-appearing skin [28]. Other quantitative studies showed that a decreased sweating response to moderate thermal stimulus was common in either dry-appearing or normal-appearing skin [29]. Later quantitative study with the use of sudomotor axon reflex test showed that sweating responses to cholinergic stimulation as evaluated by the latency time and sweat volume were retarded and impaired, respectively, in AD patients as compared with those in nonatopic controls [30]. A consensus has emerged from these studies that sweating responses are impaired in AD patients, particularly in dry-appearing skin, and retarded. Unfortunately, however, such conflicting data would have diverted the research interest away from investigating the role for sweating responses in the pathogenesis of AD. In light of such conflicting reports, we were interested in quantitatively determining the capacity of individual sweat glands/ducts to produce and deliver sweat to the skin surface by using IMT, by which sweating responses can be quantitatively evaluated in a well-defined location.

One possible explanation of previous contradictory findings on sweating defects in AD could be that this may have been a function of the time point in the stage progression when sweating tests were performed. To investigate how disease process and sweating defects could interact with each other and progress from early asymptomatic stages to the onset of clinically apparent disease, we suppose that sweating responses in AD patients should be carefully investigated and analyzed depending on the clinical phenotypes and stages. All patients analyzed by us had mild-to-severe disease with typical eczematous skin lesions and elevated serum IgE levels. Thus, patients with adult-type AD were categorized into two groups, based on the clinical phenotypes and stages, acute and chronic. Adult patients with active dermatitis characterized by scaling erythematous papules, plaques, lichenoid papules, and crusting were evaluated as acute AD: most of them had exudate lesions in the flexural areas, usually within 5 years after onset. In contrast, patients characterized by systemic dry skin and relative sparing of eczematous lesions in the flexural areas were evaluated as chronic AD. There was no significant difference in the severity of disease assessed by scoring atopic dermatitis (SCORAD) index between the two groups at the time of enrollment. The mean age of acute AD was significantly younger in acute AD ($n = 12$, 23 ± 1.2 years) than in chronic AD ($n = 15$, 35.5 ± 2.3 years). Twelve unrelated, sex- and age-matched, healthy subjects with no history or family history of AD were enrolled in our study and served as healthy controls.

Sweating responses were induced by two means: the first means was immersion of both legs for 30 min in a water bath maintained at 43 °C. The other means was the injection with 500 μL of acetylcholine (Ach). Sweating responses thus induced were evaluated by the IMT, as described previously [17–20]. Sweat droplets in healthy controls under baseline conditions before thermal stimulus were distributed evenly and usually occupied each dermal fold in the forearm and abdomen, in which no significant difference can be found. Because there was an intimate association between the SSH levels and numbers or sizes of sweat droplets detected at the folds, but not those at the ridges, it is likely that the SSlH levels under quiescent baseline conditions would be determined by these basal levels of sweating (insensible sweating). These results suggest that dry skin in AD patients would largely result from the impaired "insensible" sweating in the ducts/glands at the folds. After thermal stimulus, sweat droplets were also detected at the ridges and increased in number and size with time.

In the normal-appearing uninvolved skin of acute AD, the number of sweat droplets observed at the folds was dramatically decreased not only before thermal stimulus (Fig. 11.4a) but also 15–30 min after thermal stimulus: this trend was evident even at the earliest acute stage, in which skin surface structure as evaluated by the surface topography of the skin was not disrupted yet by the disease process (Shimoda Y. et al. manuscript submitted). In the involved skin of acute AD, the number of sweat droplets at the folds was also profoundly decreased, while the size of sweat droplets was larger, particularly those at the ridges, than those in healthy controls: larger sizes of the droplets could be interpreted as implicating compensatory hyperhidrosis to maintain thermoregulatory function. The compensatory hyperhidrosis became most apparent at the ridges in the uninvolved skin sites of acute AD. In contrast, sweat droplets observed in chronic AD were much less numerous in number and smaller in size than those in acute AD and controls. The severity of disease as assessed by SCORAD was positively related to the number of sweat droplets at the ridges in acute AD, while that was inversely related to those at the folds in chronic AD. Thus, hyperhidrosis could be preferentially observed in the sweat glands/ducts at the ridges in acute AD, while systemic hypohidrosis observed either at the folds or ridges in chronic AD could contribute to the progression to the full development of chronic AD characterized by systemic dry skin.

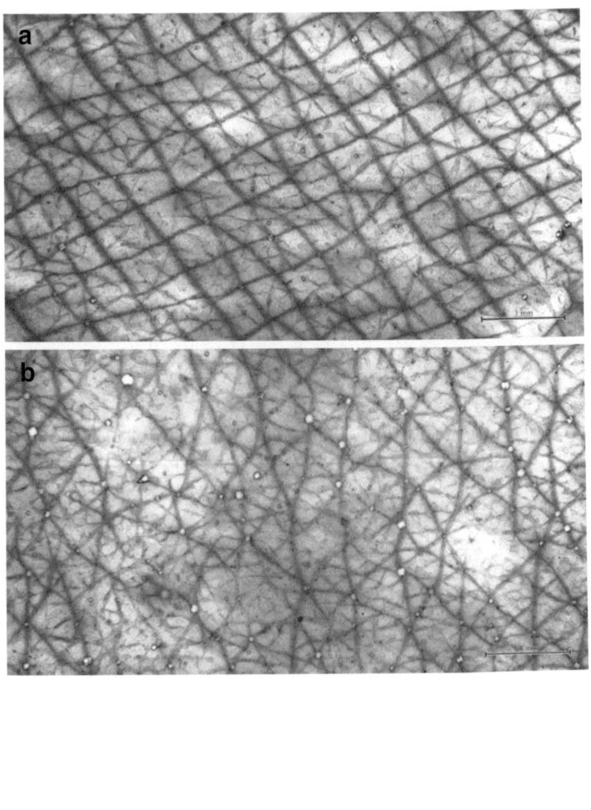

Fig. 11.4 Insensible sweating responses in the forearm of the earliest asymptomatic stage of acute AD evaluated by IMT before and after treatment of 3 FTU of a moisturizer. (**a**) The number of sweat droplets at the folds before treatment, i.e., insensible sweating responses, is profoundly decreased despite no significant changes of the surface topography. (**b**). One week after treatment with 3 FTU of a moisturizer, the number of sweat droplets located at the folds, i.e., insensible sweating responses, is markedly increased

We next asked whether decreased sweating in AD patients could be due to their inability to produce sweat or to deliver sweat to the skin surface. According to our previous studies [18, 19], the presence of sweat in the skin outside the sweat glands/ducts can be immunohistochemically identified by staining the specimens with anti-DCD Abs. In healthy controls, DCD antigen was solely detected in the cytoplasm of dark cells in the sweat glands and sweat. In the acute AD lesions, DCD antigen was also detected in the cytoplasm of dark cells in the sweat glands of the involved skin of acute AD at much higher intensity than those in healthy controls, excluding the possibility that decreased sweating responses in AD patients could be due to their inability to produce sweat. We reasoned that if it were possible to detect the presence of DCD in the dermis or epidermis outside sweat glands/ducts after thermal stimulus, then the leakage of sweat from the sweat glands/ducts could be the cause of both the profound decrease in sweating responses and inflammation. To test the possibility, we immunohistochemically identified DCD antigen in the skin lesions of AD after thermal stimulus. Surprisingly, DCD antigen was detected not only within the glands/ducts but also in the dermal tissue adjacent to the glands/ducts (Fig. 11.5), indicating leakage of sweat either from the glands or ducts into the dermis. These findings could be interpreted as indicating that in AD patients sweat, instead of pouring out and being removed from the skin surface, may diffuse in the dermal tissue around the grands/ducts and that, as a result, the ability to deliver sweat into the surface could be impaired. Because sweat has been shown to contain various inflammatory cytokines [12–15, 31–33], it is likely that leakage of sweat into the dermis could initiate a complex sequence of events that promotes eczematous inflammation. In view of a recent observation that the areas of anhidrosis on thermoregulatory sweat testing correspond to their symptomatic areas such as itching and strange sensation [34], itching and strange sensation frequently detected in

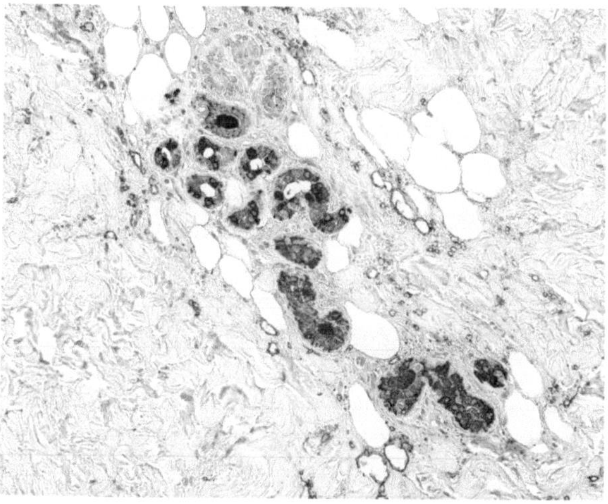

Fig. 11.5 DCD expression can be detected not only in the cytoplasm of dark cells in the sweat glands of an AD patient but also in the dermal tissues around the glands

AD lesions could now be explained by leakage of sweat into the dermis associated with anhidrosis, rather than by small-fiber neuropathy.

Sweating responses to Ach were also significantly decreased in sweat glands/ducts at the folds in acute AD as compared with those in healthy controls, a finding similar to those after thermal stimulus. These results suggest that sweating defects observed in AD patients would be due to dysfunction of sweat glands/ducts themselves. Our finding indicate that leakage of sweat into the dermal tissue around sweat glands/ducts was most evident in the involved skin of acute AD and that this leakage of sweat may represent the actual early events that presumably occur well before patients have typical dry skin: the sweat duct fragility may be related to putative defective function of tight junction (TJ), which can prevent the free diffusion of macromolecules.

Factors involved in the initiation of AD are unknown, although both genetic and environmental factors have been implicated. Due to its location within the skin, sweating defects provide an opportunity to directly detect the alterations during the course of disease. Based on our observations on sweating defects observed in AD patients, we propose a three-stage model for the pathogenesis of AD that involves three temporally overlapping stages. According to the three-stage model, AD would initially arise from a localized defect in sweating responses from some sweat glands/ducts located at the folds: this defect could start with leakage of sweat from the glands/ducts probably due to the genetic fragility of TJ. The leakage was not associated with portal occlusion. At this stage, those at the ridges remain fully functional or more productive. Leakage of sweat not only provides an inflammatory milieu but also results in the profound decrease in skin hydration. Because this disease process begins days or weeks before the development of clinically apparent AD lesions, sweating defects would develop in the absence of clinically apparent skin lesions. As a next step, compensatory hyperhidrosis would occur preferentially in the sweat glands/ducts at the ridges, which may exacerbate the inflammatory responses. In the final stage, patients eventually manifest the phenotype with systemic hypohidrosis not associated with compensatory hyperhidrosis. This model provides an explanation for why conflicting results with respect to sweating defects have been reported in AD patients. In the three-stage model, needed is careful distinction between primary events and those occurring secondary to inflammation or its treatment.

Therapies directed at restoring the sweating defects at early times may prove efficacious for the prevention of further progression to the disease.

11.6 Role of Sweating in Aggravation of AD

AD patients often complain of itching and exacerbation of their skin symptoms after sweating. In addition, AD lesions often show marked predilection to flexural areas characterized by increased sweating, such as cubital and popliteal fossa. These findings suggest the important role of sweating in aggravation of the disease. Nevertheless, there have been few reports describing the possible mechanism(s) by which sweating contribute to the pathogenesis of AD. Without proving the presence

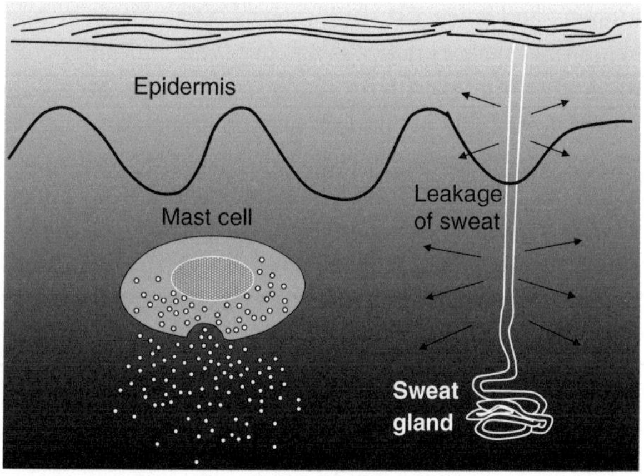

Fig. 11.6 Dermal mast cells would be sensitized to autologous sweat by repeated leakage of sweat into the dermis and epidermis in AD patients

of sweat in the epidermis and dermis outside the glands/ducts, migration of sweat containing specific IgE antibodies to allergens and various proteolytic enzymes has been long thought to play a role in modifying various inflammatory dermatoses [7]. Consistent with this view, immediate-type skin lesions to autologous sweat have been reported to develop in AD patients [35, 36]. Support for this view also comes from the recent finding that immediate-type skin reactions to autologous sweat correlate with the clinical severity of AD and serum total and specific IgE levels [37]. Although the mechanisms causing sensitization to autologous sweat in AD patients are at present speculative, it has been suggested that the component of sweat could penetrate deep into the skin and come into contact with skin resident cells such as keratinocytes and mast cells in AD lesions through the disruption of epidermal barrier by intense scratching [37]. In addition to this mechanism, leakage of sweat into the dermis and epidermis from the glands/ducts would contribute to the sensitization to sweat (Fig. 11.6) because it has been proven to occur upon thermal stimulus in vivo [19, 20]. As to the antigens to which AD patients can react, Hide's group reported that basophils from AD patients release histamine in response to sweat samples from AD patients in vitro [38] and that fungal protein MGL_1304 is a major allergen in human sweat that can elicit histamine release via specific IgE [39], suggesting the possibility that sweat seeping through the fragile or damaged epithelial lining of the sweat duct could cause not only chronic inflammation associated with itching sensation but also dry skin. Thus, leakage of sweat into the dermis and epidermis starts a vicious cycle.

11.7 Management of AD Patients with Sweating Defects

None of AD guidelines have not provided consistent recommendations regarding how to maintain the normal functioning of sweating. As described above, climate factors such as low humidity negatively affect sweating function, thereby serving to increase the prevalence of AD. The effect of dry environment was investigated in humans and mice [3]. In humans, office workers reported significantly less skin symptoms such as itch and AD in higher humidity conditions [40], and skin symptoms also improved with increasing relative humidity [41]. In addition, a higher prevalence of AD in children born during autumn and winter has been reported than spring and summer [42, 43]: from the sweat's viewpoint, a plausible explanation is that a high humidity environment has evolved the capacity to sweat in children, thereby preventing genetically susceptible children from developing AD. With respect to the protective effects of high humidity on the development of contact hypersensitivity, we have recently demonstrated that epicutaneously applied hapten, either lipid soluble or water soluble, can penetrate more readily through the stratum corneum with lower water content than that with higher water content [3]. These findings suggest that humidification of indoor air, particularly in places where exposure to allergens at high risk, may help decrease the likelihood of developing allergic diseases. In support of this view, children with AD living in a subtropical climate have been shown to have a lower prevalence of filaggrin (*FLG*) mutations compared with those living in colder and drier parts of Japan [44]. In addition, the global rise in AD prevalence in most industrialized countries and severity suggests that urbanization and Westernized lifestyle could be contributing.

There have been great variations in standard recommendations for skin care in AD, such as optimal bathing practices and the application of moisturizers. In this regard, Scholtz advocated the concept that bathing may aggravate AD: based on the concept, he recommended bathing avoidance and emollient application [45]. In contrast, Gutman and Kligman recommended daily bathing followed by immediate smearing of a topical steroid ointment during intensive therapy and an emollient during maintenance [46]. Although both groups argued in favor of their own research, no research has quantitatively analyzed the effect of bathing and subsequent usage of emollient on skin hydration and sweating responses. In this regard, Chiang et al. reported that bathing followed by moisturizer application provides modest hydration benefits, though less than that of simply applying moisturizer alone [47]. Although this study quantified skin hydration status at 90 min postintervention, effects of these regimens on skin hydration should have been analyzed over a longer time point. Clinicians involved in the care of AD patients characterized by various degrees of sweating defects need to be aware of the great potential of sweat to increase skin hydration. Thus, it is likely that these regimens can have a major impact primarily on sweating response, thereby increasing skin hydration. Indeed, our recent unpublished data indicate that skin hydration in a quiescent basal condition is largely dependent on the "insensible" sweating from sweat glands/ducts at the folds. Future studies are certainly required to address the effect of frequent or daily bathing followed by immediate application of moisturizers or a steroid ointment.

We have recently demonstrated that a moisturizer, heparinoid, can improve not only AD lesions but also lichen planus lesions and lichen amyloidosis (LA) lesions refractory to various treatment modalities including topical corticosteroids, particularly used under occlusion, by markedly restoring sweating responses, especially those at the folds [20]. Importantly, such restoration of sweating responses was associated with improvement of the skin surface topography of the skin. Histological analyses of the resolved LA lesions disclosed elimination of amyloid deposition, which was associated with the appearance of pore opening in the "hub" corresponding to the center of LA papules [20]. Leakage of sweat was frequently observed in nontreated LA lesions, but not in the completely resolved LA lesions treated with a moisturizer under occlusive dressing. These results clearly indicate that treatment of such inflammatory dermatoses characterized by sweating defects should be primarily directed at preventing the leakage of sweat into the dermis and epidermis.

In our ongoing experiment, we compared the effects of a moisturizer, heparinoid, on "insensible" sweating responses with those of petrolatum and corticosteroids under baseline conditions. Various topical agents, such as 1 and 3 fingertip unit (FTU) of a moisturizer, petrolatum, and corticosteroids, were applied twice daily on different sites of the forearm of healthy volunteers for 14 days. Individual sweat gland/duct activity to sweat was evaluated by measurements of IMT and SSH. One and three FTU of a moisturizer significantly improved the skin surface topography and increased SSH levels better than petrolatum or corticosteroids. Importantly, IMT analyses showed that 3 FTU of a moisturizer most markedly increased "insensible" sweating responses (Fig. 11.4b) than other topical agents and 1 FTU of the moisturizer. Based on these findings, we recommend that sweating defects in AD be primarily treated with a high dose (probably >3FTU) of the moisturizer, heparinoid, but not with petrolatum and corticosteroids. Together with these skin care regimens, daily immersion of legs in warm water is strongly recommended as a practical implication for efficiently restoring not only "insensible" sweating but also thermoregulatory "sensible" sweating responses in AD patients.

Conclusion

Sweating defects in AD patients have been apparently underestimated. The fact that sweating defects in the glands/ducts at the folds can be initially detected even in normal-appearing skin at the earliest asymptomatic stage of AD suggests that we should start therapies directed at restoring the sweating defects at early times in the earliest asymptomatic stage of AD patients while ameliorating inflammatory responses. What is important for the management for AD is to realize that leakage of sweat into the dermis and epidermis could represent the actual early events that trigger inflammation and cause itching and tingling sensation in AD lesions. Impaired ability to sweat results in failure to dissipate heat sufficiently, predisposing individuals to the development of AD. Prompt recognition and proper treatment for sweating defects are absolutely needed, especially for AD patients aggressively treated with topical corticosteroids and petrolatum, which may impair sweating responses. The efficacy of topical agents should be evaluated not only for anti-inflammatory effects but also the effects on sweating responses 4521.

Acknowledgment This work was supported in part by grants from the Ministry of Education, Culture, Sports, Science and Technology (to TS) and the Health and Labour Sciences Research Grants (Research on Intractable Diseases) from the Ministry of Health, Labour and Welfare of Japan (to TS).

References

1. Augustin J, Franzke N, Augustin M, Kappas M. Does climate change affect the incidence of skin and allergic disease in Germany? J Dtsch Dermatol Ges. 2008;6:632–8.
2. Engebretsen KA, Johansen JD, Kazic S, et al. The effect of environmental humidity and temperature on skin barrier function and dermatitis. J Eur Acad Dermatol Venereol. 2016;30:223–49.
3. Doi T, Mizukawa Y, Shimoda Y, et al. Importance of water content of the stratum corneum in mouse models for contact hypersensitivity. J Invest Dermatol. 2017;137:151–8.
4. Vocks E, Busch R, Fröhlich C, Borelli S, Mayer H, Ring J. Influence of weather and climate on subjective symptom intensity in atopic eczema. Int J Biometeorol. 2001;45:27–33.
5. Krämer U, Weidinger S, Darsow U, Möhrenschlager M, Ring J, Behrendt H. Seasonality in symptom severity influenced by temperature or grass pollen: results of a panel study in children with eczema. J Invest Dermatol. 2005;124:514–23.
6. Goldsmith LA. Biology of eccrine and apocrine sweat glands. In: Fitzpatrick TB, editor. Dermatology on general medicine. New York: McGraw-Hill; 1998. p. 155–64.
7. Cui C-Y, Schlessinger D. Eccrine sweat gland development and sweat secretion. Exp Dermatol. 2015;24:644–50.
8. Sato K, Kang WH, Saga K, Sato KT. Biology of sweat glands and their disorders. I. Normal sweat gland function. J Am Acad Dermatol. 1989;20:537–63.
9. Sato K, Kang WH, Saga K, Sato KT. Biology of sweat glands and their disorders. II. Disorders of sweat gland function. J Am Acad Dermatol. 1989;20:713–26.
10. Watabe A, Sugawara T, Kikuchi K, Yamasaki K, Sakai S, Aiba S. Sweat constitutes several natural moisturizing factors, lactate, urea, sodium, and potassium. J Dermatol Sci. 2013;72:177–82.
11. Rieg S, Steffen H, Seeber S, Humeny A, Kalbacher H, Dietz K, et al. Deficiency of dermcidin-derived antimicrobial peptides in sweat of patients with atopic dermatitis correlates with an impaired innate defense of human skin in vivo. J Immunol. 2005;174:8003–10.
12. Sato K, Sato F. Interleukin-1 alpha in human sweat is functionally active and derived from the eccrine sweat gland. Am J Physiol. 1994;266:R 950–9.
13. Jones AP, Webb LM, Anderson AO, Leonard EJ, Rot A. Normal human sweat contains interleukin-8. J Leukoc Biol. 1995;57:434–7.
14. Li HH, Zhou G, Fu XB, Zhang L. Antigen expression of human eccrine sweat glands. J Cutan Pathol. 2009;36:318–24.
15. Dai X, Okazaki H, Hanakawa Y, Murakami M, Tohyama M, Shirakata Y, et al. Eccrine sweat contains IL-1α, IL-1β and IL-31 and activates epidermal keratinocytes as a danger signal. PLoS One. 2013;8:e67666.
16. Wenzel FG, Horn TD. Non-neoplastic disorders of the eccrine glands. J Am Acad Dermatol. 1998;38:1–17.
17. Shiohara T, Sato Y, Komatsu Y, Ushigome Y, Mizukawa Y. Sweat as an efficient natural moisturizer. Curr Probl Dermatol. 2016;51:30–41.
18. Shiohara T, Doi T, Hayakawa J. Defective sweating responses in atopic dermatitis. Curr Probl Dermatol. 2011;41:68–79.
19. Ushigome Y, Sato Y, Shimoda Y, et al. Localized hypohidrosis is an unrecognized sequela of herpes zoster. J Am Acad Dermatol. 2017;76:160–2.
20. Shimoda-Komatsu Y, Sato Y, Yamazaki Y, et al. Lichen amyloidosis as a sweat gland/duct disorder: resolution associated with restoration of sweating disturbance. Br J Dermatol. 2017;176:1308–15.
21. Peng Y, Cui X, Liu Y, et al. Systematic review focusing on the excretion and protection roles of sweat in the skin. Dermatology. 2014;228:115–20.
22. Biehe-Hulette SJ, Kailler JM, Elstun IT, et al. Thermoregulatory vs. event sweating- comparison of clinical methodologies, physiology and results. Int J Cosmet Sci. 2014;36:102–8.
23. Sulzberger MB, Herrmann F, Zak FG. Studies of sweating : preliminary report with particular emphasis of a sweat retention syndrome. J Invest Dermatol. 1947;9:221–42.

24. Lobitz WC Jr, Campbell CJ. Physiologic studies in atopic dermatitis(disseminated neurodermatitis) I. The local cutaneous response to intradermally injected acetylcholine and epinephrine. Arch Dermatol Syphilol. 1953;67:575–89.
25. Rovensky J, Saxl O. Differences in dynamics of sweat secretion in atopic children. J Invest Dermatol. 1964;43:171–6.
26. Warndorff JA. The response of sweat gland to acetylcholine in atopic subjects. Br J Dermatol. 1970;83:306–11.
27. Murphy GM, Smith SE, Smith SA, et al. Autonomic function in cholinergic urticarial and atopic eczema. Br J Dermatol. 1984;110:581–6.
28. Kiistala R. Cholinergic and adrenergic sweating in atopic dermatitis. Acta Derm Venereol. 1992;72:106–8.
29. Candas V, Libert JP, Vogt JJ. Human skin wittedness and evaporative efficiency of sweating. J Appl Physiol. 1979;46:522–8.
30. Eishi K, Lee JB, Bae SJ, Takenaka M, Katayama I. Impaired sweating function in adult atopic dermatitis: results of the quantitative sudomotor axon reflex test. Br J Dermatol. 2002;147:683–8.
31. Ahmed AA, Nordlind K, Schultzberg M, Lidén S. Proinflammatory cytokines and their corresponding receptor proteins in eccrine sweat glands in normal and cutaneous leishmaniasis human skin. An immunohistochemical study. Exp Dermatol. 1996;5:230–5.
32. Faulkner SH, Spilsbury KL, Harvery J, Jackson A, Huang J, Platt M, et al. The detection and measurement of interleukin-6 in venous and capillary blood samples, and in sweat collected at rest and during exercise. Eur J Appl Physiol. 2014;114:1207–16.
33. Marques-Deak A, Cizza G, Eskandari F, Torvik S, Christie IC, Sternberg EM, et al. Measurement of cytokines in sweat patches and plasma in healthy women: validation in controlled study. J Immunol Methods. 2006;315:99–109.
34. Flores S, Davis MD, Pittelkow MR, Sandroni P, Weaver AL, Fealey RD. Abnormal sweating patterns associated with itching, burning and tingling of the skin indicate possible underlying small-fibre neuropathy. Br J Dermatol. 2015;172:412–8.
35. Adachi K, Aoki T. IgE antibody to sweat in atopic dermatitis. Arch Derm Venereol Suppl (Stockh). 1989;144:83–7.
36. Jung K, Schlenvogt G, Ladwig K, et al. The sweat of patients with atopic dermatitis contains specific Ig E antibodies to inhalant allergens. Clin Exp Dermatol. 1996;21:347–50.
37. Ilves T, Virolainen A, Harvima IT. Immediate wheal reactivity to autologous sweat in atopic dermatitis is associated with clinical severity, serum total and specific IgE and sweat tryptase activity. Int Arch Allergy Immunol. 2016;170:84–91.
38. Hide M, Tanaka T, Yamamura Y, et al. IgE-mediated hypersensitivity against human sweat antigen in patients with atopic dermatitis. Acta Derm Venereol. 2002;82:335–40.
39. Hiragun T, Ishii K, Hiragun M, et al. Fungal protein MGL_1304 in sweat is an allergen for atopic dermatitis patients. J Allergy Clin Immunol. 2013;132:608–15.
40. Reinikainen LM, Jaakola JJ. The effect of air humidification on symptoms and perception of indoor air quality in office workers: a six-period cross-over trial. Arch Environ Health. 1992;47:8–15.
41. Reinikainen LM, Jaakola JJ. Significance of humidity and temperature on skin and upper airway symptoms. Indoor Air. 2003;13:344–52.
42. Nilsson L, Bjorksten B, Hattevig G, et al. Season of birth as predictor of atopic manifestations. Arch Dis Child. 1997;76:341–4.
43. Kusunoki T, Asai K, Harazaki M, et al. Month of birth and prevalence of atopic dermatitis in school children: dry skin in early infancy as a possible etiologic factor. J Allergy Clin Immunol. 1999;103:1148–52.
44. Sasaki T, Furusyo N, Shiohama A, Takeuchi S, Nakahara T, Uchi H, et al. Filaggrin loss-of-function mutations are not a predisposing factor for atopic dermatitis in an Ishigaki Island under subtropical climate. J Dermatol Sci. 2014;76:10–5.
45. Scholtz J. Management of atopic dermatitis. A preliminary report. Calif Med. 1964;100:103–5.

46. Gutman A, Kligman A, Sciacca A, et al. Soak and smear. A standard technique revisited. Arch Dermatol. 2005;141:1556–9.
47. Chiang C, Eichenfield LF. Quantitative assessment of combination bathing and moisturizing regimens on skin hydration in atopic dermatitis. Pediatr Dermatol. 2009;26:273–8.

12 Microbiome, Dysbiosis, and Atopic Dermatitis

Keiji Iwatsuki, Osamu Yamasaki, and Shin Morizane

Abstract

The loss of diversity in a normal skin microbiome known as dysbiosis is observed in most patients with atopic dermatitis (AD). In particular, staphylococcal colonization is correlated with the severity of AD, and it is thought to be a possible trigger for AD. However, the questions of whether staphylococcal colonization precedes the development of AD, and whether the colonization of commensal microbiota is protective against the occurrence of eczema have been controversial. In addition to the genetic skin barrier dysfunctions, virulence factors generated by *Staphylococcus* species may enhance the impairment of barrier functions, and they may induce allergic inflammation via innate and adaptive immunity. This chapter summarizes the current knowledge on the pathogenic link between the skin microbiome and AD.

Keywords

Skin microbiome • Microbiota • *Staphylococcus* • Quorum sensing • Skin barrier Defensin • Cathelicidin

12.1 Introduction

Both genetic and environmental factors are responsible for the development of atopic dermatitis (AD). The skin microbiome and especially staphylococcal colonization are thought to comprise one of the triggering factors for AD, and they are correlated with the severity of AD. In fact, *Staphylococcus aureus* (*S. aureus*) is heavily colonized in the skin of many patients with AD. Almost all *S. aureus* strains have the ability to

K. Iwatsuki (✉) • O. Yamasaki • S. Morizane
Department of Dermatology, Okayama University Graduate School of Medicine, Dentistry and Pharmaceutical Sciences, Okayama City, Okayama, Japan
e-mail: keijiiwa@cc.okayama-u.ac.jp

I. Katayama et al. (eds.), *Evolution of Atopic Dermatitis in the 21st Century*,
https://doi.org/10.1007/978-981-10-5541-6_12

secrete a group of enzymes including exotoxins, nucleases, proteases, lipases, hyaluronidase, and collagenase, some of which may affect skin barrier functions, and these strains induce allergic inflammation via innate and adaptive immunity. In addition to these microbial products, some strains produce one or more exotoxins targeting the specific molecules that constitute the cell adhesion and host immune system: exfoliative toxins (ETs) that can cleavage desmoglein 1, toxic shock syndrome toxin-1 (TSST-1), Panton-Valentine leukocidin (PVL), and others.

12.2 Commensal Microbiota and Dysbiosis

12.2.1 Age- and Body Site-Related Commensal Microbiota

Big data on the skin microbiome have revealed the diversity and abundance of each habitat's signature microbes even in healthy subjects and the strong niche specialization of microbiota both within and among individuals [1]. Other studies demonstrated the body site-specific colonization of skin commensal bacteria, probably due to cutaneous conditions including regional skin anatomy, moisture, lipid content, sweating, pH, sebum, and other factors [2, 3]. *Staphylococcus* and *Corynebacterium* species are major commensals on the moist areas, and *Propionibacterium* species are dominantly detected in the sebaceous regions. Recent studies concerning the site-specific bacterial colonization indicate that innate lymphoid cells (ILCs), in particular interleukin (IL)-22-producing cells, regulate the selective containment of lymphoid-resident bacteria to prevent the systemic inflammation associated with chronic diseases [4, 5].

Newborns harbor a rather uniform microbiome influenced by the mode of delivery: vaginally delivered infants acquire bacterial communities resembling their own mother's vaginal microbiota, dominated by *Lactobacillus*, *Prevotella*, or *Sneathia* spp., and cesarean-section infants harbor bacterial communities similar to those found on the skin surface, dominated by *Staphylococcus*, *Corynebacterium*, and *Propionibacterium* spp. [6]. In contrast, a birth cohort study based on the longitudinal sampling of bacterial 16S rRNA gene sequences has shown that the delivery mode and the feeding method (breast, formula, or combination) had little effect on skin bacterial colonization [7]. In addition, those authors have reported that early colonization with commensal staphylococci at 2 months postdelivery is associated with a lower risk of AD at 1 year and that 1-year-old infants with AD were not colonized with *S. aureus* before having AD. A comparative cohort study in Japan on 1- and 6-month-old infants noted that the 6-month-old infants with *S. aureus* colonization showed a higher risk of developing AD compared to those without colonization (odds ratio 4.351, $p = 0.002$) [8].

12.2.2 Commensal Staphylococci

The skin microbiome closely interacts with the local immune system in both health and disease. As described above, the skin microbiota differs greatly among the topographic locations. AD preferentially involves the antecubital and popliteal fossae, where microbial populations are highly diverse in healthy individuals. In patients with AD, however, the temporal loss of diversity with predominant staphylococcal colonization (i.e., dysbiosis) is a common feature upon a disease flare, and the diversity is restored after successful anti-inflammatory treatment [9].

One of commensal bacteria, *S. epidermidis*, is believed to play a protective role by influencing the innate immune response of keratinocytes through Toll-like receptors (TLRs) signaling. For example, the activation of TLR-2 by *S. epidermidis* enhances the tight junction barrier in epidermal keratinocytes [10] and the generation of antimicrobial peptides such as β-defensins 2 and 3 [11]. *S. epidermidis* suppresses TLR3-mediated inflammation due to skin injury by stimulating TLR2 with lipoteichoic acid (LTA) [12].

Serine proteases secreted from a subset of *S. epidermidis* inhibit biofilm formation and nasal colonization by *S. aureus*. Furthermore, *S. epidermidis*-secreted proteases enhance the susceptibility of *S. aureus* to antimicrobial peptides such as human β-defensin 2 [13].

The unique peptides produced by *S. epidermidis* known as phenol-soluble modulin (PSM)γ and PSMδ may serve as an antimicrobial peptides (AMPs) on the normal skin surface due to their molecular structures containing both hydrophobic and cationic amino acids mimicking classic AMPs such as LL-37 [14]. These peptides selectively exhibited bactericidal activity against skin pathogens, such as *S. aureus*, Group A *Streptococcus*, and *Escherichia coli*, whereas they are not active against *S. epidermidis*. This selective activity is likely to be an important part of a normal microbial defense strategy against the colonization of pathogenic microbiota. However, further studies are needed to establish whether colonization with commensal staphylococci modulates skin immunity and attenuates the development of AD.

12.2.3 Genetic Skin Barrier Functions and Dysbiosis

Normal skin is composed of physiological barriers including cornified cell envelope, filaggrin, and tight junctions that function to retain moisture and to prevent the penetration of allergens and microbes (Fig. 12.1). The development of the AD phenotype was associated with gene mutations related to the skin barrier functions including filaggrin (*FLG*) and with the serine protease inhibitor Kazal-type 5 (*SPINK-5*) which encodes the protease inhibitor lymphoepithelial Kazal-type-related inhibitor (LEKTI). The latter has been shown to be responsible for Netherton syndrome, which is characterized by a severe form of AD and trichorrhexis invaginata (bamboo hair) [15, 16].

12.2.3.1 *FLG* Mutations

FLG mutations account for 30% of the AD population in European countries, and they are associated with the early onset of AD. *FLG* mutations in Japan are unique from those found in European-origin populations [17]. A high-throughput *FLG*

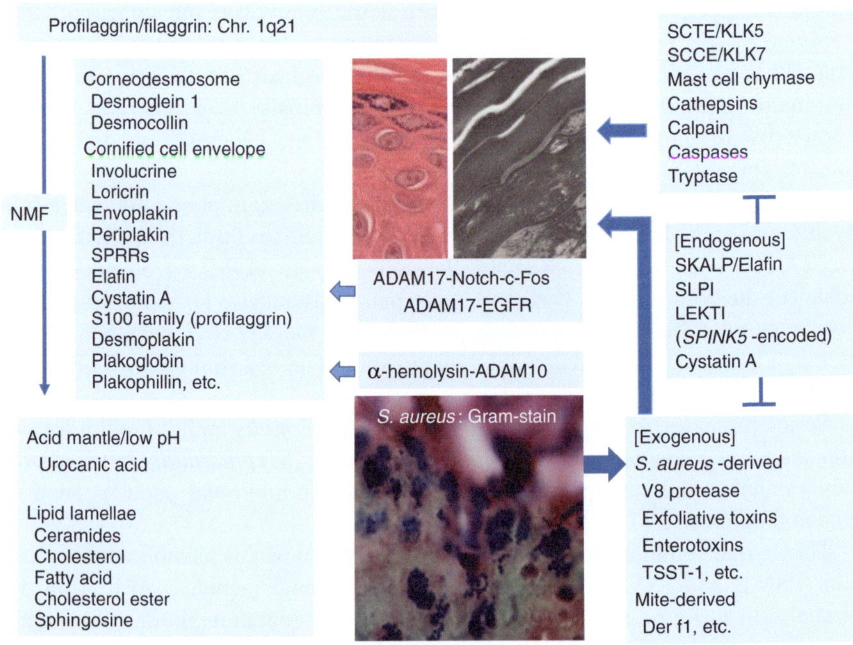

Fig. 12.1 Homeostasis of physiological skin barrier and *S. aureus*-derived virulence factors. *KLK* kallikrein, *LEKTI* lymphoepithelial Kazal-type-related inhibitor, *NMF* natural moisturizing factor, *SCCE* stratum corneum chymotryptic enzyme, *SCTE* stratum corneum tryptic enzyme, *SKALP* skin-derived antileukoprotease, *SLPI* secretory leukocyte protease inhibitor, *SPINK-5* serine protease inhibitor Kazal-type 5, *SPRR proteins* small proline-rich proteins, *TSST-1* toxic shock syndrome toxin-1

mutation detection test revealed that 89 individuals out of the 820 participants were heterozygous for one of the ten *FLG* mutations, and two individuals were compound heterozygous for two of the ten mutations [18]. A recent study indicates that individuals with bi-allelic *FLG* mutations do not always have severe AD, and it confirmed that not all individuals with bi-allelic *FLG* mutations have AD [19].

The *FLG* mutation-induced disruption of barrier functions in horny layers allows increased epicutaneous penetration of exogenous allergens [20], with subsequent sensitization to the allergens, which results in the development of AD and food allergy [21]. *FLG* mutations might be involved in the pathogenesis of wheat-dependent exercise-induced anaphylaxis [22]. However, a current study did not identify a close relationship between peanut allergy and loss-of-function variants in the *FLG* mutations in children with AD [23].

12.2.3.2 *SPINK-5* Mutations and Kallikreins (KLKs)

The balance of activity between proteases and their inhibitors is essential to maintain skin barrier functions. As exemplified in Netherton syndrome, a loss-of-function mutation of *SPINK-5* attenuates the activity of a protease inhibitor, LEKTI, which in turn results in the enhancement of KLK protease activity. It was demonstrated that the levels of KLKs are increased in the horny layers of AD [24].

The enhancement of protease activity through increased KLK7 expression by T helper cell 2 (Th2) cytokines such as IL-4 and IL-13 might be an important factor for mechanical and chemical epidermal barrier dysfunction in patients with AD [25]. These observations indicate that endogenous KLK activity is increased in the skin lesions of AD, suggesting an association between polymorphism in *SPINK-5* and AD [26]. The impairment of skin barrier functions due to endogenous serine proteases such as KLKs increases the risk of *S. aureus* colonization of the skin, and exogenous proteases released by *S. aureus* alter the skin barrier functions.

12.3 Staphylococcal Colonization and Virulence

More than 90% of patients with AD are colonized with *S. aureus* in the lesional skin, whereas most healthy individuals do not harbor this pathogen. Upon colonization of *S. aureus* in the skin, virulence factors released from *S. aureus* further damage the skin barrier functions and induce a Th2-skewed inflammatory milieu, which suppresses the innate immune system.

12.3.1 Quorum-Sensing Signals

12.3.1.1 *agr* Signaling

Cell density-dependent gene regulation known as "quorum sensing" has a crucial role in virulence genes' expression (Fig. 12.2). The *S. aureus agr* quorum-sensing cascade includes the RNAIII-dependent and RNAIII-independent pathways, and the RNAII-dependent transcription of *agrB*, *agrD*, *agrC*, and *agrA* genes [27]. Among these pathways, all of the phenol-soluble modulins (PSMs), except for the *hld* gene encoding δ-toxin, are upregulated through the RNAIII-independent pathway. The RNAIII-dependent pathway upregulates the expression of proteases, lipase, urease, enterotoxin, leukocidins, α-toxin, and mecA, whereas it downregulates the generation of protein A, SarH1, oligopeptide, and fibronectin-binding proteins.

12.3.1.2 *agr* Mutation

A recent cohort study demonstrated that dysfunctional mutations in the *agr* locus, especially in *agr*C gene, were detected only in the strains from the infants without AD [8]. The *agr* quorum-sensing circuit may thus be involved in the development of AD, and low levels of RNAIII expression caused by the *agr*C mutations may reduce staphylococcal colonization, thereby blocking the development of AD.

12.3.2 Virulence Factors

Almost all *S. aureus* strains have the ability to secrete virulence group of enzymes and exotoxins, including four hemolysins (α-, β-, δ-, and γ-toxins), nucleases, proteases, lipases, hyaluronidase, and collagenase (Fig. 12.2).

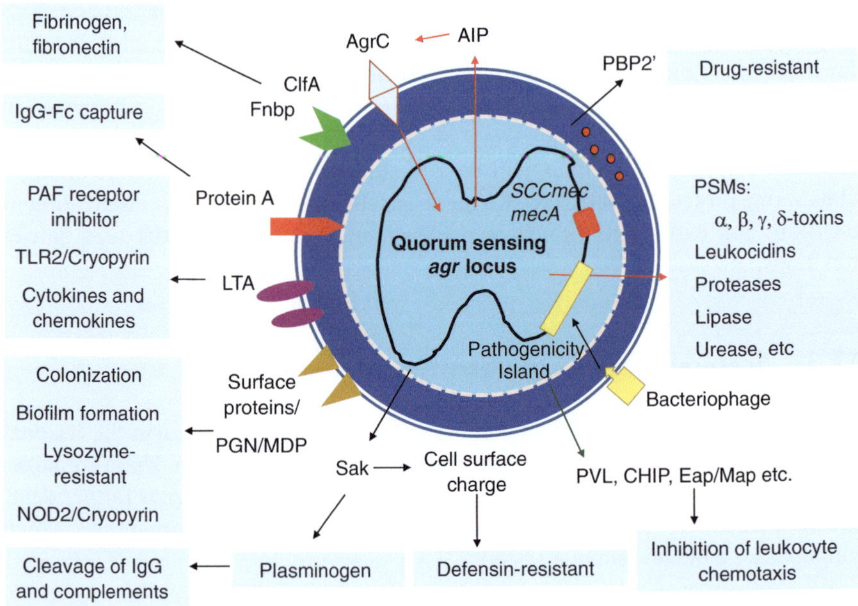

Fig. 12.2 Staphylococcal virulence factors and quorum-sensing circuit. The agr RNAIII-dependent pathway upregulates the expression of virulence factors including proteases, lipase, urease, enterotoxin, leukocidins, α-toxin, and mecA. *Agr* accessory gene regulator, *AIP* autoinducing peptide, *CHIP* chemotaxis inhibitory protein of staphylococci, *ClfA* clumping factor A, *Eap* extracellular adherens protein, *ET* exfoliative toxin, *LTA* lipoteichoic acid, *Map* major histocompatibility class II analogue protein, *MDP* muramyl dipeptide, *NOD2* nucleotide-binding oligomerization domain 2, *PAF* platelet-activating factor, *PGN* peptidoglycan, *PSM* phenol-soluble modulin, *PVL* Panton-Valentine leucocidin, *Sak* staphylokinase, *SCC* staphylococcal cassette chromosome, *SE* staphylococcal enterotoxin, *TLR* Toll-like receptor

In addition to these microbial products, some strains produce one or more exotoxins targeting the specific molecules that constitute the cell adhesion and host immune systems. Some of these staphylococcal products have biological properties that are harmful to physiological and immunological skin barriers against pathogens.

12.3.2.1 Disruption of Physiological Skin Barriers

The staphylococcal V8 serine protease increases desquamation of the epidermis, and the exfoliative toxins A and B (ETA/B) cleave desmoglein-1, a desmosomal adhesion protein. Excess shedding of corneocytes leads to a disrupted skin barrier and increased bacterial invasion. *S. aureus*-derived ceramidase increases the permeability of the stratum corneum [28]. Vulnerability to bacterial colonization in the skin of patients with AD is associated with reduced levels of a natural antimicrobial agent, sphingosine, which results from decreased levels of ceramides [29]. In addition to the protease-induced skin barrier defects, possible physiological factors leading to staphylococcal colonization and dysbiosis include a decrease in antimicrobial peptides and sweat containing IgA and dermcidin, and increased skin pH, moisture, lipid content, and more [30–33].

Previous studies have demonstrated that lipoteichoic acid (LTA) and surface proteins of *S. aureus* are responsible for colonization on the nasal mucosa [34, 35]. Staphylococcal LTA manifests its immunomodulatory effects via the platelet-activating factor receptor (PAF-R), which leads to the production of IL-10 [36]. A toxin-receptor complex, such as the Hla (pore-forming α-hemolysin)-ADAM10 complex, disrupts a cell adhesion molecule, E-cadherin [37]. Furthermore, mice lacking ADAM17 in the epidermis induced AD-like dermatitis [38, 39], and naturally occurring dysbiosis with dominant colonization of *S. aureus* and *Corynebacterium bovis* induced eczematous dermatitis [40]. It has been demonstrated that the ADAM17-Notch-c-Fos and/or the ADAM17-EGFR signaling pathways play an essential role to sustain the homeostasis of skin barrier functions [38, 39].

12.3.2.2 Disruption of Immunological Skin Barriers

The subsequent cellular events induced by *S. aureus* colonization include the activation of phospholipase A2, phosphatidylinositol hydrolysis, the production of nitric oxide, prostaglandin (PG) E2, PGI2 and thromboxane A2, the activation of NF-kB, and the upregulation of various inflammatory cytokines [41, 42]. It has been postulated that bacterial toxins stimulate Rho-family GTPases that activate the downstream signaling pathways affecting the expression of inflammatory mediators and defensins [43].

It was demonstrated that *S. aureus*-derived δ-toxin is capable of the degranulation of mast cell granules and that *S. aureus* isolates recovered from AD patients produced large amounts of δ-toxin [44]. In addition, δ-toxin promotes allergic skin inflammation via IgE and IL-4 production. PSMs of *S. aureus* have various biological properties: antimicrobial function, the recruitment of leukocytes, and the induction of IL-18 and IL-17 cascades [45, 46].

S. aureus induces the expression of the skin-homing receptor cutaneous lymphocyte-associated antigen (CLA) on T cells. Keratinocyte-derived chemokines, thymic stromal lymphopoietin (TSLP), and IL-31 secretion are induced and augmented by *S. aureus* enterotoxins [47].

12.3.3 Th2 Immunity and Group 2 Innate Lymphoid Cells

Skin barrier dysfunction allows the penetration of immune stimuli which drive dendritic cells to enhance Th2 polarization [48]. The resultant Th2-skewed immune response, characterized by IL-4/IL-13 production, damages the physiological skin barriers by downregulation of filaggrin [49], loricrin, involucrin [50], desmoglein 3 [51], and ceramide [52]. TSLP has also emerged as a key cytokine in the pathogenesis of Th2 cell-associated AD [53]. Early studies have shown that TSLP overexpression in keratinocytes leads to the spontaneous development of AD-like disease in mice [54].

12.3.3.1 Th2 Immunity and the Microbiome

Upon *Staphylococcus* colonization, a Th2 inflammatory response and persistent IL-18 secretion from keratinocytes are induced by wall LTA and protein A, respectively [36, 55]. *Staphylococcus* enterotoxins A (SEA) and B (SEB) stimulate the expressions of ICAM-1 and HLA-DR in normal human keratinocytes, and over 50% of AD patients have specific IgE antibodies to SEA and/or SEB in their serum [56]. Epicutaneous sensitization with SEB elicits a local, cutaneous inflammatory response characterized by dermal infiltration with eosinophils and mononuclear cells and an increased mRNA expression of the Th2 cytokine IL-4 but not of the Th1 cytokine IFN-γ.

Cutaneous and systemic bacterial infections are exacerbated by IL-4 signaling because IL-4 hampers neutrophil expansion and migration by antagonizing G-CSF and chemokine receptor-mediated signals via CXCR2-CXCR4 [57]. The level of cytokine IL-22, often coproduced by IL17-secreting cells, is often elevated in AD skin lesions. IL-22 is important for limiting the growth of *S. aureus* on mechanically injured skin. The blockade of IL-23 and IL-22 may enhance susceptibility to staphylococcal skin infection [5].

12.3.3.2 Superantigens and Regulatory T Cells

Superantigens mediate direct cross-linking of major histocompatibility complex class II (MHCII) molecules on antigen-presenting cells with T-cell receptors, and they induce a strong proliferative response followed by the clonal deletion of a substantial portion of defined Vβ T-cells [58]. Epicutaneous exposure to superantigens skews the immune response toward Th2 cells, leading to the allergic skin inflammation and increased IgE synthesis that are characteristics of AD [59]. Patients with AD have significantly increased numbers of regulatory T (Treg) cells with normal immunosuppressive activity. However, after superantigen stimulation, Treg cells lose their immunosuppressive activity [60].

12.3.3.3 Group 2 Innate Lymphoid Cells

Innate lymphoid cells (ILCs) are divided into three different subsets based on their different cytokine expression patterns and transcription factors. ILC1 cells produce type 1 cytokines such as IFN-γ upon stimulation with IL-12, IL-15, and IL-18, and they express a transcription factor, T-bet. ILC2 cells produce Th2 cytokines such as IL-4, IL-5, IL-9, and IL-13 upon stimulation with IL-33, IL-25, TSLP, eicosanoids, and IL-1β, and they express GATA-3. ILC3 produces type 3 cytokines such as IL-17A and IL-22 upon stimulation with IL-1β and IL-23, and they express RORγτ. These cells play a crucial role in defense against extracellular pathogens such as staphylococcal infections [61, 62]. A recent study demonstrated that AD skin contained not only ILC2 cells but also prominent aryl hydrocarbon receptor $(AHR)^+$ ILC3 cells [63].

12.4 Susceptibility to Cutaneous Infections

Keratinocytes serve as the first line of defense against cutaneous pathogens and are able to stimulate an immune response by releasing cytokines and antimicrobial cationic peptides such as defensins and LL-37 to eradicate pathogens. However, despite the upregulation of antimicrobial peptide generation, mice lacking three components of the cornified cell envelope, including envoplakin, periplakin, and involucrin, show an AD phenotype with increased skin bacterial load [64].

12.4.1 Staphylococcal Infections

Human β-defensins (HBD) are present at significantly lower levels in the inflamed skin lesions of AD patients [65, 66] (Fig. 12.3), although a disturbed skin barrier may trigger defensin induction in AD and psoriasis [67]. HBD2 has a less bactericidal activity against Gram-positive cocci such as *S. aureus* than HBD3 [68]. However, endogenous HBD2 expression was required and sufficient for protection against *S. aureus* protease SspA/V8-mediated integrity damage, probably via IL-1β-induced protective factors derived from epidermal keratinocytes [69].

Patients with hyperimmunoglobulin E (IgE) syndrome, type 1 caused by *STAT3* mutations, also present with AD-like eczema and recurrent abscess formation because of susceptibility to *S. aureus* infections [70]. Defects of Th17 cell development due to the defective IL-6 signaling and induced regulatory T (iTreg) cell generation due to defective IL-10 signaling account for the cutaneous pathology at least in part [71].

As ADAM10 cleaves multiple cellular substrates such as E-cadherin, it is of interest to understand the potential role of this protein in staphylococcal disease pathogenesis. Implication of ADAM10 in the development of AD suggests that the Hla (a pore-forming α-hemolysin)-ADAM10 complex may contribute to staphylococcal colonization and invasion [37, 72].

12.4.2 Eczema Herpeticum

Herpes simplex virus type 1 (HSV-1), F35 strains, is clearly associated with eczema herpeticum [73]. A previous study has shown that Th2 predominance and Th1

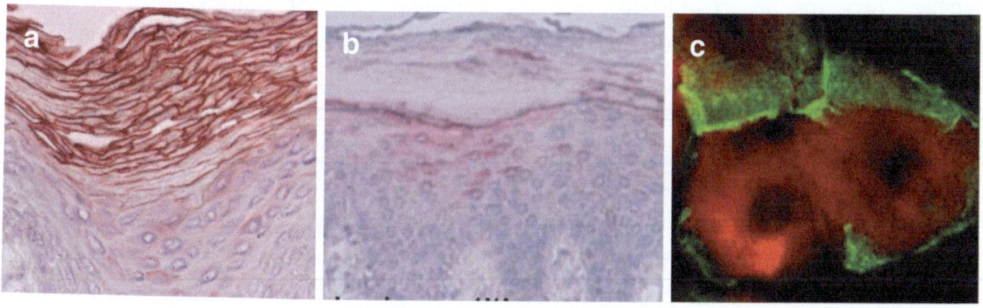

Fig. 12.3 Expression of human β-defensin 2 (HBD2) in psoriasis and atopic dermatitis (Ref. [66]). (**a**) Increased expression of HBD2 in psoriasis vulgaris, whereas (**b**) low expression in the atopic dermatitis. (**c**) HBD2 (*green fluorescence*) is expressed as surrounding the corneocytes (*red fluorescence*)

deficiency are much more pronounced in the subgroup of AD patients at risk for eczema herpeticum [74]. A murine model of eczema herpeticum with an impaired skin barrier demonstrated a critical role of defective NK activities in the development of severe HSV-1-induced skin lesions [75]. Other pathways related to the susceptibility to eczema herpeticum in AD include the inhibition of the IRF2, IRF3, and IRF7 innate immune pathways [76, 77], the expression of indoleamine 2,3-dioxygenease 1 (IDO1) [78], FLG mutations [79], TSLP [80], *S. aureus* α-toxin [81], and abnormalities in IFN-γ response [82].

Vitamin D levels are significantly lower in children with moderate or severe AD compared to children with mild AD. Children with AD with eczema herpeticum also displayed significantly lower vitamin D levels compared to those with AD alone [83, 84]. Further clinical trials are needed to provide conclusive evidence regarding the involvement of vitamin D in AD.

12.5 Therapeutic Approach Against Microbiota

Antibiotics temporarily reduce *S. aureus* colonization on the skin. Without signs of infection, oral antibiotics generally have a minimal therapeutic effect on the dermatitis [85]. Apart from their indication for overt secondary bacterial infections, antibiotics (by both systemic and topical applications) should not be recommended for the management of AD because no effect has been observed in clinical improvement or the sparing of steroids [86] and due to the risk of increasing prevalence of antibiotic resistance [87]. Since the production of virulence factors of *Staphylococcus* species may induce impairment of skin barrier functions and inflammation, there is no doubt that targeting the quorum-sensing signaling pathway and/or anti-toxin therapy is a promising approach for managements of dysbiosis.

12.5.1 Managements of Dysbiosis

Inhibition of bacterial adherence and colonization is the first line of prevention of bacterial infections. Previous studies have indicated that staphylococcal LTA and surface proteins are responsible for the establishment of colonization on nasal mucosa. *S. aureus* colonizes persistently in approximately 20% of the population and transiently in 60% and never colonizes in the remaining 20% [35]. It is clear that the differences in the individual defense mechanisms on the nasal mucosa are a key to preventing colonization in the host.

Therapeutic procedures to selectively eradicate pathogenic *S. aureus*, with a simultaneous protection of *S. epidermidis*, have been used clinically. These procedures include the application of a low pH cream and a gluco-oligosaccharide that inhibits the attachment of *S. aureus* cells on the epithelial surfaces [88].

In AD patients successfully treated with emollients, the patients' dysbiosis with dominant staphylococcal colonization is recovered with the overall diversity of the commensal, with the abundance of *Stenotrophomonas* species [89]. The application of moisturizers significantly reduced the relapse of inflammation in AD patients [90]. These data support the importance of emollients and moisturizers in the management of AD.

12.5.2 Vaccination

A number of investigations are focusing on active or passive immunization against *S. aureus* infections, using a capsular polysaccharide vaccine [91] and humanized monoclonal antibodies [92]. A prophylactic *S. aureus* four-antigen vaccine (SA4Ag) is under development for the prevention of invasive *S. aureus* disease [93].

12.5.3 Anti-exotoxin and Anti-biofilm Therapy

Bacterial glycocalyx is a polysaccharide-containing material produced by bacteria. Bacteria that adhere to implanted medical devices or damaged tissue can become the cause of persistent infections. These bacteria encase themselves in a hydrated matrix of polysaccharide and protein, forming a slimy layer known as a biofilm. Since *S. aureus* can generally produce a biofilm on damaged skin tissue, antimicrobial agents may not eradicate *S. aureus* without the help of neutrophils. The *S. aureus* glycocalyx may play a crucial role in colonization and adherence to damaged skin tissue [94].

Infection with *agr* or *hla* (pore-forming toxin α-hemolysin, Hla) deletion mutants, loss of the Hla receptor ADAM10, or neutralization of Hla significantly attenuate virulence in mouse models of skin and soft tissue infections [37]. The blocking of staphylococcal autoinducing peptide 4 (AIP4) in *agr*-signaling provides a defensive effort against *S. aureus* virulence [95]. Recent advances in understanding the molecular mechanisms underlying toxin-induced tissue injury and host immune reactions have enabled us to develop a new approach to antitoxin treatments: the direct neutralization of exotoxins and the inhibition of the *agr* quorum-sensing pathway to produce exotoxins.

References

1. Human Microbiome Project Consortium. Structure, function and diversity of the healthy human microbiome. Nature. 2012;486:207–14.
2. Grice EA, et al. Topographical and temporal diversity of the human skin microbiome. Science. 2009;324(5931):1190–2.
3. Costello EK, et al. Bacterial community variation in human body habitats across space and time. Science. 2009;326(5960):1694–7.
4. Sonnenburg GF, et al. Innate lymphoid cells promote anatomical containment of lymphoid-resident commensal bacteria. Science. 2012;336(6086):1321–5.
5. Malhotra N, et al. IL-22 derived from γδ T cells restricts Staphylococcus aureus infection of mechanically injured skin. J Allergy Clin Immunol. 2016;138:1098–107.
6. Dominguez-Bello MG, et al. Delivery mode shapes the acquisition and structure of the initial microbiota across multiple body habitats in newborns. Proc Natl Acad Sci U S A. 2010;107:11971–5.

7. Kennedy EA, et al. Skin microbiome before development of atopic dermatitis: early colonization with commensal staphylococci at 2 months is associated with a lower risk of atopic dermatitis at 1 year. J Allergy Clin Immunol. 2017;139(1):166–72.
8. Nakamura Y et al. Evolutionary risk management of agr locus is important for S. aureus adaptation in the skin of atopic dermatitis. 41 JSID program issue 2016 (abstract).
9. Kong HH, et al. Temporal shifts in the skin microbiome associated with disease flares and treatment in children with atopic dermatitis. Genome Res. 2012;22(5):850–9.
10. Yuki T, et al. Activation of TLR2 enhances tight junction barrier in epidermal keratinocytes. J Immunol. 2011;187(6):3230–7.
11. Lai Y, et al. Activation of TLR2 by a small molecule produced by Staphylococcus epidermidis increases antimicrobial defense against bacterial skin infections. J Invest Dermatol. 2010;130(9):2211–21.
12. Lai Y, et al. Commensal bacteria regulate Toll-like receptor 3-dependent inflammation after skin injury. Nat Med. 2009;15(12):1377–82.
13. Dubin G, et al. Molecular cloning and biochemical characterisation of proteases from Staphylococcus epidermidis. Biol Chem. 2001;382:1575–82.
14. Cogan AL, et al. Selective antimicrobial action is provided by phenol-soluble modulins derived from Staphylococcus epidermidis, a normal resident of the skin. J Invest Dermatol. 2010;130(1):192–200.
15. Chavanas S, et al. Mutations in SPINK5, encoding a serine protease inhibitor, cause Netherton syndrome. Nat Genet. 2000;25(2):141–2.
16. Komatsu N, et al. Elevated stratum corneum hydrolytic activity in Netherton syndrome suggests an inhibitory regulation of desquamation by SPINK5-derived peptides. J Invest Dermatol. 2002;118(3):436–43.
17. Nomura T, et al. Unique mutations in the filaggrin gene in Japanese patients with ichthyosis vulgaris and atopic dermatitis. J Allergy Clin Immunol. 2007;119:434–40.
18. Kono M, et al. Comprehensive screening for a complete set of Japanese-population-specific filaggrin gene mutations. Allergy. 2014;69:537–40.
19. Sekiya A, et al. Compound heterozygotes for filaggrin gene mutations do not always show severe atopic dermatitis. J Eur Acad Dermatol Venereol. 2017;31:158–62.
20. Kawasaki H, et al. Altered stratum corneum barrier and enhanced percutaneous immune responses in filaggrin-null mice. J Allergy Clin Immunol. 2012;129(6):1538–46.
21. Brown SJ, et al. Loss-of-function variants in the filaggrin gene are a significant risk factor for peanut allergy. J Allergy Clin Immunol. 2011;127(3):661–7.
22. Mizuno O, et al. Loss-of-function mutations in the gene encoding filaggrin underlie a Japanese family with food-dependent exercise-induced anaphylaxis. J Eur Acad Dermatol Venereol. 2015;29(4):805–8.
23. Brough HA, et al. Atopic dermatitis increases the effect of exposure to peanut antigen in dust on peanut sensitization and likely peanut allergy. J Allergy Clin Immunol. 2015;135(1):164–70.
24. Komatsu N, et al. Human tissue kallikrein expression in the stratum corneum and serum of atopic dermatitis patients. Exp Dermatol. 2007;16(6):513–9.
25. Morizane S, et al. TH2 cytokines increase kallikrein 7 expression and function in patients with atopic dermatitis. J Allergy Clin Immunol. 2012;130(1):259–61.
26. Nishio Y, et al. Association between polymorphisms in the SPINK5 gene and atopic dermatitis in the Japanese. Genes Immun. 2003;4(7):515–7.
27. Queck SY, et al. RNAIII-independent target gene control by the agr quorum-sensing system: insight into the evolution of virulence regulation in Staphylococcus aureus. Mol Cell. 2008;32(1):150–8.
28. Ohnishi Y, et al. Ceramidase activity in bacterial skin flora as a possible cause of ceramide deficiency in atopic dermatitis. Clin Diagn Lab Immunol. 1999;6(1):101–4.
29. Arikawa J, et al. Decreased levels of sphingosine, a natural antimicrobial agent, may be associated with vulnerability of the stratum corneum from patients with atopic dermatitis to colonization by Staphylococcus aureus. J Invest Dermatol. 2002;119(2):433–9.

30. Imayama S, et al. Reduced secretion of IgA to skin surface of patients with atopic dermatitis. J Allergy Clin Immunol. 1994;94:195–200.
31. Kimata H. Increase in dermcidin-derived peptides in sweat of patients with atopic eczema caused by a humorous video. J Psychosm Res. 2007;62(1):57–9.
32. Rieg S, et al. Deficiency of dermcidin-derived antimicrobial peptides in sweat of patients with atopic dermatitis correlates with an impaired innate defense of human skin in vivo. J Immunol. 2005;174(12):8003–10.
33. Hata TR, Gallo RL. Antimicropeptides, skin infections, and atopic dermatitis. Semin Cutan Med Surg. 2008;27(2):144–50.
34. Weidenmaier C, et al. Role of teichoic acid in *Staphylococcus aureus* nasal colonization, a major risk factor in nosocomial infections. Nat Med. 2004;10(3):243–5.
35. Foster TJ. Immune evasion by staphylococci. Nat Rev Microbiol. 2005;3:943–58.
36. Zhang Q, et al. Staphylococcal lipoteichoic acid inhibits delayed-type hypersensitivity reaction via the platelet-activating factor receptor. J Clin Invest. 2005;115(10):2855–61.
37. Inoshima N, et al. Genetic requirement for ADAM10 in severe Staphylococcus aureus skin infection. J Invest Dermatol. 2012;132(5):1513–6.
38. Murthy A, et al. Notch activation by the metalloproteinase ADAM17 regulates myeloproliferation and atopic barrier immunity by suppression epithelial cytokine synthesis. Immunity. 2012;36:105–19.
39. Franzke CW, et al. Epidermal ADAM17 maintains the skin barrier by regulating EGFR ligand-dependent terminal keratinocyte differentiation. J Exp Med. 2012;209(6):1105–19.
40. Kobayashi T, et al. Dysbiosis ad Staphylococcus aureus colonization drives inflammation in atopic dermatitis. Immunity. 2015;42:756–66.
41. Dragneva Y, et al. Subcytocidal attack by staphylococcal alpha-toxin activates NF-kappaB and induces interleukin-8 production. Infect Immun. 2001;69(4):2630–5.
42. Rose F, Dahlem G, Guthmann B, et al. Mediator generation and signaling events in alveolar epithelial cells attacked by *S. aureus* alpha-toxin. Am J Physiol Lung Cell Mol Physiol. 2002;282:L207–14.
43. Boquet P, Lemichez E. Bacterial virulence factors targeting Rho GTPases: parasitism or symbiosis? Trends Cell Biol. 2003;13:238–46.
44. Nakamura Y, et al. Staphylococcus δ-toxin induces allergic skin disease by activating mast cells. Nature. 2013;503(7476):397–401.
45. Syed AK, et al. Staphylococcus aureus phenol-soluble modulins stimulate the release of proinflammatory cytokines from keratinocytes and are required for induction of skin inflammation. Infect Immun. 2015;83(9):3428–37.
46. Nakagawa S et al. Staphylococcus PSMa induces IL-17-dependent skin inflammation through IL-36 and IL-1 secretion from keratinocytes. 41st JSID program issue 2016 (abstract).
47. Bieber T. Atopic dermatitis. N Engl J Med. 2008;358(14):1483–94.
48. Hamman H, Lambrecht BN. Barrier epithelial cells and the control of type 2 immunity. Immunity. 2015;43(1):29–40.
49. Howell MD, et al. Cytokine modulation of atopic dermatitis filaggrin skin expression. J Allergy Clin Immunol. 2007;120(1):150–5.
50. Kim BE, et al. Loricrin and involucrin expression is down-regulated by Th2 cytokines through STAT-6. Clin Immunol. 2008;126(3):332–7.
51. Kobayashi J, et al. Reciprocal regulation of permeability through a cultured keratinocyte sheet by IFN-gamma and IL-4. Cytokine. 2004;28:186–9.
52. Hatano Y, et al. Interleukin-4 suppresses the enhancement of ceramide synthesis and cutaneous permeability barrier functions induced by tumor necrosis factor-alpha and interferon-gamma in human epidermis. J Invest Dermatol. 2005;124(4):786–92.
53. Ziegler SF, Artis D. Sensing the outside world: TSLP regulates barrier immunity. Nat Immunol. 2010;11(84):289–93.
54. Li M, et al. Retinoid X receptor ablation in adult mouse keratinocytes generates an atopic dermatitis triggered by thymic stromal lymphopoietin. Proc Natl Acad Sci U S A. 2005;102:14795–800.

55. Nakano H, et al. Persistent secretion of IL-18 in the skin contributes to IgE response in mice. Int Immunol. 2003;15:611–21.
56. Morishita Y, et al. Possible influences of Staphylococcus aureus on atopic dermatitis: the colonization features and the effects of staphylococcal enterotoxins. Clin Exp Allergy. 1999;29:1110–7.
57. Woytschak J, et al. Type 2 interleukin-4 receptor signaling in neutrophils antagonizes their expansion and migration during infection and inflammation. Immunity. 2016;45(1):172–84.
58. Wang ZQ, et al. Staphylococcal enterotoxin B-induced T-cell anergy is mediated by regulatory T cells. Immunology. 1998;94(3):331–9.
59. Laouini D, et al. Epicutaneous sensitization with superantigen induces allergic skin inflammation. J Allergy Clin Immunol. 2003;112(5):981–7.
60. Ou LS, et al. T regulatory cells in atopic dermatitis and subversion of their activity by superantigens. J Allergy Clin Immunol. 2004;113(4):756–63.
61. Morita H, et al. Innate lymphoid cells in allergic and nonallergic inflammation. J Allergy Clin Immunol. 2016;138(85):1253–64.
62. Moro K, et al. Interferon and IL-27 antagonize the function of group 2 innate lymphoid cells and type 2 innate immune responses. Nat Immunol. 2016;17(1):76–86.
63. Bruggen MC, et al. In situ mapping of innate lymphoid cells in human skin: evidence for remarkable differences between normal and inflamed skin. J Invest Dermatol. 2016;136(12):2396–405.
64. Natsuga K, et al. Increased bacterial load and expression of antimicrobial peptides in skin of barrier-deficient mice with reduced cancer susceptibility. J Invest Dermatol. 2016:99–106.
65. Ong PY, et al. Endogenous antimicrobial peptides and skin infections in atopic dermatitis. N Engl J Med. 2002;347(15):1151–60.
66. Huh WK, et al. Dynamic alteration of human beta-defensin 2 localization from cytoplasm to intercellular space in psoriatic skin. J Mol Med. 2002;80(10):678–4.
67. Harder J, et al. Enhanced expression and secretion of antimicrobial peptides in atopic dermatitis and after superficial skin injury. J Invest Dermatol. 2010;130(5):1355–64.
68. Sakagami-Yasui Y, et al. Two arginine residues in the COOH-terminal of human β-defensin-3 constitute an essential motif for antimicrobial activity and IL-6 production. Exp Dermatol. 2017; doi:10.1111/exd.13361.
69. Wang B, et al. IL-1 β-induced protection of keratinocytes against Staphylococcus aureus-secreted proteases is mediated by human β-defensin 2. J Invest Dermatol. 2017;137(81):95–105.
70. Minegishi Y, et al. Dominant-negative mutations in the DNA-binding domain of STAT3 cause hyper-IgE syndrome. Nature. 2007;448:1048–52.
71. Minegishi Y, Saito M. Cutaneous manifestations of hyperIgE syndrome. Allergy Int. 2012;61(2):191–6.
72. Maretzky T, et al. ADAM10-mediated E-cadherin release is regulated by proinflammatory cytokines and modulates keratinocyte cohesion in eczematous dermatitis. J Invest Dermatol. 2008;128(7):1737–46.
73. Yoshida M, Umene K. Close association of predominant genotype of herpes simplex virus type 1 with eczema herpeticum analyzed using restriction fragment length polymorphism of polymerase chain reaction. J Virol Methods. 2003;109(1):11–6.
74. Peng WM, et al. Risk factors of atopic dermatitis patients for eczema herpeticum. J Invest Dermatol. 2007;127(5):1261–3.
75. Kawakami Y, et al. Defective natural killer cell activity in a mouse model of eczema herpeticum. J Allergy Clin Immunol. 2017;139(3):997–1006.e10.
76. Gao PS, et al. Genetic variants in interferon regulatory factor 2 (IRF2) are associated with atopic dermatitis and eczema herpeticum. J Invest Dermatol. 2012;132:650–7.
77. Bin L, et al. Identification of novel gene signatures in patients with atopic dermatitis complicated by eczema herpeticum. J Allergy Clin Immunol. 2014;134(4):848–55.

78. Staudacher A, et al. Exaggerated IDO1 expression and activity in Langerhans cells from patients with atopic dermatitis upon viral stimulation: a potential predictive biomarker for high risk of eczema herpeticum. Allergy. 2015;70(11):1432–9.
79. Gao PS, et al. Filaggrin mutations that confer risk of atopic dermatitis confer greater risk for eczema herpeticum. J Allergy Clin Immunol. 2009;124(3):507–13.
80. Gao PS, et al. Genetic variants in thymic stromal lymphopoietin are associated with atopic dermatitis and eczema herpeticum. J Allergy Clin Immunol. 2010;125(6):1403–7.
81. Bin L, et al. Staphylococcus aureus α-toxin modulates skin host response to viral infection. J Allergy Clin Immunol. 2012;130(3):683–91.
82. Leung DY, et al. Human atopic dermatitis complicated by eczema herpeticum is associated with abnormalities in IFN-γ response. J Allergy Clin Immunol. 2011;127(4):965–73.
83. Albenali LH, et al. Vitamin D and antimicrobial peptide levels in patients with atopic dermatitis and atopic dermatitis complicated by eczema herpeticum: a pilot study. J Allergy Clin Immunol. 2016;138(6):1715–9.
84. Kim MJ, et al. Vitamin D status and efficacy of vitamin D supplementation in atopic dermatitis: A systematic review and meta-analysis. Nutrients. 2016;8(12.) pii:E789
85. Hanifin J, et al. Guidelines of care for atopic dermatitis, developed in accordance with the American Academy of Dermatology (AAD)/American Academy of Dermatology Association "Administrative Regulations for Evidence-Based Clinical Practice Guidelines". J Am Acad Dermatol. 2004;50(3):391–404.
86. Ring J, et al. Guidelines for treatment of atopic eczema (atopic dermatitis) part I. J Eur Acad Dermatol Venereol. 2010;26(8):1045–60.
87. Niebuhr M, et al. Antibiotic treatment of cutaneous infections with Staphylococcus aureus in patients with atopic dermatitis: current antimicrobial resistances and susceptibilities. Exp Dermatol. 2008;17(11):953–7.
88. Akiyama H, et al. Actions of gluco-oligosaccharide against Staphylococcus aureus. J Dermatol. 2002;29(9):580–6.
89. Seite S, et al. Microbiome of affected and unaffected skin of patients with atopic dermatitis before and after emollient treatment. J Drugs Dermatol. 2014;13(11):1365–72.
90. Kawashima M, et al. The usefulness of moisturizers for maintenance of remission in atopic dermatitis. Jpn J Dermatol. 2007;117:1139–45. (In Japanese with English abstract)
91. Fattom A, et al. Safety and immunogenicity of a booster dose of Staphylococcus aureus type 5 and 8 capsular polysaccharide conjugate vaccine (Staph VAX) in hemodialysis patients. Vaccine. 2004;23(5):656–63.
92. Domanski PJ, Patel PR, Bayer AS, et al. Characterization of a humanized monoclonal antibody recognizing clumping factor A expressed by Staphylococcus aureus. Infect Immun. 2005;73(8):5229–32.
93. Frenck RW Jr, et al. Safety, tolerability, and immunogenicity of a 4-antigen Staphylococcus aureus vaccine (SA4Ag): results from a first-in-human randomised, placebo-controlled phase 1/2 study. Vaccine. 2017;35(2):375–84.
94. Akiyama H, et al. Confocal laser scanning microscopic observation of glycocalyx production by Staphylococcus aureus in mouse skin: does *S. aureus* generally produce a biofilm on damaged skin? Br J Dermatol. 2002;147(5):879–85.
95. O'Rourke JP, et al. Development of a mimotope vaccine targeting the Staphylococcus aureus quorum sensing pathway. PLoS One. 2014;9(811):e111198.

Psychological Stress in Atopic Dermatitis 13

Mayuko Nakano-Tahara, Hiroyuki Murota,
and Ichiro Katayama

Abstract

Accurately evaluating the factors that exacerbate atopic dermatitis is helpful in management of this skin condition. Psychological stress is a major exacerbating factor and often aggravates atopic dermatitis. The most common symptoms of atopic dermatitis themselves can also act as secondary stressors and lead to a deterioration in quality of life. Moreover, patients with atopic dermatitis may also suffer from other mental disorders such as depression and anxiety. It is known that psychological stress is associated with abnormal skin barrier function and a shift toward cytokine expression in T-helper 2 cells. The stress response affects three systems: the hypothalamic-pituitary-adrenal axis, which regulates the release of adenocorticotropin and cortisol; the sympathoadrenal medullary axis, which regulates the release of catecholamines; and the neurotrophin neuropeptide axis, which regulates the release of substance P. Therefore, treatment for psychological stress is quite important for controlling skin barrier function and inhibiting immune activation in cases of atopic dermatitis. Treatments for psychological stress include pharmacotherapy, such as topical corticosteroids, and psychotherapy, such as relaxation exercises, coping skills training, and stress management instruction.

Keywords

Atopic dermatitis • Psychological stress • Hypothalamic-pituitary-adrenal axis • Sympathoadrenal medullary axis • Neurotrophin neuropeptide axis

M. Nakano-Tahara, M.D., Ph.D. (✉) • H. Murota, M.D., Ph.D. • I. Katayama, M.D., Ph.D.
Department of Dermatology, Osaka University Graduate School of Medicine,
2-2 Yamadaoka, Suita, Osaka 565-0871, Japan
e-mail: 104tahara@derma.med.osaka-u.ac.jp

I. Katayama et al. (eds.), *Evolution of Atopic Dermatitis in the 21st Century*,
https://doi.org/10.1007/978-981-10-5541-6_13

13.1 Environmental Triggers

Exacerbating factors for atopic dermatitis (AD) include a low humidity environment, seasonal changes, xerosis, psychological stress, sleep loss, house dust, pollen, cigarette smoke, certain foods, rapid temperature changes, and perspiration [1, 2]. Psychological stress is a major exacerbating factor that results in a protracted course or recurrence of AD symptoms [2–5]. Lammintausta et al. reported that psychological stress is the most commonly cited factor provoking relapses of dermatitis or aggravating the symptoms in 801 patients with AD (22–41 years old) [3]. The degree of psychological stress largely depends on one's interpretation of circumstances and daily life events. In particular, adult patients with AD who have suffered from the disease over a long period of time become refractory and difficult to manage medically because of the stress of regular hospital visits and high anxiety caused by usage of topical steroids. In our own experience, psychological stress and sleep loss are the prominent exacerbating factors (Nakano-Tahara, submitted for publication). In 2013 and 2014, we administered questionnaires consisting of questions regarding potential aggravating factors to first-year students ($n = 6839$) at Osaka University. We focused on the aggravating factors and performed linear regression analysis on the data between the remission course and symptomatic courses. The results indicate that the exacerbating factors predisposing a patient toward a protracted course are psychological stress, sleep loss, house dust, pollen, temperature, sweat, and air dryness. Psychological stress has the highest impact on the clinical course of adolescent AD. Subjects with AD consider both the effort of medication usage and AD symptoms as major sources of psychological stress. The frequency of psychological stress in students suffering from AD does not significantly correlate with the disease severity as determined by SCORAD scores. Kijima et al. also reported that a high anxiety level is not solely the result of disease severity [6]. We also followed students who presented with symptoms of AD at a medical checkup in 2012 ($n = 288$) for 4 years and determined how their level of psychological stress had changed throughout college life with questionnaires assessing frequency of psychological stress, skin symptoms, and treatment information (Fig. 13.1). Figure 13.2 shows fluctuations in symptoms of AD. The number of students without any treatment and regular clinic visits gradually decreased, and the number of cured students increased every year. The frequency of stress in a group of students attending regular clinic visits was higher than in a group of cured students in 2015 (Fig. 13.3). The frequency of stress significantly decreased in both of these groups throughout the 4 years of college life.

There are three psychosocial factors that affect AD symptoms. (1) Emotional factors can determine the natural course of the disease from onset through recurrence and protraction in some cases [2, 4]. Psychosocial stress (stressors) and poor coping mechanisms exacerbate AD. (2) The loss of sleep, appearance of diseased skin, intractable clinical course, and burden of treatment secondary to

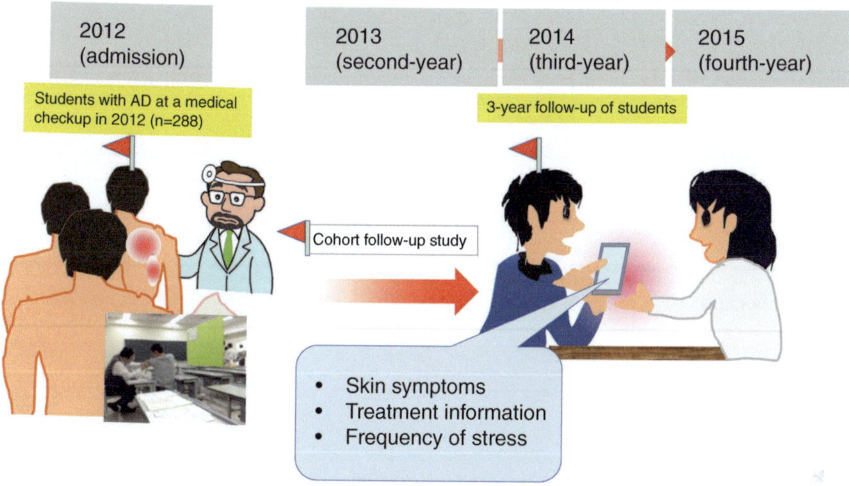

Fig. 13.1 Cohort questionnaire study of Osaka University students with AD (n = 288) who were followed for 4 years from 2012 to 2016

disabling pruritus may elevate the patient's level of psychological stress. The psychosocial problems derived from AD contribute to an impaired quality of life [7]. (3) Patients with AD may suffer from other mental disorders, such as depression and anxiety [8]. Overall, studies indicate that AD is a skin disease associated with increased anxiety levels [9].

13.2 Assessment of Psychological Stress

Psychosomatic evaluation is very important for patients with AD because the ability to cope with psychological stress varies among individuals. Personalized psychological treatment based on an exact evaluation may be effective in successfully treating the dermatitis. Several important psychosomatic scales and measures of coping with stress are described below.

13.2.1 Psychosomatic Scales

The Psychosomatic Scale for Atopic Dermatitis (PSS-AD) is a 12-item scale consisting of the following three factors: exacerbation triggered by stress, disturbances due to AD, and ineffective control [10].

The Depression-Anxiety-Stress Scale (DASS) is a 42-item self-reporting instrument designed to measure the three related negative emotional states of depression, anxiety, and tension/stress [11].

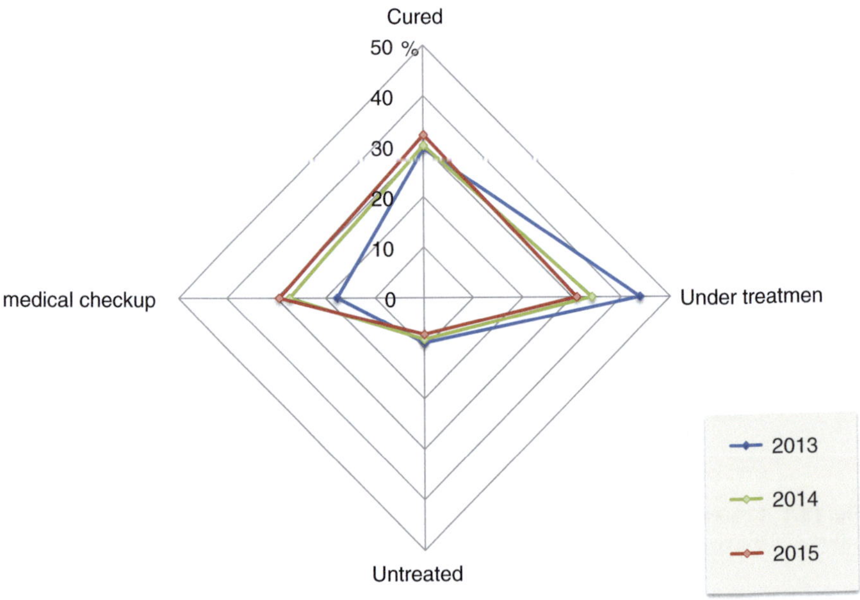

Fig. 13.2 The change in patient symptoms of AD from 2013 to 2015. This diagram indicates the ratio of students with AD who were cured, under treatment, untreated, and without medical checkup

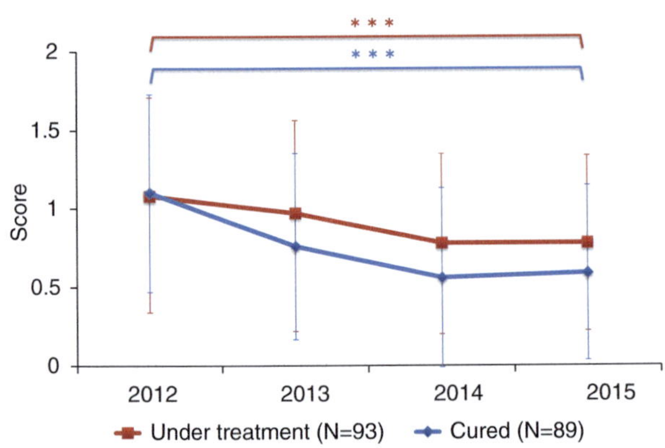

Fig. 13.3 The frequency of psychological stress through college life. The frequency of stress was scored as follows: 0, very little; 1, sometimes; 2, often; and 3, always. Each bar represents the mean ± SD. Key (***) $P < 0.001$ by paired t-test

The Inventory of Stress Symptoms for Adults Lipp (ISSL) assesses symptoms of stress, the patients' stress level (alarm, resistance, near exhaustion, and exhaustion), and the kind of predominant symptoms present (physical or psychological) in the preceding 24 h, the preceding week, and the preceding month [12].

The Trier Inventory for the Assessment of Chronic Stress (TICS) consists of 57 items to evaluate different aspects of chronic stress in the following nine subscales:

work overload, social overload, excessive demands from work, lack of social recognition, work discontent, social tension, pressure to perform, social isolation, and chronic worrying [13].

The Screening Scale for Chronic Stress (SSCS) consists of 12 items to assess the following five aspects of the experience of chronic stress: chronic worrying, work overload, social overload, excessive demands from work, and lack of social recognition [13].

13.2.2 Measure of Coping Skills

The Brief COPE tool assesses the following 14 dimensions of effective and ineffective coping strategies: self-distraction, active coping, denial, substance use, use of emotional support, use of instrumental support, behavioral disengagement, venting, positive reframing, planning, humor, acceptance, religion, and self-blame [14].

13.3 Influence of Stress on Skin Function and Immunity

13.3.1 Influence of Stress on Skin Function

Stressful events influence cutaneous functions. Stressful life events preceding the onset of itching were found in >70% of the patients with AD [15]. Aioi et al. demonstrated that stress induces impairment of the barrier function and water retention property in stratum corneum in mice [16]. This impairment is concomitant with a decline in ceramide and pyrrolidone carboxylic acids, which are intensely hygroscopic amino acids. Moreover, Garg et al. reported that psychological stress delays recovery of the skin barrier [17].

13.3.2 Influence of Stress on Immunity

The systemic stress response affects two central biological systems. One system is the hypothalamic-pituitary-adrenal axis (HPA), in which various neuroendocrine mediators (i.e., adrenocorticotropin, β-endorphin, and cortisol) are produced in response to stress [18]. The other system is the sympathoadrenal medullary system, which regulates the release of epinephrine and norepinephrine [18]. Catecholamines and cortisol, which are stress hormones, mediate the differentiation of T-helper (Th) cells to Th2 cells. This differentiation results in an increased allergic inflammatory response [19, 20]. IL-31, which is produced by activated Th2 cells, causes pruritus [21, 22]. Elias et al. reported that an increase in endogenous glucocorticoids disrupts the barrier function of the skin, stratum corneum cohesion, and epidermal antimicrobial function [23].

Nerve terminals in cutaneous sensory nerves release neuropeptides, such as calcitonin gene-related peptide (CGRP) and substance P (SP), both of which have a variety of effects on the local inflammatory response [24, 25]. Mast cell stimulation by

SP and corticotropin-releasing hormone (CRH), which are secreted under stress and regulate the HPA, results in the release of proinflammatory cytokines [26, 27]. Mast cells also play a central role in neurogenic inflammation [28]. SP increases expression of functional CRH receptor-1 [27]. The correlation between neurotransmitters in psychodermatological pathways and skin inflammation is now well known, and mast cells, CRH, and SP have been implicated in a brain-skin connection [27]. Some degree of brain-skin connection underlies any inflammatory skin disease [18, 29]. Moreover, SP was shown to be involved in stress-induced hair loss in mice [30].

13.4 Treatment

Most treatments of AD, such as topical corticosteroid, oral antihistamines, and phototherapy for skin inflammation, have been prescribed using a standard medical approach. Adherence to treatment is difficult for a patient during the chronic course of AD, which has frequent flare-ups, but can be improved with a good relationship between the doctor and patient. Supportive psychotherapy by a clinician, with respect, acceptance, and empathy, is widely used with standard psychological therapy. To achieve success with this approach, the patient needs to clarify the level of his or her stress and what he or she defines as stressors. Using this information, the doctor analyzes the coping behavior of the patient and advises the patient regarding what would be an effective coping mechanism. For example, relaxation exercises may be of help in preventing habitual rubbing and improving symptoms of skin inflammation [31].

Identifying and avoiding the exacerbating factors of AD that influence the clinical course of this disease are important for long-term management of AD symptoms. The goal of psychodermatological treatment is to not only improve the condition of the skin but also to give advice to patients regarding how to cope with exacerbating factors using relaxation exercises, coping skills training, and stress management. This combined regimen leads to increased resilience against psychological stress.

References

1. Leung DY. New insights into atopic dermatitis: role of skin barrier and immune dysregulation. Allergol Int. 2013;62(2):151–61.
2. Kijima A, Murota H, Takahashi A, et al. Prevalence and impact of past history of food allergy in atopic dermatitis. Allergol Int. 2013;62:105–12.
3. Lammintausta K, Kalimo K, Raitala R, et al. Prognosis of atopic dermatitis. A prospective study in early adulthood. Int J Dermatol. 1991;30:563–8.
4. Morren MA, Przybilla B, Bamelis M, et al. Atopic dermatitis: triggering factors. J Am Acad Dermatol. 1994;31:467–73.
5. Chida Y, Hamer M, Steptoe A. A bidirectional relationship between psychosocial factors and atopic disorders: a systematic review and meta-analysis. Psychosom Med. 2007;70:102–16.
6. Kijima A, Murota H, Matsui S, et al. Abnormal axon reflex-mediated sweating correlates with high state of anxiety in atopic dermatitis. Allergol Int. 2012;61:469–73.

7. Higaki Y, Kawamoto K, Kamo T, et al. The Japanese version of Skindex-16: a brief quality-of-life measure for patients with skin diseases. J Dermatol. 2002;29:693–8.
8. Shirata K, Nishitani Y, Fujino Y, et al. The importance of mental support to the patients with adult atopic dermatitis. Osaka City Med J. 1996;42:45–52.
9. Hashizume H, Horibe T, Ohshima A, et al. Anxiety accelerates T-helper 2-tilted immune responses in patients with atopic dermatitis. Br J Dermatol. 2005;152:1161–4.
10. Ando T, Hashiro M, Noda K, et al. Development and validation of the psychosomatic scale for atopic dermatitis in adults. J Dermatol. 2006;33:439–50.
11. Turkoglu O, Mutlu HH. Evaluation of stress scores throughout radiological biopsies. Iran J Radiol. 2016;13:e37978.
12. Santos MA, Nakano TC, Mendes FA, et al. Emotional stress evaluation of patients with moderate and severe sleep apnea syndrome. Int Arch Otorhinolarygol. 2017;21:28–32.
13. Kuhlmann SM, Huss M, Burger A, et al. Coping with stress in medical students: results of a randomized controlled trial using a mindfulness-based stress prevention training (MediMind) in Germany. BMC Med Educ. 2016;16:316.
14. Carver CS. You want to measure coping but your protocol's too long: consider the brief COPE. Int J Behav Med. 1997;4:92–100.
15. Faulstich ME, Willamson DA. An overview of atopic dermatitis: toward a bio-behavioural integration. J Psychosom Res. 1985;29:647–54.
16. Aioi A, Okuda M, Matsui M, et al. Effect of high population density environment on skin barrier function in mice. J Dermatol Sci. 2001;25:189–97.
17. Garg A, Chren MM, Sands LP, et al. Psychological stress perturbs epidermal permeability barrier homeostasis: implications for the pathogenesis of stress-assiciated skin disorders. Arch Dermatol. 2001;137:53–9.
18. Arck PC, Slominski A, Theoharides TC, et al. Neuroimmunology of stress: skin takes center stage. J Invest Dermatol. 2006;126:1697–704.
19. Tausk F, Elenkov I, Moynihan J. Psychoneuroimmunology. Dermatol Ther. 2008;21:22–31.
20. Elnekov IJ. Glicocorticoids and the Th1/Th2 balance. Ann N Y Acad Sci. 2004;1024:138–46.
21. Dillon SR, Sprecher C, Hammond A, et al. Interleukin 31, a cytokine produced by activated T cells, induces dermatitis in mice. Nat Immunol. 2004;5:752–60.
22. Sonkoly E, Muller A, Lauerma AI, et al. IL-31: a new link between T cells and pruritus in atopic skin inflammation. J Allergy Clin Immunol. 2006;117:411–7.
23. Elias PM, Sun R, Eder AR, et al. Treating atopic dermatitis at the source: corrective barrier repair therapy based upon new pathogenic insights. Expert Rev Dermatol. 2013;8:27–36.
24. Toyoda M, Nakamura M, Makino T, et al. Nerve growth factor and substance P are useful plasma markers of disease activity in atopic dermatitis. Br J Dermatol. 2002;147:71–9.
25. Pavlovic S, Liezmann C, Blois SM, et al. Substance P is a key mediator of stress- induced protection from allergic sensitization via modified antigen presentation. J Immunol. 2011;186:848–55.
26. Fukudo S. Hypothalamic-pituitary-adrenal axis in gastrointestinal physiology. Chapter 28, section II: neuro-gastroenterology. Wood JD Section Editor. In: Johnson L, editor. Physiology of the gastrointestinal tract. 5th ed. Oxford, UK: Elsevier; 2012. p. 795–815.
27. Asadi S, Alysandratos KD, Angelidou A, et al. Substance P (SP) induces expression of functional corticotropin-releasing hormone receptor-1 (CRHR-1) in human mast cells. J Invest Dermatol. 2012;132:324–9.
28. Baldwin AL. Mast cell activation by stress. Methods Mol Biol. 2006;315:349–60.
29. Senra MS, Wollenberg A. Psychodermatological aspects of atopic dermatitis. Br J Dematol. 2014;170:38–43.
30. Arck PC, Handjiski B, Kuhlmei A, et al. Mast cell deficient and neurokinin-1 receptor knockout mice are protected from stress-induced hair growth inhibition. J Mol Med. 2005;83:386–96.
31. Ehlers A, Stangier U, Gieler U. Treatment of atopic dermatitis: a comparison of psychological approaches to relapse prevention. J Consult Clin Psycho. 1995;63:624–35.

Evolution of Animal Models of Atopic Dermatitis

14

Ichiro Katayama, Kohsuke Yamaga, and Hiroyuki Murota

Abstract

Historically, several atopic dermatitis (AD) models have been introduced and applied for the understanding of human AD and evaluation of the clinical effect of new drugs.

After the establishment of transgenic technology, several transgenic or knock-out mouse lines expressing atopic dermatitis-like phenotypes have been reported with promising results. However, it remains unclear as to whether Th2-type cytokines, IL-4, IL-5, or IL-13, play an essential role in the induction of the IgE-mediated reaction or if impaired skin barrier functions with abnormal itch perception play a more fundamental role in human atopic dermatitis.

Another point of discussion is whether IgE antibody itself induces spongiotic eczematous reactions occasionally observed in acute phases of human atopic dermatitis.

Keywords

Atopic dermatitis • Animal model • Monoclonal IgE antibody • Transgenic/knockout mouse

14.1 Introduction

Atopic dermatitis (AD) has been recognized as a representative, multifactorial allergic disease influenced by genetic factors since Besnier's first description in 1892 [1]. Dry skin, immunological dysfunction, increased IgE production, or autonomous nervous system imbalance is frequently observed in atopic dermatitis patients with bronchial

I. Katayama (✉) • K. Yamaga • H. Murota
Department of Dermatology, Course of Integrated Medicine, Graduate School of Medicine, Osaka University, 2-2 Yamada-Oka, Suita, Osaka 565-0871, Japan
e-mail: katayama@derma.med.osaka-u.ac.jp

I. Katayama et al. (eds.), *Evolution of Atopic Dermatitis in the 21st Century*, https://doi.org/10.1007/978-981-10-5541-6_14

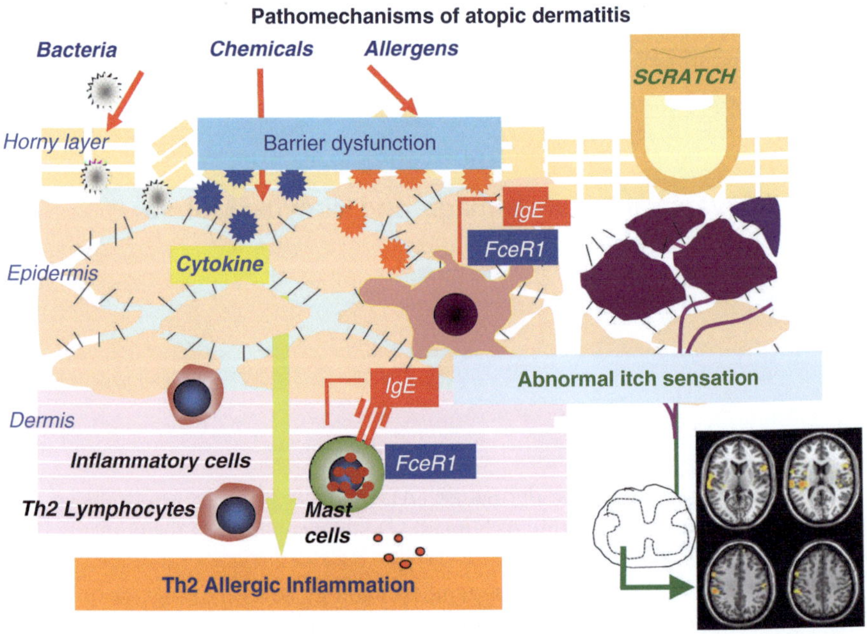

Fig. 14.1 Pathomechanisms of atopic dermatitis. Environmental allergens trigger the overproduction of IgE antibody when they come in through barrier-disrupted sensitive, atopic skin, while chemical or bacterial factors induce epidermal keratinocytes and fibroblasts to release several cytokines and predispose the skin to inflammation. Uncontrolled scratching behavior due to aberrant itch perception in the central nervous system is closely related with barrier-disrupted sensitive skin and Th2-skewed allergic inflammation

asthma or pollenosis closely related with genetic factors. Uncontrolled scratching behavior due to aberrant itch perception in the central nervous system is closely related with barrier-disrupted sensitive skin and Th2-skewed allergic inflammation. In 2006, Palmer et al. reported that common loss-of-function variants of the epidermal barrier protein filaggrin are a major genetic factor for the risk of atopic dermatitis [2]. Subsequently, these mutations have also been linked to atopic dermatitis, [3–5], asthma [6, 7], and allergies [8], and environmental factors initiate allergic diseases through penetrating the barrier-disrupted skin. However, induction mechanisms of eczema in AD and the relationships between overproduction of IgE and skin barrier dysfunctions, and abnormal itch perception, have been the matter of discussion since the nomenclature of AD was proposed by Hill and Sulzberger in 1933 (Fig. 14.1) [9].

14.2 Pathogenesis of Atopic Dermatitis

The skin of a patient with AD is often very susceptible to allergy and is called atopic skin [9]. Such vulnerability of the skin may result in a combination of genetic and environmental factors [10]. Environmental allergens trigger the overproduction of IgE antibody when they come in through the barrier-disrupted sensitive, atopic skin, while chemical or bacterial factors induce epidermal keratinocytes and fibroblasts to release several types of cytokines, which predisposes one to Th2-type skin inflammation. External ointments, cosmetics, and shampoos can also cause allergic contact dermatitis in some people, in addition to irritating atopic skin.

Recently, filaggrin (a keratohyalin granule-related small protein controlling skin barrier function) mutations have been reported to be closely associated with the risk of AD development and bronchial asthma in Icelandic and Japanese populations. Since the suggestion by Sulzberger that AD may be associated with the overproduction of IgE antibodies, IgE has been considered to play an important role in the pathogenesis of AD. However, the details of the involvement of IgE antibodies in the onset of AD remain unknown. Elevation of IgE levels in aggravated AD and elevated IgE titers in proportion to the disease duration in AD have been clinically observed. Experimental studies have demonstrated that FcεRI (+) Langerhans cells in the skin of patients with AD are more active in presenting antigens inducing the production of Th2 cytokines from T cells [11, 12]. These findings demonstrate that Th2 immune response with hyperproduction of IgE contributes to the development and progression of AD [13–15].

14.3 Animal Model of Atopic Dermatitis

To clarify this fundamental question, several AD models have been introduced, namely, the IgE transfer model [16]; topical sensitization models of protein antigens, such as ovalbumin [17]; *Dermatophagoides*-derived antigen (Dfb) [18]; or repeated hapten application models [19] and the spontaneous atopic dermatitis model [20, 21].

After the establishment of transgenic technology, several transgenic or knockout mouse lines expressing atopic dermatitis-like phenotypes have been reported with promising results. These include the Th2 or innate cytokine overexpression model [22–26], IgE transgenic model [27], and skin barrier-related protein-specific knockout mouse (Table 14.1) [28, 29]. We also previously reported a murine atopic eczema/dermatitis (AD)-model, with histopathological eczematous reactions [30–32]. Mast cells and inflammatory cells other than T cells are thought to play an important role in these IgE-mediated biphasic reactions [30]. However, it remains unclear as to whether Th2-type cytokines, IL-4, IL-5, or IL-13, play an essential role in the induction of the IgE-mediated reaction or if impaired skin barrier functions with abnormal itch perception play a more fundamental role in human atopic dermatitis.

It has been reported that scratching behavior itself is induced by itch perception and truly represents the behavior triggered by itch-induced brain sensitization [32]. Shimada et al. reported that wiping of the face with the forepaws represents hair grooming and scratching with the hind paws represents behavioral response to itch perception in rodents (Fig. 14.2) [33]. Another point of discussion is whether IgE antibody itself induces spongiotic eczematous reactions occasionally observed in acute phases of human atopic dermatitis. To address this question, we reported the passive transfer model of monoclonal anti-IgE antibody in retinoic acid-treated mice, as described below [30]. It is also an important issue as to whether the

Table 14.1 Summary of animal models of atopic dermatitis

Animal model	Authors	Year	Journals	Phenotypes
Anti-DNP IgE-induced dermatitis	Ray MC et al. [16]	1983	J Immunol	Biphasic skin reactions
Retinoic acid pretreatment and anti-DNP IgE-induced dermatitis	Katayama I et al. [30]	1990	Int Arch Allerg appl Immunol	Eczematous biphasic reactions
IL-4 transgenic mouse model	Tepper RI et al. [22]	1990	Cell	Eczematous reaction
Repeated hapten application model	Kitagaki H et al. [19]	1995	J Immunol	Th2-type skin reactions
Ovalbumin-painted model	Spergel JM et al. [17]	1998	J Clin Invest	Eosinophilic dermatitis
Keratinocyte-specific IL-18 transgenic mouse	Konshi H et al. [23]	2002	Proc Nat Acad Sci	Eczematous reaction
TSLP transgene expression model	Yoo J [24]	2005	J Exp Med	Spontaneous atopic dermatitis
IgE transgenic mouse	Mukai K [27]	2006	Immunity	Very-late-phase skin reaction
Flaky tail mouse model	Moniaga CS [28]	2010	Am J Pathol	Human atopic dermatitis-like phenotype
IL-33 keratinocyte-specific transgenic mouse	Imai Y [25]	2013	Proc Nat Acad Sci	Spontaneous itchy dermatitis
Linoleic acid (LA)-fed mouse	Fuji M [29]	2015	Exp Derm	Atopic dermatitis-like pruritic inflammation
Claudin-1 expression model in keratinocyte	Tokumasu R et al. [34]	2016	Proc Nat Acad Sci	Evolutional features of AD
IL-23-injected model	Ewald DA et al. [26]	2016	JACI	Morphological features of AD
Spontaneous occurrence of dermatitis				
Canine atopic dermatitis	Butler JM et al· [21]	1983		Dermatitis, asthma
Nc/Nga mouse	Matsuda H et al. [20]	1997		Spontaneous pruritic dermatitis

To clarify this fundamental question, several AD models have been introduced: the IgE transfer model [16], the topical sensitization model of protein antigens such as ovalbumin [17] or *Dermatophagoides*-derived antigen [18], the repeated hapten application models [19], and the spontaneous atopic dermatitis model [20, 21]. After the establishment of transgenic technology, several transgenic or knockout mice expressing atopic dermatitis-like phenotypes have been reported with promising results. These include the Th2 or innate cytokine overexpression model [22–26], IgE transgenic model [27], and the skin barrier-related protein-specific knockout mouse [28, 29]

Numbers are references in the text

evolution of skin manifestations are reproduced in animal models of atopic dermatitis. Recently, we reported that claudin-1 (CLDN1) knockout mice develop evolutional features of human AD (Fig. 14.2) [34]. To establish the evolution model of AD, we established several claudin-1 (CLDN1)-expressing mouse models. The

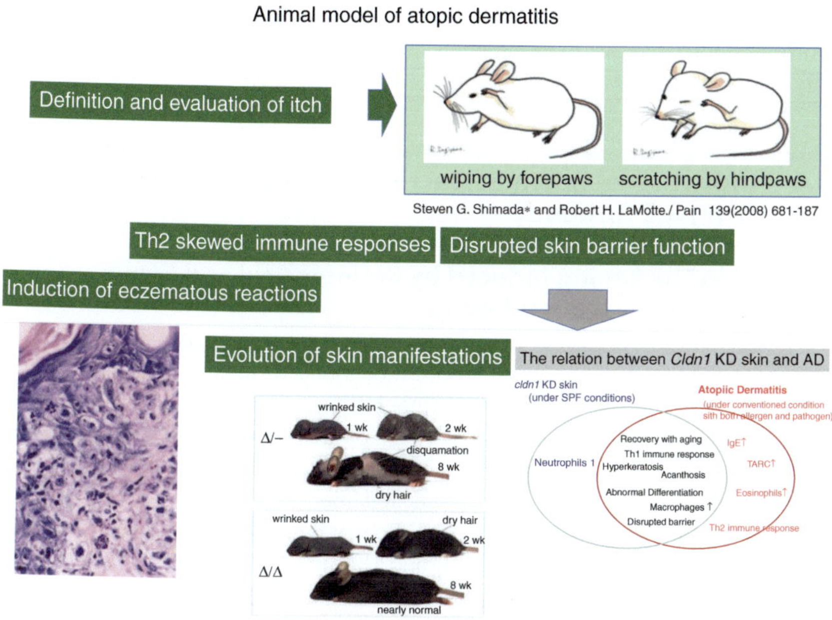

Fig. 14.2 Animal model of atopic dermatitis. Shimada et al. reported that wiping of the face with the forepaws represents hair grooming and scratching with the hind paws represents the behavioral response to itch perception in rodents [33]. Monoclonal anti-IgE antibody in retinoic acid-treated mice, as described below, induced spongiotic dermatitis mimicking human AD [30]. Claudin-1 knockout mice develop evolutional features of human AD [34]. The levels of CLDN1 were significantly lower in the skin of AD patients compared with controls

survival rate at 8 weeks was over 80% for Cldn1$^{+/+}$ and 0% for Cldn1$^{-/-}$ mice. Among the Cldn1 mutant mice, the Cldn1$^{\Delta//\Delta}$ and Cldn1Δ/- mice exhibited age-dependent changes in their skin appearance. Cldn1Δ/Δ and Cldn1Δ/- mice exhibited wrinkled skin at 1 week, abnormal dry hair at 2 weeks, and were nearly normal at 8 weeks. The Cldn1Δ/- mice, which usually did not survive beyond weaning, demonstrated more severe skin phenotypes, with severe desquamation and wrinkled skin at 2 wks; this phenotype had improved, but was still apparent at 8 wks, and only the Cldn1Δ/- mice, of all the mutant genotypes, still exhibited a different severity of skin lesions from WT at 8 wks by dermatitis score. The levels of CLDN1 were significantly lower in the skin of AD patients compared with controls. In skin samples from the trunk and limbs of human AD patients, after removing the outlier CLDN1 signals, we found that the number of macrophages was significantly inversely correlated with the CLDN1 signal. On the other hand, we found no correlation between the CLDN1 level and the thickness of the epidermis, the severity of AD by Eczema Area and Severity Index, or the serum level of defined AD factors including leukocytes, eosinophils, IgE, or thymus- and activation-regulated chemokine (TARC). Koomen et al. reported that mite antigens were more effectively presented by Langerhans cells that contained IgE antibodies on their surfaces [11]. Recent studies have reported that as FcεRI was not expressed on Langerhans cells of mice [35], their antigen presentation systems may be different from those in humans. Some reports demonstrated that mouse models using mite antigens are not appropriate for analyses of human atopic allergies [36].

14.4 Induction of Eczema Reactions by Monoclonal (Anti-DNP) IgE Antibody

14.4.1 Skin Thickening Induced by Retinoic Acid and Eczema Induced by IgE Antibodies

It was reported that eczema reactions could be induced by mite antigen patch tests in human AD patients [37] and that eosinophilic eczema reactions are induced by mite-specific IgE antibodies. For the purpose of analyzing these reactions, the following experiment was performed: monoclonal (anti-DNP) IgE antibody was intravenously administered to BALB/c mice and then DNCB was applied on their auricles and skin reactions were observed. In this case, bimodal reactions were observed: one early reaction after 30 min, and a late reaction after 24 h. Histologically, only moderate edema and mild invasion of mononuclear cells were observed, which were thought to be a kind of LPR reaction. Epidermal reactions were mild as well. As the epidermal layers of mouse skin are only 1 or 2 layers, histopathological findings observed in contact dermatitis, such as spongiosis of the epidermis or small round cell infiltrations, are not observed in mice. Therefore, retinoic acid (vitamin A) was applied five times to make the mouse skin more similar to human skin. After 10 days from the final application, inflammation reactions had disappeared and only thickening of the epidermis was observed. At this time, epidermis layers had thickened to 4–5 layers from 1–2 layers, and tissue mast cells had increased to almost twice as many as usual. In this condition, it was possible to observe eczema reactions, such as spongiosis of the epidermis or small round cell infiltrations, and even degranulation of tissue mast cells and invasion of eosinophils were observed. These results demonstrated that IgE antibodies could induce edema reactions by themselves. From another viewpoint, it could also be interpreted that in cases of plaques only exhibiting skin thickening without inflammation, which is often observed in AD patients, edema reactions could easily be induced by the activation of mast cells.

It is generally thought that in seemingly normal skin tissues of atopic dermatitis patients, cell adhesion molecules, such as intercellular adhesion molecule-1 (ICAM-1), which are expressed in keratinocytes of the epidermis or vessel endothelial cells, or vascular cell adhesion molecule-1 (VCAM-1), which is generated in vessel endothelial cells, are easily induced by scratching or other causes to make the preliminary conditions for inflammation [38].

As expression of ICAM-1 was observed in keratinocytes of the epidermis for a relatively longer time during the pretreatment with retinoic acid, certain reactions that are generally observed in atopic dermatitis patients may have occurred on the skin of the retinoic acid pretreated mice.

14.5 NC/Nga Mice Model Induced by Topical *Dermatophagoides farinae* Body (Dfb) Extract Application

After introduction of the spontaneous AD mouse model induced at conventional but not SPF conditions by Matsuda [20], the Nc/Nga mouse has been widely used for the analysis of pathomechanisms of AD or as a human AD model for the evaluation of newly developed anti-AD drugs. More recently, a mite antigen-induced AD model in Nc/Nga was reported at SPF conditions which enabled us to analyze more precise DP antigen-dependent skin reactions and to perform more accurate and convincing studies of the clinical effects of new drugs. For the application of this mouse model, we evaluated the effects of the anti-allergic drug, olopatadine, on scratching behavior induced by topical application of the mite allergen [39]. In daily practice, control of itch is an important issue in the treatment of AD. Itch is mediated by a variety of pruritogens, including histamine, and promoted by neurite outgrowth in the epidermis of AD patients, probably due to the release of nerve growth factor. Effects on mite antigen-induced skin manifestations in Nc/Nga mice are shown in Fig. 14.3. As shown, olopatadine markedly improved skin reactions due to decreased scratching behaviors (Fig. 14.4). Furthermore, olopatadine inhibited neurite infiltration into the epidermis, which may enhance itch perception (Fig. 14.5c, d) [39]. In contrast, topical tacrolimus markedly suppressed scratching behavior in this system, although neurite infiltration into the skin was observed (Fig. 14.5e). Recently, decreased production of the axonal guidance molecule semaphorin 3A in the lesional skin of AD resulting in increased epidermal innervation and itch perception was reported [40, 41]. Our study demonstrated that olopatadine robustly enhanced

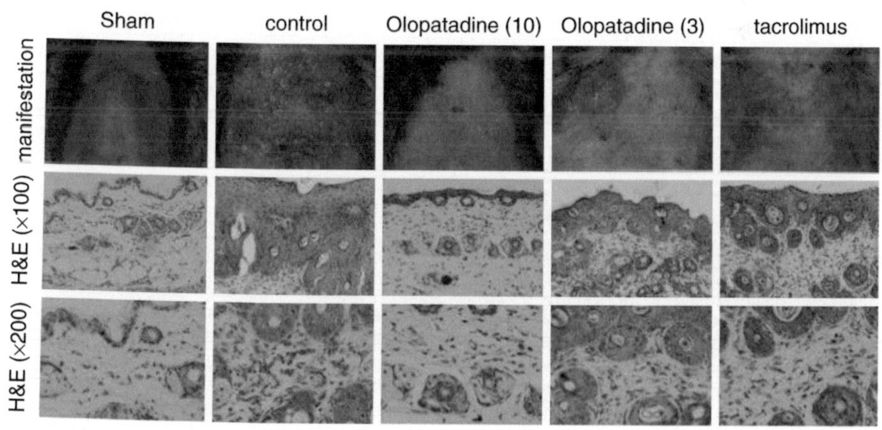

Fig. 14.3 Effects of olopatadine hydrochloride on Dfb-induced dermatitis in Nc/Nga mice: skin manifestations and histopathological findings. The gross appearance of the involved skin in the control group exhibited dryness, desquamation, erythema, crusts, and excoriation; these manifestations were relatively attenuated in the olopatadine and tacrolimus groups. Olopatadine markedly improved skin reactions due to decreased scratching behaviors with decreased mast cell infiltration to the eczematous skin lesions

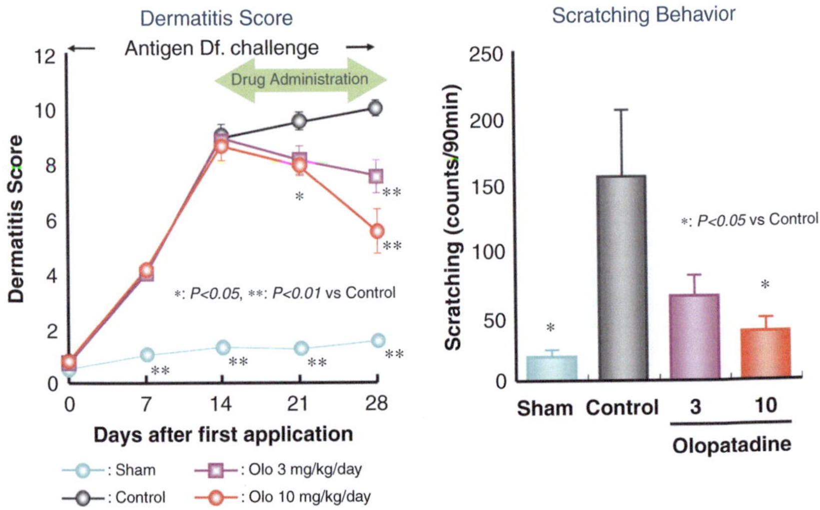

Fig. 14.4 Effects of olopatadine hydrochloride on Dfb-induced dermatitis and scratching behavior in Nc/Nga mice. Dfb treatment for 2 weeks elicited severe dermatitis. Although the dermatitis scores of the DDW group (control group) increased, those of the olopatadine (10 mg/kg/day) group significantly decreased beginning 1 week after the initial administration (day 21). After 2 weeks (day 28), the dermatitis score of the olopatadine group demonstrated a significant improvement. Olopatadine markedly improved skin reactions with decreased scratching behavior

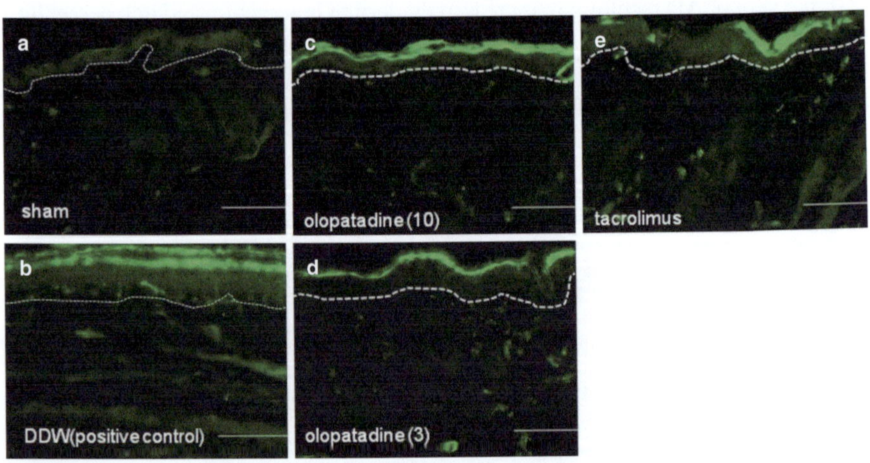

Fig. 14.5 Effects of olopatadine hydrochloride on Dfb-induced dermatitis in Nc/Nga mice: PGP9.5 immunostaining. Mite antigen-induced neurite infiltration into the epidermis with chronic hyperplastic epidermis (**b**). Olopatadine-inhibited mite antigen-induced neurite infiltration into the epidermis, which may enhance itch perception (**c, d**) [39]. Topical tacrolimus markedly suppressed scratching behavior in this system with decreased neurite infiltration into the skin (**e**). Sham refers to control skin without mite antigen application (**a**)

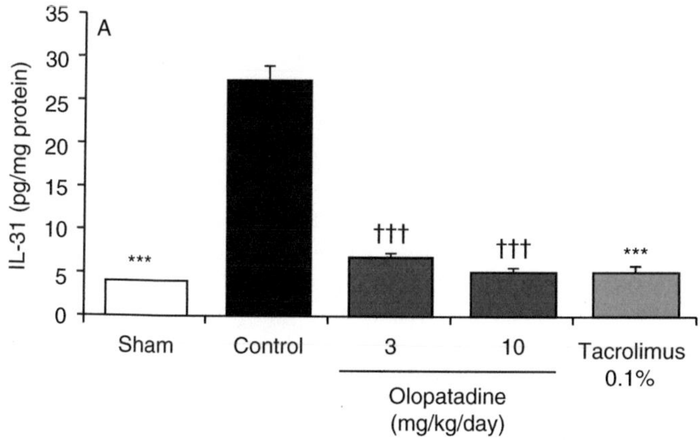

Fig. 14.6 Effects of olopatadine hydrochloride on IL-31 level in Dfb-induced dermatitis in Nc/Nga mice. IL-31 levels were significantly increased in mice that received Dfb application ($n = 10$) compared with sham-treated mice ($n = 6$). Olopatadine at 3 and 10 mg/kg/day ($n = 10$ each) significantly suppressed this increase in IL-31 levels by 88.1% and 94.5%, respectively. Tacrolimus ointment also significantly suppressed the increase in IL-31 production by 94.3% in the sham-, control-, and olopatadine-treated groups [43]

semaphorin 3A (Table 14.1). We also demonstrated that olopatadine decreased the pruritogenic cytokine [42], IL-31, expression in this Nc/Nga mouse [43]. IL-31 levels were significantly increased in mice that received Dfb application ($n = 10$) compared with sham-treated mice ($n = 6$). Olopatadine at 3 and 10 mg/kg/day ($n = 10$ each) significantly suppressed this increase in IL-31 levels by 88.1% and 94.5%, respectively. Tacrolimus ointment also significantly suppressed the increase in IL-31 production by 94.3%. In the sham-treated control and olopatadine-treated groups, IL-31 correlated positively with the tissue concentrations of several inflammatory and pruritus mediators including NGF, IL-1β, E-selectin, and amphiregulin ($r = 0.7574$, $r = 0.7324$, $r = 0.8368$, and $r = 0.6970$, respectively) [43] (Fig. 14.6, Table 14.2).

14.6 STAT6 Decoy Oligodeoxynucleotides (ODNs) on IgE-Induced Mouse AD Model

We used STAT6-deficient ($STAT6^{-/-}$) mice model [44] to demonstrate that STAT6 plays a central role in IL-4- and IL-13-mediated biological responses [31]. In an attempt to clarify the role of Th2-type cytokines, especially IL-4 and IL-13, in the IgE-mediated biphasic reaction, we examined the IgE-mediated response in the $STAT6^{-/-}$ mice in which the IL-4 and IL-13 signaling pathways has been completely abolished. To determine the inhibition of decoy ODN against STAT6 based on the response induced by anti-DNP IgE antibody, ear swelling response challenged by DNFB was examined with or without STAT6 decoy ODN or scrambled

Table 14.2 Summary of pharmacological effects of olopatadine hydrochloride on Dfb-induced dermatitis

	Control	Olopatadine
Number of scratching	↑	↓
Acanthosis	↑	↓
Neural invasion into the epidermis	↑	↓
IL-4, IFNγ	↓	→
TARC, IL-13	→	→
IL-1β, TNF-α, TSLP	↑	↓
Substance P, histamine	↑	↓
GM-CSF, E-selectin	↑	↓
NGF, amphiregulin	↑	↓
Semaphorin 3A	↓	↑
IgE	↑	↓

Olopatadine at 3 and 10 mg/kg/day ($n = 10$ each) significantly suppressed the increase in IL-31 levels by 88.1% and 94.5%, respectively. IL-31 correlated positively with the tissue concentrations of several inflammatory and pruritus mediators including NGF, IL-1β, E-selectin, and amphiregulin ($r = 0.7574$, $r = 0.7324$, $r = 0.8368$, and $r = 0.6970$, respectively). Olopatadine also decreased the tissue levels of substance P, histamine, TNF-α, and TSLP but did not decrease TARC [39, 43]

decoy ODN. STAT6 decoy ODN weakly inhibited the early phase response but not significantly, whereas the late-phase response was markedly inhibited by STAT6 decoy ODN, in line with Kaneda's report [45]. Next, we compared the effects of STAT6 decoy ODN between several injection routes. Interestingly, both the subcutaneous and intramuscular injection of STAT6 decoy ODN were effective; however, neither the intraperitoneal injection nor intravenous injection (data not shown) was effective. In the inhibitory study of STAT6 decoy ODN in different mice strains, STAT6 decoy ODN suppressed the late-phase response in BALB/c, C3H/He, and C57BL/6 mice; however, it was inhibited most strongly in BALB/c mice because BALB/c mice may be Th2-dominant mice. These data are consistent with the response of the late-phase reaction in STAT6$^{-/-}$ mice. In a preliminary study, we applied STAT6 decoy ointment to the refractory AD after ethical approval. A significant improvement of skin scores and pruritus were observed in four cases. Clinical studies are currently under way and will provide more information about the proper clinical use, indications, side effect, and usefulness in daily clinical practice in the near future.

Conclusions

Although considerable progress has been made in elucidating the mechanism of AD, the cellular and molecular mechanisms regulating AD still remain obscure. Summarized progress of the understanding of pathomechanisms of AD using animal AD models will provide new insights for the development of more evolutional therapies or drugs for the management of human AD, namely, evolutional clinical manifestations from infant to elderly patients with AD.

References

1. Holloway JW, Yang IA, Holgate ST. Genetics of allergic disease. J Allergy Clin Immunol. 2010;125(Suppl 2):S81–94.
2. Palmer CN, Irvine AD, Terron-Kwiatkowski A, Zhao Y, Liao H, Lee SP, Goudie DR, Sandilands A, Campbell LE, Smith FJ, O'Regan GM, Watson RM, Cecil JE, Bale SJ, Compton JG, DiGiovanna JJ, Fleckman P, Lewis-Jones S, Arseculeratne G, Sergeant A, Munro CS, El Houate B, McElreavey K, Halkjaer LB, Bisgaard H, Mukhopadhyay S, McLean WH. Common loss-of-function variants of the epidermal barrier protein filaggrin are a major predisposing factor for atopic dermatitis. Nat Genet. 2006;38:441–6.
3. Sandilands A, Sutherland C, Irvine AD, McLean WH. Filaggrin in the frontline: role in skin barrier function and disease. J Cell Sci. 2009;122:1285–94.
4. Baurecht H, Irvine AD, Novak N, Illig T, Buhler B, Ring J, et al. Toward a major risk factor for atopic eczema: meta-analysis of filaggrin polymorphism data. J Allergy Clin Immunol. 2007;120:1406–12.
5. Nomura T, Akiyama M, Sandilands A, Nemoto-Hasebe I, Sakai K, Nagasaki A, Ota M, Hata H, Evans AT, Palmer CN, Shimizu H, McLean WH. Specific filaggrin mutations cause ichthyosis vulgaris and are significantly associated with atopic dermatitis in Japan. J Invest Dermatol. 2008;128:1436–4.
6. Henderson J, Northstone K, Lee SP, Liao H, Zhao Y, Pembrey M, Mukhopadhyay S, Smith GD, Palmer CN, McLean WH, Irvine AD. The burden of disease associated with filaggrin mutations: a population-based, longitudinal birth cohort study. J Allergy Clin Immunol. 2008;121:872–7.
7. Weidinger S, O'Sullivan M, Illig T, Baurecht H, Depner M, Rodriguez E, Ruether A, Klopp N, Vogelberg C, Weiland SK, WH ML, von Mutius E, Irvine AD, Kabesch M. Filaggrin mutations, atopic eczema, hay fever, and asthma in children. J Allergy Clin Immunol. 2008;121:1203–9.
8. Marenholz I, Nickel R, Rüschendorf F, Schulz F, Esparza-Gordillo J, Kerscher T, Grüber C, Lau S, Worm M, Keil T, Kurek M, Zaluga E, Wahn U, Lee YA. Filaggrin loss-of-function mutations predispose to phenotypes involved in the atopic march. J Allergy Clin Immunol. 2006;118:866–71.
9. Hill LW, Sulzberger MB. Evolution of atopic dermatitis. Arch Dermatol Syphilol. 1935;32:451–63.
10. Andersen RM, Thyssen JP, Maibach HI. Qualitative vs. quantitative atopic dermatitis criteria–in historical and present perspectives. J Eur Acad Dermatol Venereol. 2016;30:604–18.
11. Grewe M, Bruijnzeel-Koomen CA, Schöpf E, Thepen T, Langeveld-Wildschut AG, Ruzicka T, Krutmann J. A role for Th1 and Th2 cells in the immunopathogenesis of atopic dermatitis. Immunol Today. 1988;19:359–61.
12. Bieber T. Fc epsilon RI on human Langerhans cells: a receptor in search of new functions. Immunol Today. 1994;15:52–3.
13. Vestergaard C, Bang K, Gesser B, Yoneyama H, Matsushima K, Larsen CG. A Th2 chemokine, TARC, produced by keratinocytes may recruit CLA+CCR4+lymphocytes into lesional atopic dermatitis skin. J Invest Dermatol. 2000;115:640–6.
14. Masuoka M, Shiraishi H, Ohta S, Suzuki S, Arima K, Aoki S, Toda S, Inagaki N, Kurihara Y, Hayashida S, Takeuchi S, Koike K, Ono J, Noshiro H, Furue M, Conway SJ, Narisawa Y, Izuhara K. Periostin promotes chronic allergic inflammation in response to Th2 cytokines. J Clin Invest. 2012;122:2590–600.
15. Soumelis V, Reche PA, Kanzler H, Yuan W, Edward G, Homey B, Gilliet M, Ho S, Antonenko S, Lauerma A, Smith K, Gorman D, Zurawski S, Abrams J, Menon S, McClanahan T, de Waal-Malefyt RR, Bazan F, Kastelein RA, Liu YJ. Human epithelial cells trigger dendritic cell mediated allergic inflammation by producing TSLP. Nat Immunol. 2002;3:673–80.
16. Ray MC, Tharp MD, Sullivan TJ, Tigelaar RE. Contact hypersensitivity reactions to dinitrofluorobenzene mediated by monoclonal IgE anti-DNP antibodies. J Immunol. 1983;131:1096–102.

17. Spergel JM, Mizoguchi E, Brewer JP, Martin TR, Bhan AK, Geha RS. Epicutaneous sensitization with protein antigen induces localized allergic dermatitis and hyperresponsiveness to methacholine after single exposure to aerosolized antigen in mice. J Clin Invest. 1998;101:1614–22.
18. Yamamoto M, Haruna T, Yasui K, Takahashi H, Iduhara M, Takaki S, Deguchi M, Arimura A. A novel atopic dermatitis model induced by topical application with dermatophagoides farinae extract in NC/Nga mice. Allergol Int. 2007;256:139–48.
19. Kitagaki H, Ono N, Hayakawa K, Kitazawa T, Watanabe K, Shiohara T. Repeated elicitation of contact hypersensitivity induces a shift in cutaneous cytokine milieu from a T helper cell type 1 to a T helper cell type 2 profile. J Immunol. 1997;159:2484–91.
20. Matsuda H, Watanabe N, Geba GP, Sperl J, Tsudzuki M, Hiroi J, Matsumoto M, Ushio H, Saito S, Askenase PW, Ra C. Development of atopic dermatitis-like skin lesion with IgE hyperproduction in NC/Nga mice. Int Immunol. 1997;9:461–6.
21. Butler JM, Peters JE, Hirshman CA, White CR Jr, Margolin LB, Hanifin JM. Pruritic dermatitis in asthmatic basenji-greyhound dogs: a model for human atopic dermatitis. J Am Acad Dermatol. 1983;8:33–8.
22. Tepper RI, Levinson DA, Stanger BZ, Campos-Torres J, Abbas AK, Leder P. L-4 induces allergic-like inflammatory disease and alters T cell development in transgenic mice. Cell. 1990;62:457–67.
23. Konishi H, Tsutsui H, Murakami T, Yumikura-Futatsugi S, Yamanaka K, Tanaka M, Iwakura Y, Suzuki N, Takeda K, Akira S, Nakanishi K, Mizutani H. IL-18 contributes to the spontaneous development of atopic dermatitis-like inflammatory skin lesion independently of IgE/stat6 under specific pathogen-free conditions. Proc Natl Acad Sci U S A. 2002;99:11340–5.
24. Yoo J, Omori M, Gyarmati D, Zhou B, Aye T, Brewer A, Comeau MR, Campbell DJ, Ziegler SF. Spontaneous atopic dermatitis in mice expressing an inducible thymic stromal lymphopoietin transgene specifically in the skin. J Exp Med. 2005;202:541–9.
25. Imai Y, Yasuda K, Sakaguchi Y, Haneda T, Mizutani H, Yoshimoto T, Nakanishi K, Yamanishi K. Skin-specific expression of IL-33 activates group 2 innate lymphoid cells and elicits atopic dermatitis-like inflammation in mice. Proc Natl Acad Sci U S A. 2013;2110:13921–6.
26. Ewald DA, Noda S, Oliva M, Litman T, Nakajima S, Li X, Xu H, Workman CT, Scheipers P, Svitacheva N, Labuda T, Krueger JG, Suárez-Fariñas M, Kabashima K, Guttman-Yassky E. Major differences between human atopic dermatitis and murine models, as determined by using global transcriptomic profiling. J Allergy Clin Immunol. 2016;139(2):562–71.
27. Mukai K, Matsuoka K, Taya C, Suzuki H, Yokozeki H, Nishioka K, Hirokawa K, Etori M, Yamashita M, Kubota T, Minegishi Y, Yonekawa H, Karasuyama H. Basophils play a critical role in the development of IgE-mediated chronic allergic inflammation independently of T cells and mast cells. Immunity. 2005;23:191–202.
28. Moniaga CS, Egawa G, Kawasaki H, Hara-Chikuma M, Honda T, Tanizaki H, Nakajima S, Otsuka A, Matsuoka H, Kubo A, Sakabe J, Tokura Y, Miyachi Y, Amagai M, Kabashima K. Flaky tail mouse denotes human atopic dermatitis in the steady state and by topical application with Dermatophagoides pteronyssinus extract. Am J Pathol. 2010;176:2385–93.
29. Fujii M, Shimazaki Y, Muto Y, Kohno S, Ohya S, Nabe T. Dietary deficiencies of unsaturated fatty acids and starch cause atopic dermatitis-like pruritus in hairless mice. Exp Dermatol. 2015;24:108–13.
30. Katayama I, Tanei R, Nishioka K, Dohi Y. Induction of eczematous skin reaction in experimentally induced hyperplastic skin of BALB/c mice by monoclonal anti-DNP-IgE antibody: possible implication for skin lesion formation in atopic dermatitis. Int Arch Allergy Appl Immunol. 1990;93:148–54.
31. Yokozeki H, Ghoreishi M, Takagawa S, Takayama K, Satoh T, Katayama I, Takeda K, Akira S, Nishioka K. Signal transducer and activator of transcription 6 is essential in the induction of contact hypersensitivity. J Exp Med. 2000;191:995–1004.
32. Ikoma A, Steinhoff M, Ständer S, Yosipovitch G, Schmelz M. The neurobiology of itch. Nat Rev Neurosci. 2006;7:535–47.

33. Shimada SG, LaMotte RH. Behavioral differentiation between itch and pain in mouse. Pain. 2008;139:681–7.
34. Tokumasu R, Yamaga K, Yamazaki Y, Murota H, Suzuki K, Tamura A, Bando K, Furuta Y, Katayama I, Tsukita S. Dose-dependent role of claudin-1 in vivo in orchestrating features of atopic dermatitis. Proc Natl Acad Sci U S A. 2016;113:E4061–8.
35. Hayashi S, Matsuda H, Okumura K, Ra C. Mouse Langerhans cells do not express the high-affinity receptor for IgE. Arch Dermatol Res. 1999;291:241–3.
36. Turner H, Kinet JP. Signalling through the high-affinity IgE receptor Fc epsilonRI. Nature. 1999;402(6760 Suppl):B24–30.
37. Mitchell EB, Crow J, Chapman MD, Jouhal SS, Pope FM, Platts-Mills TA. Basophils in allergen-induced patch test sites in atopic dermatitis. Lancet. 1982;1(8264):127–30.
38. Matsunaga T, Katayama I, Yokozeki H, Nishioka K. ICAM-1 expression on keratinocytes in mechanically-injured skin of a patient with atopic dermatitis. J Dermatol Sci. 1996;12:219–26.
39. Murota H, El-latif MA, Tamura T, Amano T, Katayama I. Olopatadine hydrochloride improves dermatitis score and inhibits scratch behavior in NC/Nga mice. Int Arch Allergy Immunol. 2010;153:121–32.
40. Tominaga M, Ogawa H, Takamori K. Decreased production of semaphorin 3A in the lesional skin of atopic dermatitis. Br J Dermatol. 2008;158:842–4.
41. Takamatsu H, Takegahara N, Nakagawa Y, Tomura M, Taniguchi M, Friedel RH, Rayburn H, Tessier-Lavigne M, Yoshida Y, Okuno T, Mizui M, Kang S, Nojima S, Tsujimura T, Nakatsuji Y, Katayama I, Toyofuku T, Kikutani H, Kumanogoh A. Semaphorins guide the entry of dendritic cells into the lymphatics by activating myosin II. Nat Immunol. 2010;11:594–600.
42. Sonkoly E, Muller A, Lauerma AI, Pivarcsi A, Soto H, Kemeny L, Alenius H, Dieu-Nosjean MC, Meller S, Rieker J, Steinhoff M, Hoffmann TK, Ruzicka T, Zlotnik A, Homey B. IL31: a new link between T cell and pruritus in atopic skin inflammation. J Allergy Clin Immunol. 2006;117:411–7.
43. Murota H, Abd El-latif M, Tamura T, Katayama I. Olopatadine hydrochloride decreases tissue interleukin-31 levels in an atopic dermatitis mouse model. Acta Derm Venereol. 2014;94:78–9.
44. Takeda K, Tanaka T, Shi W, Matsumoto M, Minami M, Kashiwamura S, Nakanishi K, Yoshida N, Kishimoto T, Akira S. Essential role of Stat6 in IL-4 signaling. Nature. 1996;380:627–30.
45. Kaneda Y, Iwaki K, Uchida T. Introduction of the human insulin gene in adult rat liver. J Biol Chem. 1989;264:12126–9.

Part V

Classification

Extrinsic and Intrinsic Atopic Dermatitis 15

Yoshiki Tokura

Abstract

Atopic dermatitis (AD) can be categorized into extrinsic and intrinsic types. The serum levels of IgE are high in extrinsic AD and normal in intrinsic AD. This dichotomy also corresponds to the following terminology: mixed AD vs pure AD, allergic AD vs non-allergic AD, and classical AD vs atopiform dermatitis. While extrinsic AD is the common type with high prevalence, intrinsic AD is approximately 20% in incidence and shows apparent female predominance. Extrinsic AD is closely associated with barrier perturbation and Th2 skewing immunological condition, but the causes and mechanisms of intrinsic AD remain elusive. In extrinsic AD, antigens can penetrate through disrupted barrier, and epidermal Langerhans cells serve as antigen-presenting cells to Th2 cells. In intrinsic AD, nonprotein antigens, such as metals and haptens, and Th1/Th17 cells participate as well as Th2 cells. Notably, intrinsic AD shows significantly higher percentages of positive patch test to nickel and cobalt than extrinsic AD, indicating high frequency of metal allergy in intrinsic AD.

Keywords

Atopic dermatitis • Extrinsic • Intrinsic • Filaggrin • Barrier • Stratum corneum Langerhans cell • Keratinocyte • T cell • Metal

Y. Tokura, M.D., Ph.D.
Department of Dermatology, Hamamatsu University School of Medicine, 1-20-1 Handayama, Hihashi-ku, Hamamatsu 431-3192, Japan
e-mail: tokura@hama-med.ac.jp

I. Katayama et al. (eds.), *Evolution of Atopic Dermatitis in the 21st Century*,
https://doi.org/10.1007/978-981-10-5541-6_15

15.1 Introduction

Several criteria have been widely approved for the definition of atopic dermatitis (AD). However, there still exist variations in the diagnosis of AD because of its heterogeneous aspects. The clinical phenotype of AD has been classified into the extrinsic and intrinsic types [1, 2] (Fig. 15.1). Historically, this dichotomy was first used for asthma. The terminology of extrinsic or allergic asthma was first introduced by Rackemann in 1947 on the basis of the triggering role of allergens. As counterpart, he described intrinsic or non-allergic asthma, which is characterized by later onset in life, female predominance, higher degree of severity, and more frequent association with nasosinusal polyposis. Intrinsic asthma was not improved by conventional treatments and was considered as a non-allergic type [3].

In AD, the extrinsic and intrinsic types began to be adopted in the late 1980s [4]. Historically, this dichotomy has also been represented by different terminology: mixed AD vs pure AD, allergic AD vs non-allergic AD, and classical AD vs

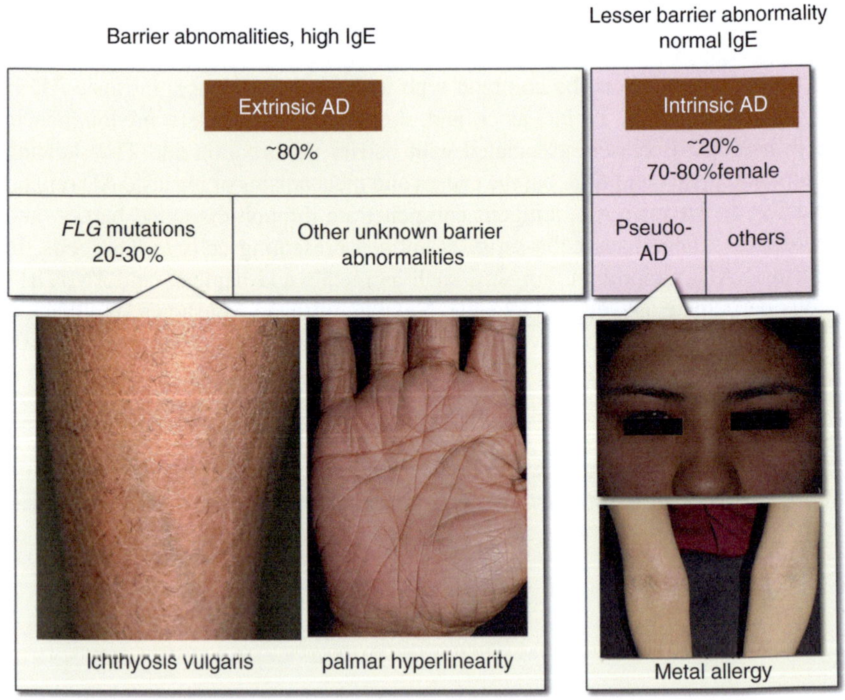

Fig. 15.1 AD spectrum encompassing extrinsic and intrinsic AD. AD can be divided into barrier-disrupted, high-IgE extrinsic type and barrier-preserved, normal-IgE intrinsic type. Some of the patients with extrinsic AD have *FLG* mutations and exhibit ichthyosis vulgaris and palmar hyperlinearity. Intrinsic AD affects mainly women and shows metal allergy in a considerable percentage of patients

atopiform dermatitis. The "mixed" type means concomitant occurrence of respiratory allergies [5]. The original concept of the non-allergic nature of intrinsic AD [1] may be misleading, since intrinsic AD is not a simple non-allergic type but is induced via some immunological mechanism. Since there is still no sufficient consensus whether the intrinsic type is a distinct entity, some researchers denominate it atopiform dermatitis [6]. However, the classification into extrinsic and intrinsic AD has been widely used especially since the millennium. Recently, various kinds of clinical studies have been performed under this nomenclature in many countries, including Germany [1, 7, 8], The Netherlands [6], Hungary [9], Italy [10, 11], Korea [12, 13], and Japan [14, 15].

15.2 Definition of Extrinsic and Intrinsic AD

Extrinsic AD and intrinsic AD are defined based on IgE-mediated sensitization, namely, the presence or absence of specific IgE for environmental allergens and food allergens [13, 14, 16]. Intrinsic AD has different features from extrinsic AD (Table 15.1). According to the EAACI nomenclature task force, the term "atopic eczema/dermatitis syndrome" can be used to cover the different subtypes of AD. In this nomenclature, the intrinsic type is termed non-allergic atopic eczema/dermatitis syndrome, which shows normal IgE levels, no specific IgE, no association with respiratory diseases (bronchial asthma or allergic

Table 15.1 Characteristics of intrinsic AD

1. Definition
Normal value of total serum IgE. Absence of specific IgE for environmental and food allergens. When the serum levels of IgE specific to mite antigens are graded into seven classes (class 0–6), intrinsic AD can be defined as total IgE $\leq$ 200 kU/L or 200 < total IgE $\leq$ 400 plus class 0 or 1 of DP- or DF-IgE and extrinsic AD as 400 < total IgE or 200 < total IgE $\leq$ 400 plus class 2 or more of the specific IgE [21]
2. Incidence
Percentage of intrinsic AD in total AD 10–45% (approximately 20%)
Female predominance (70–80%)
3. Clinical features in comparison with extrinsic AD
Higher frequency of Dennie-Morgan fold (Dutch study)
Lower frequencies of ichthyosis vulgaris and palmar hyperlinearity
Lesser severity of non-specific hand or foot eczema
Lower frequency of colonization of *Staphylococcus aureus*
4. Skin barrier
Relatively preserved barrier function
Relatively lower frequency of *FLG* mutations
5. Immunological features
High percentage of circulating IFN-γ-producing T cells
6. Contact allergens
High prevalence of metal allergy (Ni and Co)

rhinitis), and negative skin prick tests to common aeroallergens or food allergens [17]. Since total serum IgE values significantly reflect the allergen-specific IgE status [18], total IgE is a clinically useful parameter to differentiate between the extrinsic and intrinsic types in both adults [7, 14] and children [18]. The reported mean values of total serum IgE in the intrinsic type are from 22.2 to 134 kU/L, or alternatively, IgE values less than 150 or 200 kU/L have been used for an indication of intrinsic AD [19]. Our study of Japanese patients also showed that the mean value of total serum IgE was 110.5 kU/L [14] or 125 kU/L [15]. Considering relatively higher serum IgE levels in Japanese than Caucasian AD patients, these IgE values in intrinsic AD are very low.

Among specific IgE antibodies, infantile AD patients are more allergic to food [13], while environmental antigens are common in adults. It should be careful that some allergens are not useful to discriminate the two types. For example, IgE to *Malassezia sympodialis* was found in patients with the intrinsic type as well as the extrinsic type [20]. IgE levels to *Dermatophagoides* (*D*) *pteronyssinus* (DP) and *D. farinae* (DF) can be used for categorization of extrinsic and intrinsic AD as well as total IgE levels [21]. When the serum levels of IgE specific to these mites are graded into seven classes (class 0–6), intrinsic AD can be defined as IgE $\leq$ 200 kU/L or 200 $<$ IgE $\leq$ 400 plus class 0 or 1 of DP- or DF-IgE and extrinsic AD as 400 $<$ IgE or 200 $<$ IgE $\leq$ 400 plus class 2 or more of the specific IgE [21].

15.3 Epidemiology of Extrinsic and Intrinsic AD

15.3.1 Frequencies of Both Types

As extrinsic AD is commonly seen, dermatologists feel its prevalence on their daily examination. On the other hand, the frequency of intrinsic AD has been a matter of investigation. Schmid-Grendelmeier et al. [19] summarized the 12 reports that had been published from 1990 to 2000 and documented the clinical features of extrinsic and intrinsic AD. According to their study, the frequency of intrinsic AD was 10–45%. More recently, the incidence of extrinsic AD and intrinsic AD was reported as follows: 73% vs 27% [22] and 63% vs 37% [18] in German children, 88% vs 12% in Hungarian adults [9], 78.2% vs 21.8% in Dutch patients at the age of 13–37 years [6], and approximately 80% vs 20% in Korean [23]. These data are in accordance with the empirical knowledge that about 20% of AD patients show normal IgE levels and lack of sensitization toward environmental allergens. The prevalence may depend on environment, as intrinsic AD was higher in incidence in East Germany than West Germany, although the exact reason is unknown [8].

15.3.2 Female Predominance of Intrinsic AD

While extrinsic AD equally affects both males and females, intrinsic AD shows female predominance [1, 6, 10, 15, 24]. Our observation disclosed that 76.5% of AD patients were female [14]. More extremely, 14 intrinsic AD patients enrolled in a study were all female [24].

15.3.3 Relation to Age

Extrinsic AD starts at infancy or early childhood and may persist at adulthood with or without transient remission. The clinical course of intrinsic AD is an issue to be clarified. A Korean group of investigators showed that the intrinsic type is more prevalent in infancy, and even the third group of the indeterminate type between the intrinsic and extrinsic ones can be identified in younger generation [13]. A prospective birth cohort study followed for 5 years by a German group demonstrated that one third of child AD was the intrinsic one and more common in female [25]. Another German group indicated the low prevalence of the intrinsic AD among adult patients [7]. They showed 6.9% of patients fulfilled the criteria of intrinsic AD, and after follow-up, the incidence was declined to 5.4% because some patients developed respiratory allergies or IgE-mediated sensitizations. These observations may suggest that the intrinsic type is more prevalent in children than adults.

However, it should be careful that a considerable number of the above infantile or juvenile intrinsic AD patients possibly develop the extrinsic type as they grow and show high levels of serum IgE. Furthermore, the later onset was reported to be a feature of intrinsic AD [6]. It is tempting to speculate that the juvenile IgE-normal AD group contains two types, the genuine intrinsic AD and the IgE level-normal stage of extrinsic AD. In addition, as we see in Japanese patients with intrinsic AD, it may occur or deteriorate after high school age.

15.4 Clinical Characteristics of Extrinsic and Intrinsic AD

The skin manifestations of the two types of AD are indistinguishable. Intrinsic AD shares the vast majority of clinical features with extrinsic AD. However, a part of AD patients have filaggrin (FLG) gene mutations (20–30% in Japanese patients), and its frequency is higher in extrinsic AD [15]. Therefore, ichthyosis vulgaris or severe dry skin and palmar hyperlinearity may be more common in extrinsic AD (Fig. 15.1). It appears that keratosis pilaris, pityriasis alba, and non-specific hand or foot eczema may be more often seen in extrinsic AD.

Brenninkmeijer et al. extensively studied the clinical features of intrinsic AD [6] and found that the Dennie-Morgan fold is significantly more often present in the intrinsic type. However, we could not find such a difference in Japanese patients with AD. The later onset of AD and milder disease severity are characteristics of intrinsic AD. The features that are negatively associated with intrinsic AD include personal or family history of atopy, recurrent conjunctivitis, palmar hyperlinearity, keratosis pilaris, pityriasis alba, non-specific hand or foot eczema, and influence of emotional or environmental factors [6]. Some of these absent features are considered to stem from the lack of barrier disruption and/or filaggrin gene mutations in intrinsic AD.

15.5 Skin Barrier Function in Extrinsic and Intrinsic AD

15.5.1 Barrier Function of Stratum Corneum

Transepidermal water loss (TEWL) and skin surface hydration (capacitance) are representative barrier assessments. Extrinsic AD patients have increased TEWL and decreased skin surface hydration compared to healthy subjects. Intrinsic AD patients have higher levels of TEWL and skin surface hydration than extrinsic AD [23]. On the antecubital fossae, however, both types of AD patients have higher TEWL and decreased capacitance. We examined the skin surface hydration and TEWL at the nonlesional forearm and lower leg of patients and normal volunteers in a comparison between the extrinsic and intrinsic types [14]. The level of skin surface hydration was significantly lower in extrinsic AD than in normal control subjects. Thus, the skin barrier function is impaired in extrinsic AD and relatively preserved in intrinsic AD. The barrier impairment may induce allergic responses to external antigen in extrinsic AD (Fig. 15.2).

The skin perception threshold of electric current stimuli is one of the indices of itch. The electric current perception threshold significantly correlates with the skin surface hydration and inversely with TEWL in intrinsic AD patients as well as healthy individuals. In contrast, extrinsic AD patients do not exhibit such a

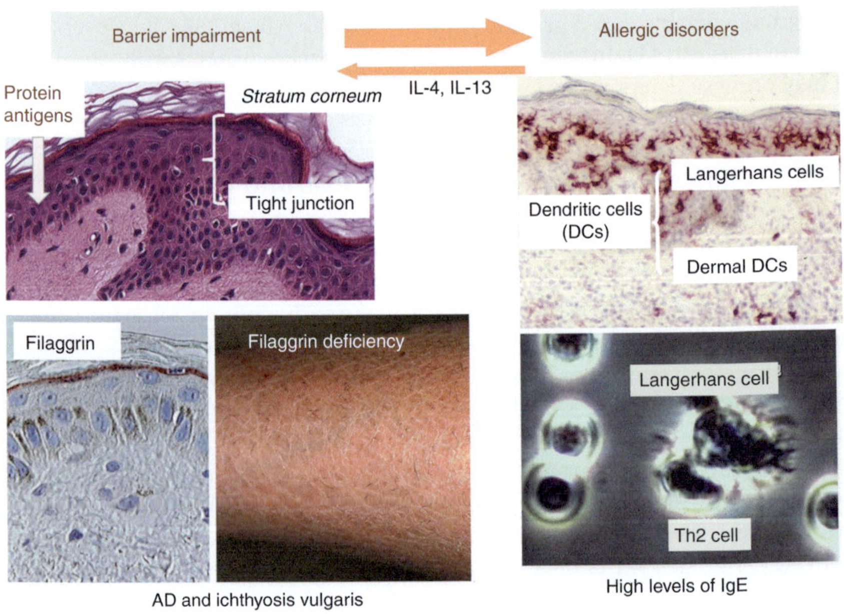

Fig. 15.2 Basic concept of extrinsic AD. In extrinsic AD, barrier impairment, which is typically associated with *FLG* mutations, induces allergic responses to external antigens, especially protein allergens. Langerhans cells (LCs) serve as antigen-presenting cells to protein antigens, and serum IgE is elevated as a result of Th2 responses

correlation. Therefore, intrinsic AD patients retain the normal barrier function and sensory reactivity to external pruritic stimuli [17]. We recently found that the frequency of sensitive skin is higher in extrinsic AD than in intrinsic AD.

15.5.2 High Frequency of *FLG* Mutations in Extrinsic AD

It is well known that loss-of-function mutation in *FLG* is a risk factor for AD [26]. These mutations also represent a strong genetic predisposing factor for atopic eczema, asthma, and allergies in various countries [27]. Profilaggrin is the major component of the keratohyalin granules within epidermal granular cells. During epidermal terminal differentiation, the profilaggrin polyprotein is dephosphorylated and rapidly cleaved by serine proteases, such as kallikrein-5 [28], to form monomeric FLG, which is further degradated into natural moisturizing factor. Perturbation of skin barrier function as a result of reduction or complete loss of FLG expression leads to enhanced percutaneous transfer of allergens (Fig. 15.2). The association of the *FLG* mutations in particular with the extrinsic type of AD was observed [15, 29].

Furthermore, *FLG* mutations are significantly associated with palmar hyperlinearity in patients with AD (Fig. 15.1), which represents a shared feature of AD and ichthyosis vulgaris (Fig. 15.1). This is in accordance with lower frequency of palmar hyperlinearity in the intrinsic type [6, 15]. We investigated *FLG* mutations in IgE-high and IgE-normal Japanese AD patients and found *FLG* mutations are less prevalent in the IgE-normal group [15, 21]. In the IgE-high patients, there was no statistical difference in SCORAD or IgE levels between the *FLG* mutation-bearing and *FLG* mutation-lacking patients. It has also been reported that *FLG* mutations predispose to early-onset and extrinsic AD [30]. Recently, we performed proteome analysis of extracts from stratum corneum of AD patients. The amounts of FLG were decreased in both extrinsic and intrinsic AD compared to healthy subjects, although the reduction tended to be more marked in extrinsic AD [31].

15.6 Immunological Abnormalities in Extrinsic and Intrinsic AD

15.6.1 Th1 and Th2 Cells

Although AD is a well-known Th2-polarized disease, there are some differences in systemic cytokine polarization between the two types of AD. In accordance with high serum IgE levels, extrinsic AD patients show high levels of Th2 cytokines, such as IL-4, IL-5, and IL-13, but intrinsic AD is linked with much lower levels of IL-4 and IL-13 [10]. Along with the elevation of IL-5 [32, 33], eosinophil counts [13] and eosinophil cationic protein levels [22] are increased in extrinsic AD. Meanwhile, there was a report demonstrating that both extrinsic and intrinsic patients had increased production of IL-5 and IL-13 [34]. However, when peripheral blood mononuclear cells were stimulated with anti-CD3 antibody, extrinsic AD patients had a decreased capacity to produce IFN-γ and GM-CSF as compared to the intrinsic AD [35]. The apoptosis of circulating memory/effector Th1 cells is confined to extrinsic AD patients, whereas intrinsic AD patients show no evidence for enhanced T-cell apoptosis in vivo [35].

Circulating IFN-γ$^+$ T-cell frequency was higher in intrinsic than extrinsic AD in our study [15]. Although not statistically significant, there was a tendency that the frequencies of circulating IL-4$^+$ or IL-5$^+$ Th2 cells were higher in extrinsic AD than in intrinsic AD. Intrinsic AD has a less Th2-skewing state but has a relatively high Th1 state, as assessed by IFN-γ-producing T cells (Fig. 15.3). The overproduction of IFN-γ may further downregulate IgE production in intrinsic AD, as suggested by our in vitro study [15].

In the skin lesions, eosinophils infiltrate in the dermis more markedly in extrinsic than intrinsic AD, and extrinsic AD exhibits more prominent deposition of eosinophil granular protein and higher staining for eotaxin [12, 36]. Although the levels of mRNA expression for IL-5, IL-13, and IL-1β are higher in both types of AD patients than nonatopic subjects, extrinsic AD shows even higher levels than intrinsic AD [36]. The expression of IFN-γ, IL-12, GM-CSF, IL-4, and IL-10 is elevated without differences between the extrinsic and intrinsic AD [35]. In the lesional skin, however, higher activation of all inflammatory axes, including Th2, was seen in intrinsic AD [37], suggesting an important role of Th2 cells in the development of intrinsic AD lesions as well as extrinsic AD lesions.

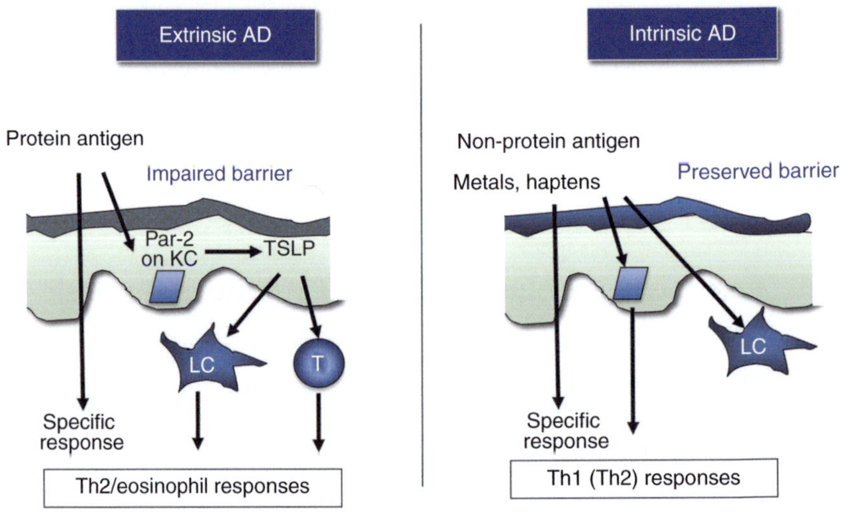

Fig. 15.3 Differences between extrinsic and intrinsic AD in the barrier status and immune responses. In extrinsic AD, the impaired stratum corneum barrier allows protein antigen to penetrate through the skin. The external stimuli via impaired barrier also stimulate keratinocytes to produce TSLP, which subsequently renders LCs to serve as antigen-presenting cells to Th2 cells. In intrinsic AD, nonprotein antigens, such as metals and haptens, can penetrate and function as antigen through the unimpaired barrier

15.6.2 Th17 Cells

We demonstrated that Th17 cells, producing IL-17A and IL-22, increased in the peripheral blood of AD and Th17 cells infiltrated in the acute skin lesions more markedly than in the chronic lesions [38]. There was a tendency that the frequency of circulating Th17 cells was higher in intrinsic AD than in extrinsic AD [15]. In the lesional skin, another group of investigators reported that positive correlations between Th17-related molecules and SCORAD scores were only found in patients with intrinsic AD, whereas only patients with extrinsic AD showed positive correlations between SCORAD scores and Th2 cytokine (IL-4 and IL-5) levels [37]. In AD, the acute skin lesion corresponds to the late phase reaction evoked by Th2 cells and eosinophils, while the chronic skin lesion corresponds to the delayed-type hypersensitivity induced by Th1/Tc1 cells [39]. Since Th17 cells exist already in the Th2-associated acute lesions, they seem to gradually disappear in the progression to the chronic lesion where Th1/Tc1 cells infiltrate.

15.6.3 Chemokines and Other Soluble Factors

Both extrinsic and intrinsic types show high serum concentration levels of Th2 chemokines, CCL17/TARC and CCL22/MDC, and high peripheral blood mononuclear cell expression of CCL17 and CCL22 at comparable levels [40]. We found that both groups had higher levels of serum CCL17 than healthy control; however, its value was significantly higher in extrinsic than intrinsic AD [15, 38]. The blood levels of soluble receptors derived from lymphocytes correlate with the activity in various diseases. There is no significant difference in the elevated amounts of sCD23, sCD25, and sCD30 between the two types [41].

15.6.4 Dendritic Cells (DCs) and Langerhans Cells (LCs)

An earlier study showed that extrinsic AD is characterized by a significantly high level of the expression of IgE high-affinity receptor (FCεR) on the CD1a^{+} DCs compared to intrinsic AD [1, 42]. When the high-affinity/low-affinity expression ratio was used as a disease marker for AD, the values for intrinsic AD fall below the diagnostic cutoff level, suggesting that intrinsic AD can be distinguished by phenotyping of epidermal LCs [1, 42]. In accordance with these data from the lesional skin, the surface expression of the high- and low-affinity receptor for IgE and the IL-4Rα chain is significantly elevated in circulating monocytes from extrinsic AD patients [3].

It is possible that epidermal LCs in the barrier-disrupted skin produce high amounts of Th2- and eosinophil-attracting chemokines. Recent accumulating evidence indicates that upon external stimulation, such as scratching and proteinases, epidermal keratinocytes produce thymic stromal lymphopoietin (TSLP), which stimulates LCs possessing TSLP receptors to promote Th2-mediated responses (Fig. 15.3) [43]. Moreover, TSLP directly stimulates Th2 cells bearing TSLP receptor to release IL-4, which leads to a vicious cycle [44]. Protein antigen is more essential than hapten as the cause of extrinsic AD. Upon epicutaneous application of ovalbumin (OVA), conditional LC depletion attenuated the development of clinical manifestations as well as serum OVA-specific IgE increase, OVA-specific T-cell proliferation, and IL-4 mRNA expression in the draining lymph nodes [45]. Consistently, even in the steady state, permanent LC depletion resulted in decreased serum IgE levels, suggesting that LCs mediate the Th2 local environment. In addition, mice deficient in TSLP receptors on LCs abrogated the induction of OVA-specific IgE levels upon epicutaneous OVA sensitization [45]. Thus, LCs initiate epicutaneous sensitization with protein antigens and induce Th2-type immune responses via TSLP signaling, suggesting that LCs play a mandatory role in extrinsic AD. In this scenario, the additional but powerful direct effect of TSLP on Th2 cells further exaggerates the response [44].

15.7 Association of Barrier Disruption with Skin Immune Responses in Extrinsic AD

15.7.1 Epidermal Cytokine and Chemokine Production in Barrier-Disrupted Skin

The skin immune status is closely associated with the disordered condition of skin barrier (Fig. 15.3). Studies using a mouse model of contact hypersensitivity (CHS) have shown that CHS responses to hapten are increased when a hapten is applied to the barrier-damaged skin [46]. Barrier disruption of the skin is experimentally performed by extraction of epidermal lipids with acetone or removal of corneocytes by tape stripping. Both procedures can induce elevated CHS responses. Not only increased permeability of hapten through the epidermis but also altered immune functions of epidermal cells potentiate T-cell activation in acute barrier disruption [46]. Such augmentation of immune reactivity may be critical to elimination of environmental noxious agents that penetrate easily into the barrier-disrupted epidermis, and it is also closely related to the mechanism underlying extrinsic AD.

Regarding epidermal chemokines of the barrier-disrupted skin, the mRNA expression levels of Th1 chemokines (CXCL10, CXCL9, and CXCL11), Th2 chemokines (CCL17 and CCL22), and eosinophil chemoattractant (CCL5) are high in the epidermal cells from Th2 response-prone mice. In particular, we found that CCL17, CCL22, and CCL5 were remarkably elevated in BALB/c mice [47]. Tape stripping induced dermal infiltration of eosinophils in BALB/c mice, and the late-phase reaction was increased with infiltration of Th2 cells as well as eosinophils, when challenged via the tape-stripped skin. Notably, Th1 chemokines (CXCL9 and CXCL10) and Th2 chemokines (CCL17 and CCL22) are derived mainly from keratinocytes and LC, respectively [47]. Therefore, it is likely that LCs serve not only as protein antigen-presenting cells [45] but also as Th2-attrracting chemokine source [48].

15.7.2 Implications for the Difference Between Extrinsic and Intrinsic AD

The above findings suggest that Th2 and eosinophil responses and resultant late-phase reaction are prone to take place in the skin with damaged barrier, providing the mechanism of Th2-polarized immunophenotype of extrinsic AD. On the contrary, LCs may not be stimulated to produce Th2 chemokines in intrinsic AD because of the presence of relatively normal stratum corneum. Protein antigens penetrating the damaged barrier further induce the Th2-shifted response in extrinsic AD, while nonprotein antigens exert the Th1 response in intrinsic AD (Fig. 15.3).

Th2 cytokine IL-4 suppresses ceramide synthesis and cutaneous permeability barrier [49]. This "outside-to-inside, back-to-outside" paradigm [50] is applicable for the pathogenesis of extrinsic AD. Neutralization of the normally acidic stratum corneum has deleterious consequences for permeability barrier homeostasis and stratum corneum integrity/cohesion attributable to serine proteases activation leading to deactivation/degradation of lipid-processing enzymes and corneodesmosomes [51]. Hyperacidification improves permeability barrier homeostasis, attributable to increased activities of two key membrane-localized, ceramide-generating hydrolytic enzymes, which correlate with accelerated extracellular maturation of stratum corneum lamellar membranes. Thus, the surface pH may be another important factor to differentiate between the extrinsic and intrinsic types of AD. These several different lines of evidence suggest the relationship between the skin barrier condition and helper T-cell polarization in AD.

15.8 Metal Allergy in Intrinsic AD

15.8.1 Patch Tests for Mite Antigens and Metals

An Italian group performed patch test with house dust mites at a concentration of 20% in petrolatum in adult extrinsic and intrinsic AD patients [11]. The patch test was positive in 47.4% of extrinsic AD and in 66.6% of intrinsic AD and in 12.2% of healthy subjects [11]. Since that extrinsic AD patients usually have high levels of IgE specific for mites, the authors wondered the reason why the patch test was highly positive in the intrinsic AD. Yet, patch tests can reflect mostly the T-cell-mediated contact sensitivity, and the IgE-high extrinsic property does not promote the patch test reactions. Rather, given that IFN-γ is produced at a higher level in the intrinsic than the extrinsic type, the higher frequency of positive reaction in the intrinsic type seems to be reasonable.

It is known in AD patients that the most frequent contact allergens are metals [52]. In 137 atopic children, 19.3% patients were positive to metals [52]. In 1965, Shanon reported that patients with metal allergy occasionally exhibit a skin manifestation indistinguishable from AD under the name of "pseudo-atopic dermatitis" [51, 52], and chrome is the causative in their report [53]. Some patients with AD were improved by intake of metal-free diet and elimination of metals [54].

The percentage of IFN-γ-producing Th1 cells is significantly higher in the peripheral blood of intrinsic AD than extrinsic AD [15]. Protein antigen is known to induce Th2 responses [43], and therefore, the impaired barrier of extrinsic AD may allow protein allergens to penetrate the barrier and to evoke Th2 responses. In this scenario, Th1-inducing nonprotein antigens, such as metals, might be causative for intrinsic AD [10]. In fact, high frequencies of positive patch test reactions to metals have been reported in AD patients [55, 56]. Nickel (Ni), cobalt (Co), and chrome (Cr) are the three major metals, and a high frequency of positive patch test to at least one of them is higher in AD patients than in non-AD patients [56]. However, the intrinsic and extrinsic types were not separately analyzed in those studies. Metals are administered orally as food and may be excreted from sweat at high concentrations as well as urine [57]. This notion raises the possibility that the concentrations of metals are high in the sweat of intrinsic AD patients.

In our study, intrinsic AD showed significantly higher percentages of positive reactions than extrinsic AD to Ni and Co (Fig. 15.1) [21]. The positivity to Co also tended to be higher in intrinsic than extrinsic AD. The prevalence of metal allergy to one or more of the three metals was more than twice higher in intrinsic AD (61.3%) than extrinsic AD (25.5%). In the IgE $\leq$ 100 group, the incidence of positive reactions to one or more of Ni, Co, and Cr was 63.6%, while the 400 $<$ IgE group exhibited 25.0% positivity. FLG deficiency may represent a risk factor for contact sensitization to allergens, such as Ni [17]. Therefore, the frequencies of positive metal patch test were analyzed in relation to *FLG* mutation. In the total patients, there was no significant difference in the patch test to the three metals between the *FLG* mutation-bearing and nonbearing groups [21]. The concentration of Ni was significantly higher in the sweat of intrinsic AD than extrinsic AD patients [21]. When the sweat Ni concentration was analyzed as the function of serum IgE values, there was an inverse correlation between them. Metals such as Ni, Co, and Cr are known to cross-react with each other [58]. Cross-reactivity may occur in patch tests depending on the concentration of metals and the moieties of vehicles. Metal allergy is one of the potential causes of intrinsic AD. Interestingly, Co allergy is more prevalent in females than males [15], which is in accordance with the female preponderance of intrinsic AD.

15.8.2 Th1-Skewing Responses of Ni and Co Allergy

Metals and haptens are representatives of nonprotein, small antigenic molecules. The mechanisms underlying Th1-polarizing action of metals remain unclear. Recently, Ni has been shown to activate toll-like receptor 4 (TLR4) signaling in antigen-presenting cells (APCs) such as DCs [59]. The same TLR4 simulation occurs with Co, and the necessity of histidines H456 and H458 of human TLR4 is evident for activation of APCs by Co [60]. Thus, metals can interact with not only major histocompatibility/self-peptide complex [61] but also with TLR4. TLR4 stimulation induces NF-κB activation and conversion of proIL-1β to IL-1β [59, 60], which has no skewing ability to Th1 or Th2 cells. Accordingly, Ni, Co, and Cr show a mixed Th1- and Th2-type cytokine response in peripheral T cells from sensitized patients [62], which is different from Th2-stimulatory protein antigens [43].

15.8.3 Significance of Metal Allergy in Intrinsic AD

Individuals highly ingesting or exposed to metals in daily life possibly develop AD via metal allergy. It has been shown that environmental Ni exposure is more important than genetic disposition, such as *FLG* mutation, in the development of Ni allergy [63]. Metals are administered with foods and applied to the skin with jewelry [57, 64]. Personal habits may increase the risk of development of contact dermatitis to metals. For example, women show a higher sensitization rate to Ni than men perhaps by wearing Ni-containing jewelry [65], which might result in the female preponderance of Ni allergy in intrinsic AD. It was reported that only piercing women in AD group had a higher incidence of sensitization to Ni but AD patient without piercing had no increased risk of Ni allergy [66].

Ni- or Co-rich food items include peanuts, hazelnuts, almond, chocolate, cocoa, sunflower seeds, beans, dried beans, porridge oats, licorice, lucerne seeds, oatmeal, and wheat bran [67–69]. Excess intake of these foods allows metal ions to be extraordinarily administered. Serum Ni levels correlate with Ni-rich food items. When Ni-allergic patients avoided Ni intake, their serum Ni levels were lowered compared to controls [65]. It is thought that metals are excreted through sweat, and therefore, sweating possibly may elicit dermatitis by serving as contactants. We found that the concentration of Ni was higher in the sweat of intrinsic than extrinsic AD patients [21], suggesting that metal allergy may be more significant in intrinsic AD. Eczematous lesions preferentially occur on the flexor aspects of the limbs and around the neck of AD patients. The degree of sweat secretion has been variously reported in AD. The possibility remains that Ni concentration is different depending on the skin sites, which might explain the predilection areas of intrinsic AD. Metal-free diet and elimination of metals improve skin eruptions in some AD patients [53, 54]. When Ni-allergic patients avoided Ni intake, their serum Ni levels were lowered compared to controls [64].

Perhaps more importantly, we recently found that Ni concentration is high in the peripheral blood of intrinsic AD patients [70]. In extrinsic and intrinsic AD patients and normal subjects, oral nickel loads were applied by using chocolate bar containing 235 μg nickel per day for 4 consecutive days. The dose of 235 μg is nearly equal to the amount of nickel that Japanese eat in daily meal. After nickel loading, the mean nickel levels (mean ± SD, ng/ml) were 3.59 ± 0.47 (intrinsic AD), 2.05 ± 2.87 (extrinsic AD), and 0 ± 0 (normal), respectively. Thus, the high serum nickel concentration in intrinsic AD was discernible as compared with extrinsic AD. Surprisingly, the nickel concentration levels before loading test were 2.79 ± 1.90 (intrinsic AD), 1.43 ± 2.15 (extrinsic AD), and 0.40 ± 0.93 (normal), respectively. Therefore, the serum nickel concentration is constitutionally high in intrinsic AD patients [70]. Serum nickel might sensitize circulating T cells, and they express skin-homing receptors upon repeated elicitation with serum nickel and migrate to the lesional skin. It is possible that the absorption or transportation of nickel in intrinsic AD patients is abnormally upregulated in a steady state.

15.9 Skin Infections in Extrinsic and Intrinsic AD

Both extrinsic and intrinsic AD patients suffer from recurrent bacterial and viral infections [71]. A higher colonization of *Staphylococcus aureus* was observed in the extrinsic (71%) versus the intrinsic children (49%) [72]. The expression of human β-defensin-3, an antimicrobial peptide, is decreased in both types of AD as compared to normal skin and psoriatic skin [71]. Therefore, skin infection with microorganisms, in particular *Staphylococcus aureus*, may be severe in the extrinsic type because of barrier perturbation, but it remains unclear whether or not the defense responses are different between the two types.

15.10 Neurotrophins and Neuropeptides in Extrinsic and Intrinsic AD

Given the original idea that external protein allergens are not causative in intrinsic AD, neurogenic inflammation induced by neuropeptides might be more important in this type [73]. Neurotrophins, nerve growth factor (NGF), and brain-derived neurotrophic factor (BDNF) are increased in both extrinsic and intrinsic AD, suggesting a similar pathophysiologic background implicating a neuroimmune network [33]. However, there is a significant correlation between BDNF and SCORAD only in intrinsic AD [33]. Maternal NGF levels were significantly higher in patients with both extrinsic and intrinsic AD than controls [41]. We measured plasma levels of SP in the two groups. The levels of SP in the IgE-high and IgE low groups were com parable [15]. In both groups, SP levels and VAS for pruritus significantly correlated with each other, indicating no dominancy of neuropeptides for intrinsic AD.

15.11 Animal Models for Intrinsic AD

Most of the mouse models of AD target extrinsic AD [74], since barrier abnormalities and/or IgE-related pruritus-prone consequences are thought to be a requirement for AD model. On the other hand, a non-IgE-associated AD model is regarded as a mode of human intrinsic AD [75]. In the mouse model of AD, IL-18 contributes the spontaneous development of AD-like skin lesions independently of IgE [76]. When the skin barrier was destroyed in the mice and protein A from *Staphylococcus aureus* was topically applied to the skin, the mice developed AD lesions with dermal infiltration of eosinophils and mast cells and showed an increase in serum levels of IL-18, but not IgE [77]. In this model, IL-18 might be important for the development of infection-associated AD by induction of IL-3 from IFN-γ- and IL-13-producing "super" Th1 cells. Since the intrinsic AD shows high levels of IFN-γ-producing cells [15, 34] and normal levels of IgE, this mouse model resembles intrinsic AD and suggests that some intrinsic AD patients may be related to infection. However, we could not find a significant elevation of serum IL-18 in our intrinsic AD patients compared to extrinsic AD patients. Thus, the IL-18 mediation remains unclear in human intrinsic AD.

Conclusions

The findings obtained from many studies suggest that intrinsic AD patients are not sensitized with protein allergens but with other antigens. Metals might be one of the strong candidates as antigens [21]. The extrinsic nature may be upmodulated as the patients grow. Therefore, the extrinsic and intrinsic types should be reevaluated at each stage of life, i.e., infancy, childhood, teenage, and adult, for the allergological management of patients, including allergen avoidance, second allergy prevention, and immunotherapy. However, the risk of an "atopy march" is significantly lower in children with the intrinsic type [17]. Again, it appears that the intrinsic type is not related to the pure Th2-dominant immunological state. Future studies on the intrinsic type of AD may clarify the pathophysiology of not only intrinsic AD but also dermatitis of unknown cause that have been called atopiform dermatitis [6] or pseudo-atopic dermatitis [54].

References

1. Novak N, Bieber T. Allergic and nonallergic forms of atopic diseases. J Allergy Clin Immunol. 2003;112:252–62.
2. Tokura Y. Extrinsic and intrinsic types of atopic dermatitis. J Dermatol Sci. 2010;58:1–7.
3. Romanet-Manent S, Charpin D, Magnan A, Lanteaume A, Vervloet D. Allergic vs nonallergic asthma: what makes the difference? Allergy. 2002;57:607–13.
4. Wuthrich B. Atopic dermatitis. Ther Umsch. 1989;46:633–40.
5. Diepgen TL, Fartasch M. Recent epidemiological and genetic studies in atopic dermatitis. Acta Derm Venereol. 1992;176:13–8.
6. Brenninkmeijer EE, Spuls PI, Legierse CM, Lindeboom R, Smitt JH, Bos JD. Clinical differences between atopic and atopiform dermatitis. J Am Acad Dermatol. 2008;58:407–14.
7. Folster-Holst R, Pape M, Buss YL, Christophers E, Weichenthal M. Low prevalence of the intrinsic form of atopic dermatitis among adult patients. Allergy. 2006;61:629–32.
8. Schafer T, Kramer U, Vieluf D, Abeck D, Behrendt H, Ring J. The excess of atopic eczema in east germany is related to the intrinsic type. Br J Dermatol. 2000;143:992–8.
9. Ponyai G, Hidvegi B, Nemeth I, Sas A, Temesvari E, Karpati S. Contact and aeroallergens in adulthood atopic dermatitis. J Eur Acad Dermatol Venereol. 2008;22:1346–55.
10. Miraglia del Giudice M, Decimo F, Leonardi S, Maioello N, Amelio R, Capasso A, et al. Immune dysregulation in atopic dermatitis. Allergy Asthma Proc. 2006;27:451–5.
11. Ingordo V, D'Andria G, D'Andria C, Tortora A. Results of atopy patch tests with house dust mites in adults with 'intrinsic' and 'extrinsic' atopic dermatitis. J Eur Acad Dermatol Venereol. 2002;16:450–4.
12. Rho NK, Kim WS, Lee DY, Lee JH, Lee ES, Yang JM. Immunophenotyping of inflammatory cells in lesional skin of the extrinsic and intrinsic types of atopic dermatitis. Br J Dermatol. 2004;151:119–25.
13. Park JH, Choi YL, Namkung JH, Kim WS, Lee JH, Park HJ, et al. Characteristics of extrinsic vs. intrinsic atopic dermatitis in infancy: correlations with laboratory variables. Br J Dermatol. 2006;155:778–83.

14. Mori T, Ishida K, Mukumoto S, Yamada Y, Imokawa G, Kabashima K, et al. Comparison of skin barrier function and sensory nerve electric current perception threshold between ige-high extrinsic and ige-normal intrinsic types of atopic dermatitis. Br J Dermatol. 2009;162(1):83–90.
15. Kabashima-Kubo R, Nakamura M, Sakabe JI, Sugita K, Hino R, Mori T, Kobayashi M, Bito T, Kabashima K, Ogasawara K, Nomura Y, Nomura T, Akiyama M, Shimizu H, Tokura Y. A group of atopic dermatitis without IgE elevation or barrier impairment shows a high Th1 frequency: possible immunological state of the intrinsic type. J Dermatol Sci. 2012;67:37–43.
16. Wollenberg A, Kraft S, Oppel T, Bieber T. Atopic dermatitis: pathogenetic mechanisms. Clin Exp Dermatol. 2000;25:530–4.
17. Wuthrich B, Schmid-Grendelmeier P. The atopic eczema/dermatitis syndrome. Epidemiology, natural course, and immunology of the IgE-associated ("extrinsic") and the nonallergic ("intrinsic") AEDS. J Investig Allergol Clin Immunol. 2003;13:1–5.
18. Ott H, Stanzel S, Ocklenburg C, Merk HF, Baron JM, Lehmann S. Total serum ige as a parameter to differentiate between intrinsic and extrinsic atopic dermatitis in children. Acta Derm Venereol. 2009;89:257–61.
19. Schmid-Grendelmeier P, Simon D, Simon HU, Akdis CA, Wuthrich B. Epidemiology, clinical features, and immunology of the "intrinsic" (non-IgE-mediated) type of atopic dermatitis (constitutional dermatitis). Allergy. 2001;56:841–9.
20. Casagrande BF, Fluckiger S, Linder MT, Johansson C, Scheynius A, Crameri R, et al. Sensitization to the yeast malassezia sympodialis is specific for extrinsic and intrinsic atopic eczema. J Invest Dermatol. 2006;126:2414–21.
21. Yamaguchi H, Kabashima-Kubo R, Bito T, Sakabe J-I, Shimauchi T, Ito T, Hirakawa S, Hirasawa N, Ogasawara K, Tokura Y. High frequencies of positive nickel/cobalt patch tests and high sweat nickel concentration in patients with intrinsic atopic dermatitis. J Dermatol Sci. 2013;72(3):240–5. (in press)
22. Ott H, Wilke J, Baron JM, Hoger PH, Folster-Holst R. Soluble immune receptor serum levels are associated with age, but not with clinical phenotype or disease severity in childhood atopic dermatitis. J Eur Acad Dermatol Venereol. 2009;24(4):395–402.
23. Choi SJ, Song MG, Sung WT, Lee DY, Lee JH, Lee ES, et al. Comparison of transepidermal water loss, capacitance and pH values in the skin between intrinsic and extrinsic atopic dermatitis patients. J Korean Med Sci. 2003;18:93–6.
24. Novak N, Kruse S, Kraft S, Geiger E, Kluken H, Fimmers R, et al. Dichotomic nature of atopic dermatitis reflected by combined analysis of monocyte immunophenotyping and single nucleotide polymorphisms of the interleukin-4/interleukin-13 receptor gene: the dichotomy of extrinsic and intrinsic atopic dermatitis. J Invest Dermatol. 2002;119:870–5.
25. Kusel MM, Holt PG, de Klerk N, Sly PD. Support for 2 variants of eczema. J Allergy Clin Immunol. 2005;116:1067–72.
26. Palmer CN, Irvine AD, Terron-Kwiatkowski A, Zhao Y, Liao H, Lee SP, et al. Common loss-of-function variants of the epidermal barrier protein filaggrin are a major predisposing factor for atopic dermatitis. Nat Genet. 2006;38:441–6.
27. Nomura T, Akiyama M, Sandilands A, Nemoto-Hasebe I, Sakai K, Nagasaki A, et al. Specific filaggrin mutations cause ichthyosis vulgaris and are significantly associated with atopic dermatitis in japan. J Invest Dermatol. 2008;128:1436–41.
28. Sakabe J, Yamamoto M, Hirakawa S, Motoyama A, Ohta I, Tatsuno K, Ito T, Kabashima K, Hibino T, Tokura Y. Kallikrein-related peptidase 5 functions in proteolytic processing of profilaggrin in cultured human keratinocytes. J Biol Chem. 2013;288:17179–89.
29. Weidinger S, Illig T, Baurecht H, Irvine AD, Rodriguez E, Diaz-Lacava A, et al. Loss-of-function variations within the filaggrin gene predispose for atopic dermatitis with allergic sensitizations. J Allergy Clin Immunol. 2006;118:214–9.
30. Weidinger S, Rodriguez E, Stahl C, et al. Filaggrin mutations strongly predispose to early-onset and extrinsic atopic dermatitis. J Invest Dermatol. 2007;127:724–6.

31. Sakabe J, Kamiya K, Yamaguchi H, Ikeya S, Suzuki T, Aoshima M, Tatsuno K, Fujiyama T, Suzuki M, Yatagai T, Ito T, Ojima T, Tokura Y. Proteome analysis of stratum corneum from atopic dermatitis patients by hybrid quadrupole-orbitrap mass spectrometer. J Allergy Clin Immunol. 2014;134:957–60.
32. Namkung JH, Lee JE, Kim E, Cho HJ, Kim S, Shin ES, et al. IL-5 and IL-5 receptor alpha polymorphisms are associated with atopic dermatitis in koreans. Allergy. 2007;62:934–42.
33. Raap U, Werfel T, Goltz C, Deneka N, Langer K, Bruder M, et al. Circulating levels of brain-derived neurotrophic factor correlate with disease severity in the intrinsic type of atopic dermatitis. Allergy. 2006;61:1416–8.
34. Simon D, Von Gunten S, Borelli S, Braathen LR, Simon HU. The interleukin-13 production by peripheral blood T cells from atopic dermatitis patients does not require CD2 costimulation. Int Arch Allergy Immunol. 2003;132:148–55.
35. Akdis M, Trautmann A, Klunker S, Daigle I, Kucuksezer UC, Deglmann W, Disch R, Blaser K, Akdis CA. T helper (Th) 2 predominance in atopic diseases is due to preferential apoptosis of circulating memory/effector Th1 cells. FASEB J. 2003;17:1026–35.
36. Jeong CW, Ahn KS, Rho NK, Park YD, Lee DY, Lee JH, et al. Differential in vivo cytokine mrna expression in lesional skin of intrinsic vs. extrinsic atopic dermatitis patients using semi-quantitative rt-pcr. Clin Exp Allergy. 2003;33:1717–24.
37. Suárez-Fariñas M, Dhingra N, Gittler J, Shemer A, Cardinale I, de Guzman Strong C, Krueger JG, Guttman-Yassky E. Intrinsic atopic dermatitis shows similar TH2 and higher TH17 immune activation compared with extrinsic atopic dermatitis. J Allergy Clin Immunol. 2013;132:361–70.
38. Koga C, Kabashima K, Shiraishi N, Kobayashi M, Tokura Y. Possible pathogenic role of Th17 cells for atopic dermatitis. J Invest Dermatol. 2008;128:2625–30.
39. Oyoshi MK, He R, Kumar L, Yoon J, Geha RS. Cellular and molecular mechanisms in atopic dermatitis. Adv Immunol. 2009;102:135–226.
40. Park CO, Lee HJ, Lee JH, Wu WH, Chang NS, Hua L, et al. Increased expression of cc chemokine ligand 18 in extrinsic atopic dermatitis patients. Exp Dermatol. 2008;17:24–9.
41. Wang IJ, Hsieh WS, Guo YL, Jee SH, Hsieh CJ, Hwang YH, et al. Neuro-mediators as predictors of paediatric atopic dermatitis. Clin Exp Allergy. 2008;38:1302–8.
42. Oppel T, Schuller E, Gunther S, Moderer M, Haberstok J, Bieber T, et al. Phenotyping of epidermal dendritic cells allows the differentiation between extrinsic and intrinsic forms of atopic dermatitis. Br J Dermatol. 2000;143:1193–8.
43. Kabashima K. New concept of the pathogenesis of atopic dermatitis: interplay among the barrier, allergy, and pruritus as a trinity. J Dermatol Sci. 2013;70:3 11.
44. Tatsuno K, Fujiyama T, Yamaguchi H, Waki M, Tokura Y. TSLP directly interacts with skin-homing Th2 cells highly expressing its receptor to enhance IL-4 production in atopic dermatitis. J Invest Dermatol. 2015;135:3017–24.
45. Nakajima S, Igyártó BZ, Honda T, Egawa G, Otsuka A, Hara-Chikuma M, Watanabe N, Ziegler SF, Tomura M, Inaba K, Miyachi Y, Kaplan DH, Kabashima K. Langerhans cells are critical in epicutaneous sensitization with protein antigen via thymic stromal lymphopoietin receptor signaling. J Allergy Clin Immunol. 2013;129:1048–55.
46. Nishijima T, Tokura Y, Imokawa G, Seo N, Furukawa F, Takigawa M. Altered permeability and disordered cutaneous immunoregulatory function in mice with acute barrier disruption. J Invest Dermatol. 1997;109:175–82.
47. Onoue A, Kabashima K, Kobayashi M, Mori T, Tokura Y. Induction of eosinophil- and th2-attracting epidermal chemokines and cutaneous late-phase reaction in tape-stripped skin. Exp Dermatol. 2009;18:1036–43.
48. Mori T, Kabashima K, Yoshiki R, Sugita K, Shiraishi N, Onoue A, et al. Cutaneous hypersensitivities to hapten are controlled by ifn-gamma-upregulated keratinocyte th1 chemokines and ifn-gamma-downregulated langerhans cell th2 chemokines. J Invest Dermatol. 2008;128:1719–27.

49. Hatano Y, Terashi H, Arakawa S, Katagiri K. Interleukin-4 suppresses the enhancement of ceramide synthesis and cutaneous permeability barrier functions induced by tumor necrosis factor-alpha and interferon-gamma in human epidermis. J Invest Dermatol. 2005;124:786–92.
50. Elias PM, Schmuth M. Abnormal skin barrier in the etiopathogenesis of atopic dermatitis. Curr Opin Allergy Clin Immunol. 2009;9:437–46.
51. Hachem JP, Roelandt T, Schurer N, Pu X, Fluhr J, Giddelo C, et al. Acute acidification of stratum corneum membrane domains using polyhydroxyl acids improves lipid processing and inhibits degradation of corneodesmosomes. J Invest Dermatol. 2010;130:500–10.
52. Giordano-Labadie F, Rance F, Pellegrin F, Bazex J, Dutau G, Schwarze HP. Frequency of contact allergy in children with atopic dermatitis: results of a prospective study of 137 cases. Contact Dermatitis. 1999;40:192–5.
53. Shanon J. Pseudo-atopic dermatitis. Contact dermatitis due to chrome sensitivity simulating atopic dermatitis. Dermatologica. 1965;131:176–90.
54. De CP, Decock PA, Shanon J. Pseudo-atopic dermatitis. An example of pseudo-nomenclature. Dermatologica. 1966;133:236–7.
55. Ruff CA, Belsito DV. The impact of various patients factors on contact allergy to nickel, cobalt, and chrome. J Am Acad Dermatol. 2006;55:32–9.
56. Dena M, Donald VB. Cutaneous delayed-type hypersensitivity in patients with atopic dermatitis. J Am Acad Dermatol. 2013;70(1):102–7.
57. Jensen CS, Menné T, Lisby S, Kristiansen J, Veien NK. Experimental systemic contact dermatitis from nickel: a dose-response study. Contact Dermatitis. 2003;49:124–32.
58. Lammintausta K, Pitkänen OP, Kalimo K, et al. Interrelationship of nickel and cobalt contact sensitization. Contact Dermatitis. 1985;13:148–52.
59. Schmidt M, Raghavan B, Müller V, Vogl T, Fejer G, Tchaptchet S, et al. Crucial role for human toll-like receptor 4 in the development of contact allergy to nickel. Nat Immunol. 2010;11:814–9.
60. Raghavan B, Martin SF, Esser PR, Goebeler M, Schmidt M. Metal allergens nickel and cobalt facilitate TLR4 homodimerization independently of MD2. EMBO Rep. 2012;13:1109–15.
61. Schram SE, Warshaw EM. Genetics of nickel allergic contact dermatitis. Dermatitis. 2007;18:125–33.
62. Minang JT, Areström I, Troye-Blomberg M, Lundeberg L, Ahlborg N. Nickel, cobalt, chromium, palladium and gold induce a mixed Th1- and Th2-type cytokine response in vitro in subjects with contact allergy to the respective metals. Clin Exp Immunol. 2006;146:417–26.
63. Thyssen JP. Nickel and cobalt allergy before and after nickel regulation: evaluation of a public health intervention. Contact Dermatitis. 2011;65(Suppl. 1):1–68.
64. Darsow U, Fedorov M, Schwegler U, Twardella D, Schaller KH, Habernegg R, et al. Influence of dietary factors, age and nickel contact dermatitis on nickel excretion. Contact Dermatitis. 2012;67:351–8.
65. Martin SF, Esser PR, Weber FC, Jakob T, Freudenberg MA, Scmidt M, et al. Mechanisms of chemical-induced innate immunity in allergic contact dermatitis. Allergy. 2011;66:1152–63.
66. Thyssen JP, Linneberg A, Engkidle K, Menné T, Johansen JD. Contact sensitization to common haptens is associated with atopic dermatitis: new insight. Br J Dermatol. 2012;166:1255–61.
67. Sharma AD. Relationship between nickel and diet. Indian J Dermatol. 2007;73:307–12.
68. Veien NK, Andersen MR. Nickel in Danish food. Acta Derm Venereol. 1986;66:502–9.
69. Christensen JM, Kristiansen J, Nielsen NH, Menne T, Byrialsen K. Nickel concentrations in serum and urine of patients with nickel eczema. Toxicol Lett. 1999;108:185–9.
70. Yamaguchi H, Hirasawa N, Asakawa S, Okita K, Tokura Y. Intrinsic atopic dermatitis shows high serum nickel concentration. Allergol Int. 2015;64:282–4.
71. Howell MD, Boguniewicz M, Pastore S, Novak N, Bieber T, Girolomoni G, et al. Mechanism of HBD-3 deficiency in atopic dermatitis. Clin Immunol. 2006;121:332–8.
72. Ricci G, Patrizi A, Neri I, Bendandi B, Masi M. Frequency and clinical role of staphylococcus aureus overinfection in atopic dermatitis in children. Pediatr Dermatol. 2003;20:389–92.

73. Pavlovic S, Liezmann C, Blois SM, Joachim R, Kruse J, Romani N, Klapp BF, Peters EM. Substance P is a key mediator of stress-induced protection from allergic sensitization via modified antigen presentation. J Immunol. 2011;186:848–55.
74. Jin H, He R, Oyoshi M, Geha RS. Animal models of atopic dermatitis. J Invest Dermatol. 2009;129:31–40.
75. Chen L, Overbergh L, Mathieu C, Chan LS. The development of atopic dermatitis is independent of immunoglobulin E up-regulation in the K14-IL-4 skh1 transgenic mouse model. Clin Exp Allergy. 2008;38:1367–80.
76. Konishi H, Tsutsui H, Murakami T, Yumikura-Futatsugi S, Yamanaka K, Tanaka M, et al. IL-18 contributes to the spontaneous development of atopic dermatitis-like inflammatory skin lesion independently of ige/stat6 under specific pathogen-free conditions. Proc Natl Acad Sci U S A. 2002;99:11340–5.
77. Terada M, Tsutsui H, Imai Y, Yasuda K, Mizutani H, Yamanishi K, et al. Contribution of IL-18 to atopic-dermatitis-like skin inflammation induced by staphylococcus aureus product in mice. Proc Natl Acad Sci U S A. 2006;103:8816–21.

Part VI

Clinical Manifestations

Infantile and Childhood AD

16

Hirokazu Arakawa

Abstract

Atopic dermatitis (AD) is a common chronic relapsing skin disease that mainly manifests as itchy eczema/dermatitis. The majority of AD patients have dry skin, and skin eczema during the healing process is accompanied by severe itchy dry skin. The onset or relapse of AD occurs at any age from infancy to adult. The course of AD may be influenced by age, season, and the environmental factors. A variety of skin manifestations can be seen when the disease takes a chronic course. Various exogenous products applied to the skin may affect AD symptoms. In addition, physical strain, mental stress, and immunoglobulin E allergic reactions can worsen the symptoms.

Keywords

Pruritus • Xerosis • Dirty neck • Dennie-Morgan folds

16.1 Introduction

Atopic dermatitis (AD) is the most common chronic, relapsing, pruritic skin disease seen in infancy and childhood (Table 16.1). Approximately 50% of patients with AD experience symptoms in the first year of life, and an additional 30% are diagnosed between 1 and 5 years of age. Clinical manifestations are often classified into three categories according to age: infancy (less than 2 years old), young children/school-age children (2–12 years old), and adolescence/adulthood (13 years old or

H. Arakawa, M.D., Ph.D.
Department of Pediatrics, Gunma University Graduate School of Medicine,
3-39-22 Showa-machi, Maebashi, Gunma 371-8511, Japan
e-mail: harakawa@gunma-u.ac.jp

I. Katayama et al. (eds.), *Evolution of Atopic Dermatitis in the 21st Century*,
https://doi.org/10.1007/978-981-10-5541-6_16

Table 16.1 Clinical manifestation of atopic dermatitis

Major features
• Pruritus
• Facial and extensor eczema in infants and children
• Flexural eczema in adolescents
• Chronic or relapsing dermatitis
• Personal or history of atopic disease
Associated features
• Xerosis
• Cutaneous infections (*Staphylococcus aureus*, group A *Streptococcus*, herpes simplex, coxsackievirus, vaccinia, molluscum, warts)
• Nonspecific dermatitis of the hands or feet
• Ichthyosis, palmar hyperlinearity, keratosis pilaris
• Nipple eczema
• White dermatographism and delayed blanch response
• Dennie lines (Dennie-Morgan infraorbital folds)
• Facial erythema or pallor
• Elevated serum immunoglobulin E levels
• Positive results of immediate-type allergy skin tests

older) [1]. The clinical course is chronic and recurrent. It is defined as chronic when skin manifestations persist for more than 2 months in infancy and more than 6 months after the infantile periods [2].

16.2 Differences in Skin Manifestations by Age Category

16.2.1 Infancy

Infants have an immature skin barrier function that weakens their skin defense against exogenous irritants [3]. In general, excessive use of body soap and shampoo for infants removes sebum from their skin, which induces dry skin and causes increased skin inflammation. In addition, drooling and finger sucking may stimulate the perioral skin and promote a barrier disruption. Although the age at AD onset varies in infancy, the majority of infants with AD naturally go into remission several months or years after onset.

A seasonal variation of AD symptoms may be observed, in which patients deteriorate during the winter and improve in the summer. In some severe cases, patients are unlikely to improve naturally, although they may live without any problems for 2–3 years after onset. Young infants show a drying of skin areas that are exposed to the outside air, such as the cheeks, forehead, and scalp, followed by skin flushing in the same region (Fig. 16.1a). As the disease activity of AD becomes stronger, the flushing becomes much worse. Itching occurs as papules appear. Scratch-injured papules become exudative and form a crust. Skin eczema can then spread across the entire face, including around the ears, perioral, cheeks, and chin (Fig. 16.1b).

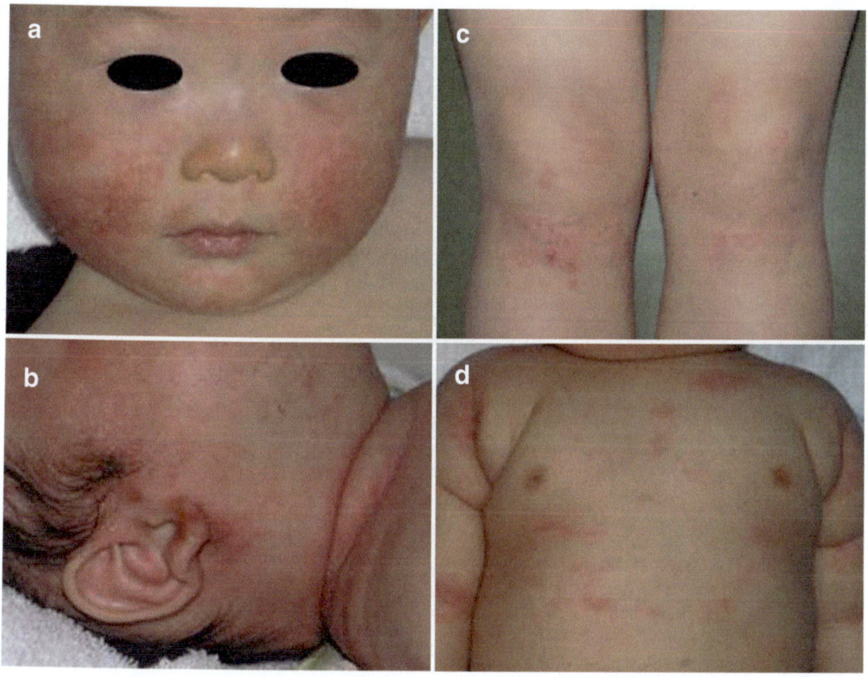

Fig. 16.1 Examples of skin manifestation of atopic dermatitis. (**a**) Face, mild desquamation and erythema; (**b**) around the ear and neck, erythema, exudation, and desquamation; (**c**) knees, mild desquamation and erythema, including partial mild lichenification; and (**d**) trunk, sparse mild erythema on the trunk and flexure areas of upper extremities (Japanese guideline for atopic dermatitis 2014 [2])

In addition to the face, the neck is also susceptible to irritation by bacterial toxins. Flexure parts, including the axillar, cubital, and popliteal fossa, are susceptible to chemical irritants such as sweat and soap. Such stimuli may induce flashing, papules, and exudation in these skin areas. Vulnerable areas including the wrist and dorsum of the hands and ankle are affected by dryness. Furthermore, eczema spreads to extensor surfaces of the extremities in season when extremities are exposed (Fig. 16.1c). In general, the trunk and diaper area are usually spared, but when disease activity is strong, a disseminated erythema appears on the chest, abdomen, back, and waist (Fig. 16.1d), and the erythema then spreads over the entire surface of the trunk (Fig. 16.2c).

16.2.2 Young and School-Age Children

As children grow from infancy to school age, their skin tends to become gradually drier due to reduced sebum secretion ability. Their scope of activities also expands from home to school. Therefore, their skin can be exposed to a variety of irritants, such as sweat, sand, and mud on playgrounds, as well as chlorine in swimming pools, leading to deterioration in AD symptoms.

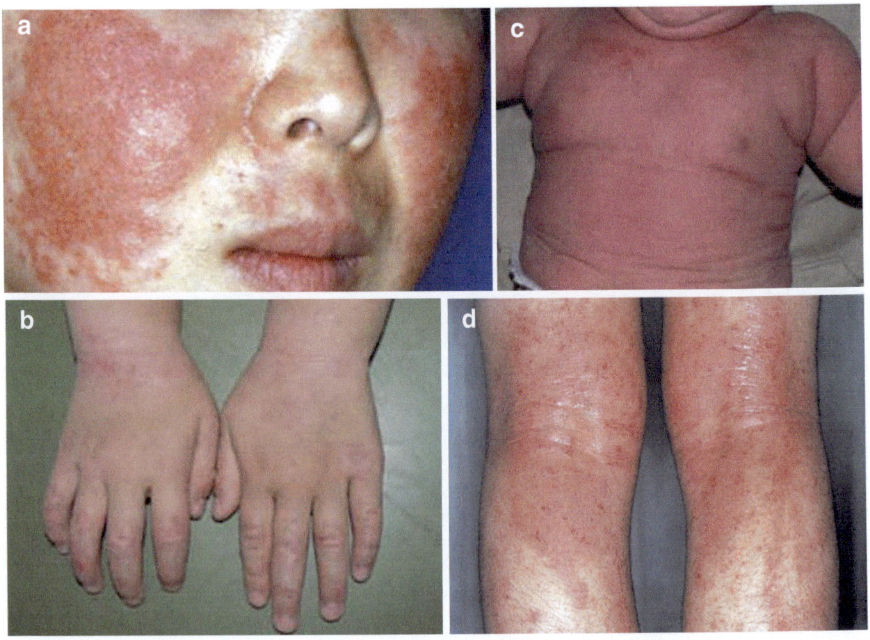

Fig. 16.2 Examples of eruption with severe inflammation includes (**a**) face, apparent erythema, desquamation, and infiltration; (**b**) fingers, apparent erythema, desquamation, and lichenification; (**c**) trunk, generalized erythema and erythroderma; and (**d**) popliteal fossa, marked erythema, desquamation, erosion, scratch marks, and lichenification (Japanese guideline for atopic dermatitis 2014 [2])

Skin symptoms may improve as children go through school, and unlike infancy, severe cases are relatively rare. Eczema on the face improves, while skin eruptions typically appear in the flexure portions including the neck, axillar cubital and popliteal fossa, inguinal, wrists, and ankles.

On the contrary, some patients complain of itching on the trunk and extremities, but their skin eruptions are unremarkable. As symptoms progress, the skin becomes dry with peeling scales and further severe excoriation (Fig. 16.2a, b). In rare severe cases, eczema spreads to the face and extremities. Erosions and blood crusts may often appear due to a repeated scratching. In addition, excessive scratching sometimes causes lichenification and prurigo nodules on the elbows, knees, and extremities (Fig. 16.2d).

16.2.3 Adolescence and Adulthood

Physical and mental growth and the lifestyle change greatly affect the clinical symptoms of AD. Particularly, stress, overwork, and anxiety associated with study and entrance exams increase. Such psychogenic factors can exacerbate AD symptoms and lead to repeated itching. In addition, social activities provide fewer opportunities to visit a medical institution, resulting in limited treatment.

After puberty, sebum secretion from the skin is increased due to sex hormones, and seborrhea and acne vulgaris are likely to occur. Skin eruptions overlap, especially on the face. During this period, eczema can extend from the neck to the upper chest region and the upper part of the back, spreading in the shape of a clothes hanger. The skin rash on the face increases again and the whole face turns red in more severe cases with AD (termed "red-faced"). Together with rashes on the face and the neck, it is distributed like a sculptural portrait (termed "portrait type").

As the secondary changes based on long-term treatment appear, the skin manifestation in puberty is much more complicated compared to that in school-age children and infants. A red/purple pigmentation, prurigo, nodules, and skin atrophy influenced by steroid ointments may sometimes be observed. In some severe cases, the skin rash and resulting erythroderma may spread over the whole body.

16.3 Eruption Emergence Site

In the patients with AD, the spread and intensity of the eruption is defined mainly by endogenous factors. Skin eruptions can appear anywhere on the body but tend to occur more intensely and earlier in region where exogenous factors may be applied, called a predilection site. Predilection sites differ slightly by age category. Skin eruptions usually appear in a left-right symmetry that becomes erythroderma if it spreads over the whole body. The impact of exogenous factors may be the reason for predilection site differences.

16.3.1 Face

Infants with an immature skin barrier function may be strongly affected by cold and dry air, especially on the scalp, forehead, and cheeks. The entire face (except the scalp) is highly affected by exposure to dust and other allergens and immunoglobulin E allergic reactions. Also, the use of body soap and shampoo greatly impacts the scalp, hairline, and around the ears. The eyelids and eyelid margins are influenced by allergic conjunctivitis as well as lacrimation. The perioral, cheeks, and lips may be impacted by drool and contact stimuli with food. The nasolabial region is influenced by blowing the nose due to allergic rhinitis.

16.3.2 Flexure Areas

The physical characteristics of infants, including a short neck and less flexibility (movement) in the extremities, may contribute to sweat retention and stimuli by *Staphylococcus aureus* in the neck; axillary, cubital, and popliteal fossa; wrist; and inguinal and ankle areas.

16.3.3 Areas Exposed by Various Irritants

Hands and fingers are influenced by moisture, sand, soap, shampoo, detergents, and finger sucking in infancy. Elbows, knees, wrists, ankles, feet, toes, and nipples are impacted by friction and pressure stimuli, while the vulva and perineum are irritated by excrement.

16.3.4 Trunk and Extremities

Skin eruptions due to endogenous factors mainly appear as a sporadic or diffuse type. Nummular dermatitis and pityriasis simplex often appear in the trunk and extremities. Nummular dermatitis occurs in ages from infancy to adulthood. It appears as an intensified inflammation, but it does not have an intense itch.

Pityriasis simplex is a skin disease that shows many dried circular depigmentation plaques flushed with a mild scale, accompanied by inflammation of the face, trunk, and extremities. It occurs between infancy and school age and does not have an intense itch. Some patients with AD have pityriasis simplex and nummular eczema.

16.4 Feature of Skin Eruptions

Skin eruptions are characteristic of eczema and dermatitis, and they can be divided into acute or chronic lesions. Xerosis, or dry skin, is the most common skin abnormality of allergic children.

Acute skin lesions are intensely pruritic with erythematous papules that occur at the onset or acute deterioration during the chronic phase. A lot of small blisters in the epidermis are erythematous exudative or serous papules. Either their progression or scratching destroys the epidermis and induces exudation from the skin, leading to dry skin, and crust formation, and scabbing. Once in the healing process, the skin is regenerated, and then an incomplete keratinization of the stratum corneum may lead to excoriation and scaling papules.

Chronic AD is characterized by lichenification, or a thickening of the skin, with accentuated surface markings and fibrotic papules (prurigo nodularis). The skin thickens in response to mechanical stimuli such as repeated scratching, leading to chronic papules (or prurigo), then lichenification, and then nodule lesions.

16.5 Impact of Itching

Itching is not just an associated symptom but could be referred to as the disease itself. Scratching and excoriation cause increased skin inflammation that contributes to the development of more pronounced eczematous skin lesions. Moreover, inflammation facilitates disease progression and remodeling.

Itching occurs during bathing, exercise, sleep, ointment application, sweating due to irritation and body warmth, frustrating, and contact with wool clothes (wool intolerance). As itching becomes more aggravated, quality of life worsens according to the degree of skin symptoms. Itching is also the biggest factor that inhibits the treatment and is generally the biggest problem associated with all respects of AD.

16.5.1 Scratching Behavior

While scratched areas are usually only those that can be reached by the hands, patients may also sometimes pull their hair and scratch using their feet. Areas covered by clothes cannot be scratched, but patients can scratch by twisting their body. When children rub their face on their mother's clothes or the collar of their own clothes, eruptions along the cheek, perioral area, or jaw worsen. Rubbing their occipital scalp with their bedding may cause hair loss. In early infants, it is possible to weaken the scratching behavior by covering the scratched site with bandage or clothes, as well as by putting gloves on their hands. However, suppressing the scratching behavior becomes difficult a few months after birth, and most young and school-age children cannot restrain themselves from scratching.

16.5.2 Impact of Scratching

As mentioned above, scratching the skin lesions may induce erythema and papules. The epidermis is mechanically destroyed by scratching, leading to small blisters in the epidermis, followed by erosion and exudation. The exudate dries to become a scab and skin regeneration occurs under the crust. Nerve entering into the recently regenerated epidermis may become sensitive to itching. Scratching also enhances pigmentation and causes hair loss, thickening of the skin, and lichenification.

16.5.3 Sleep Disorders

Skin symptoms in AD may cause sleep disorders to a greater or lesser degree. Sleep disorders seen in AD patients include difficulty falling asleep and awaking during the night. The difficulty of falling asleep is caused by an increase in itching sensitivity due to body warmth while in bed. In this case, the scratch action is considered necessary in order to erase the itch. Even if the hands were temporarily restrained and the patient completely stops the scratch, contrary to our expectation, they could not get to sleep. Diminishing the itch by scratching seems to help a patient get to sleep. It has been reported that itch irritation to the skin leads to nocturnal awakening [4]. Video camera recordings have revealed that scratching is very intense at night [5]. Night awakening is more likely to occur in the higher age group than in younger children, even at the same level of skin symptoms. It has been reported that there is a scratching behavior that is performed unintentionally but preferably, called the scratch addiction [6, 7]. If scratching is intense in situations other than well-itching situations (bathing, sleeping, mood, etc.,) in infants [8], it is necessary to consider the involvement of psychogenic stress [9].

16.6 Secondary Changes in Skin Eruptions Caused by Chronic AD (Table 16.1)

If AD symptoms persist for many years, the skin exhibits a variety of manifestations as follows:

16.6.1 White Dermographism

This is a blanching response resulting from capillary vasoconstriction after skin stroking and is more pronounced in persons with atopy. This phenomenon is one of the small criteria for diagnosis outlined by Hanifin and Rajka.

16.6.2 Keratosis Pilaris

Keratosis pilaris, often found on the extensor surfaces of the upper arms and thighs, is characterized by a roughness of the skin caused by keratin plugs lodged in the openings of hair follicles. Keratosis pilaris creates a "goose bump," "gooseflesh," or "chicken skin" appearance. It is seen in patients with atopic dermatitis and patients with very dry skin.

16.6.3 Depigmentation

Pityriasis simplex, also called pityriasis alba, has less pigment than the surrounding skin. It is noticeable after sunburn. Secondary depigmentation spots are those that become depigmented by intense scratching. It can often be seen on the wrists and the back of the feet. A part of the lip may sometimes appear whitish due to missing pigment as a result of acute or chronic cheilitis [10].

16.6.4 Pigmentation

It is possible for pigmentation to remain in the skin where there was once dermatitis. Although there are fears about the effects of steroid ointments, pigmentation is irrelevant. Skin pigmentation after inflammation may be temporary, but hyperpigmentation sometimes remains after a long duration of dermatitis. Orbital darkening is one of the examples, when dermatitis spreads over the whole body and acute cheilitis occurs, and a point-like pigmentation along with the depigmentation can sometimes be seen.

When chronic stimuli are applied to the skin, strong pigmentation remains in some patients with AD. A mesh-like black-brown pigmentation over the front of the neck to the clavicle is referred to as dirty neck or poikiloderma-like skin changes.

16.6.5 Enhancement of Folds

Chronic skin dermatitis increases skin folds; a typical example is palmar and plantar hyperlinearity. In addition, Dennie lines (Dennie-Morgan folds), which are prominent symmetric skin folds, can sometimes be seen extending in an arc from the inner canthus beneath and parallel to the lower eyelid margin. They are often accompanied by allergic shiners, which are blue-gray to purple discolorations beneath the lower eyelids that are attributed to venous stasis.

16.6.6 Hair Loss

Areas covered with itchy hair where a rash and itch exists first cause hair rupture, and then the hair becomes sparse, eventually leading to hair loss. Hair loss in the occipital region in infants and the temporal region (Fig. 16.3a) and outer half of eyebrows (Hertoghe's sign) in the school-age children can often be observed.

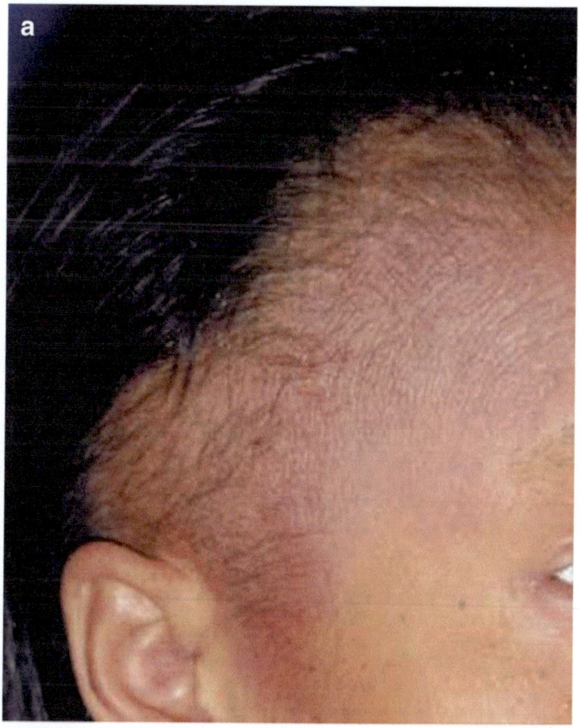

Fig. 16.3 Examples of secondary changes of skin eruption caused by chronic course includes (**a**) hear loss in the temporal region and (**b**) nail luster (Guidelines for the treatment of atopic dermatitis 2015) (in Japanese)

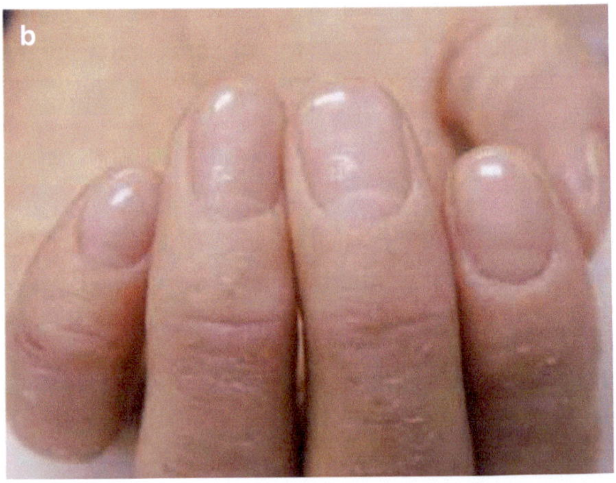

Fig. 16.3 (continued)

16.6.7 Nail Luster

When skin scratching is intense, nails exhibit a pearl-like gloss (pearly nail) (Fig. 16.3b). When zinc oxide ointment is applied to the skin, the nails are polished and nail luster becomes remarkable. Nails become thinner, and as blood capillaries under the nails appear, their ends look red.

16.6.8 Prurigo

Prurigo refers to very itchy nodules with a solitary erythema the size of a few millimeters and is therapy-resistant [11]. The pathogenesis of prurigo is unknown, but it may be caused by folliculitis because most of the rash is due to a hair follicle consistency.

16.7 Concomitant Symptoms

16.7.1 Bacterial Growth on the Skin Surface

Excluding the dried skin surface, *S. aureus* colonization (fixing) is observed in most forms of skin rash, including erythema. There are many colonies in eroded skin and in crust formations widely accompanied with desquamation. Large colony expansions may worsen the eczema [12, 13].

16.7.2 Lymph Node Enlargement

If there is some degree of skin symptoms and area spread, superficial swollen lymph nodes without pain do not necessarily mean infection. This is called dermatopathic lymphadenopathy.

16.8 Clinical Course

When observing AD patients as a group, the onset and improvement of AD occurs at infancy or later. Although the frequency of onset and improvement is reduced with age, the onset exceeds improvement in early infancy, but this is reversed up to 1 year of age. The tendency for an increase in onset over improvement can be seen in the later teen years. Infant through school-age patients with AD may have a milder form, but some of them may deteriorate again in puberty. While some patients do not show fluctuations in AD symptoms during the course of a year, others have AD symptoms depending on the season. Although the winter and summer seasons are worse for school children, improvements are generally only known to occur in the summer. In addition, some patients also exhibit annual changes in AD symptoms.

Except for early infancy, AD is difficult to cure in a short period after the initial onset. It is possible to suppress, but not cure, the temporary symptoms through therapy. Even once improved, recurrence may be seen after several months or years.

References

1. Rajka G. Essential aspect of atopic dermatitis. Berlin-Heidelberg: Springer-Verlag; 1989. p. 1.
2. Katayama I, Kohno Y, Akiyama K, Aihara M, Kondo N, Saeki H, Shoji S, Yamada H, Nakamura K, Japanese Society Of Allergology. Japanese guideline for atopic dermatitis 2014. Allergol Int. 2014;63:377–98.
3. Hoeger PH, Enzmann CC. Skin physiology of the neonate and young infant:a prospective study of functional skin parameters during early infancy. Pediatr Dermatol. 2002;19:256–62.
4. Aoki T, Kushimoto H, Hishikawa Y, et al. Nocturnal scratching and its relationship to the disturbed sleep of itchy subjects. Clin Exp Dermatol. 1991;16:268–72.
5. Ebata T, Aizawa H, Kamide R. An infrared video camera system to observe nocturnal scratching in atopic dermatitis patients. J Dermatol. 1996;23:153–5.
6. Kobayashi M. Investigation of scratching behavior in atopic dermatitis patients. Jpn J Dermatol. 2000;110:275–82.
7. Higaki Y, Arikawa J, Yoshihara N, et al. The role of scratching behavior and psychosocial stress in intractable atopic dermatitis. Jpn J Dermatol. 2001;111:837–42.
8. Suehiro Y. How to manage scratching in atopic dermatitis. J Pediat Dermatol. 2003;22:113–5.
9. Suehiro Y. How to control itch in atopic dermatitis. J Pediat Dermatol. 2003;22:86–8.
10. Hanifin JM, Rajka G. Diagnostic features of atopic dermatitis. Acta Derm Venereol (Stockh). 1980;92(Suppl):44–7.
11. Miyauchi H, Uehara M. Follicular occurrence of prurigo nodularis. J Cutan Pathol. 1988;15: 208–11.
12. Morishita Y, Tada J, Sato A, Toi Y, Kanzaki H, Akiyama H, Arata J. Possible influences of Staphylococcus aureus on atopic dermatitis-- the colonizing features and the effects of staphylococcal enterotoxins. Clin Exp Allergy. 1999;29:1110–7.
13. Tokura Y, Ishii-Ginoza M, Seo N, Ito T, Sakurai M, Furukawa F, Takigawa M. Streptococcal impetigo induces Th1-preponderant activation of T lymphocytes with subsequent anergy to superantigenic exotoxins in patients with atopic dermatitis. Br J Dermatol. 1998;138:357–8.

Clinical Manifestation: Adult-Type Atopic Dermatitis

17

Aya Takahashi, Hiroyuki Murota, and Ichiro Katayama

Abstract

Most of the patients with atopic dermatitis (AD) get better before about 10 years old. Although some patients get better and flare up once again after adolescence, some never get better and symptoms remain from childhood through to adulthood, and some have an onset after adolescence. and dirty neck are common among any type of AD of adolescent and adult, and other typical manifestations are also found.

Scratching the itchy spot for a long time and inappropriate treatment induce intractable chronic eczema. In the adolescent and adult patients of AD, the life and job environment directly affect the condition of their eruption. In addition, decreased perspiration in AD is one of the causes of skin dryness and decreased skin barrier function, so it is susceptible to complications like skin infectious disease.

Keywords

Atopic dermatitis • Adult phase • Clinical manifestation • Face erythema Dirty neck

17.1 Introduction

Internationally, the diagnostic criteria of atopic dermatitis produced by Hanifin and Rajka are commonly used [1]. While in Japan, Clinical Practice Guidelines for the Management of Atopic Dermatitis (AD) have been made by the Japanese Dermatological Association and used frequently [2, 3]. This present that we can

A. Takahashi (✉) • H. Murota • I. Katayama
Department of Dermatology, Course of Integrated Medicine, Graduate School of Medicine, Osaka University, 2-2 Yamadaoka, Suita, Osaka, Japan, 5650871
e-mail: aya529@green.ocn.ne.jp

I. Katayama et al. (eds.), *Evolution of Atopic Dermatitis in the 21st Century*,
https://doi.org/10.1007/978-981-10-5541-6_17

diagnose the patient who fulfill the three items, (1) pruritus, (2) typical morphology and distribution of the eczema, and (3) chronic or chronically relapsing course, regardless of the severity of symptoms as AD. Eruption is symmetrically distributed and frequently develops on the forehead, periorbital area, perioral area, lips, periauricular area, neck, joint areas of limbs, and trunk. Its distribution is characterized by age. Drs. Lewis Webb Hill and Marion B. Sulzberger who used the name "atopic dermatitis" first also presented that the clinical manifestations of AD change by generations in their paper [4]. Most of the AD patients get better before about 10 years old. Although some patients get better and flare up once again after adolescence, some never get better and symptoms remain from childhood through to adulthood, and some have an onset after adolescence.

17.2 Manifestations of Adult Type

When the patient feel an itching sensation, they scratch their skin and it causes symptom such as erythema or papule (Fig. 1). Scratching repeatedly with

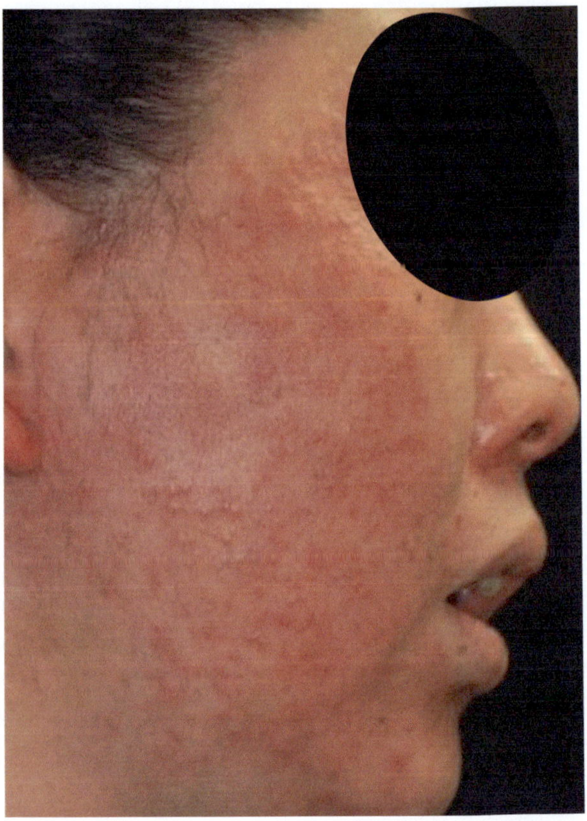

Fig. 17.1 Intractable erythema of the face: erythema of the face is a common manifestation in adult (adolescence/adulthood) phase. It is characterized by edematous erythema and many papules and is incurable

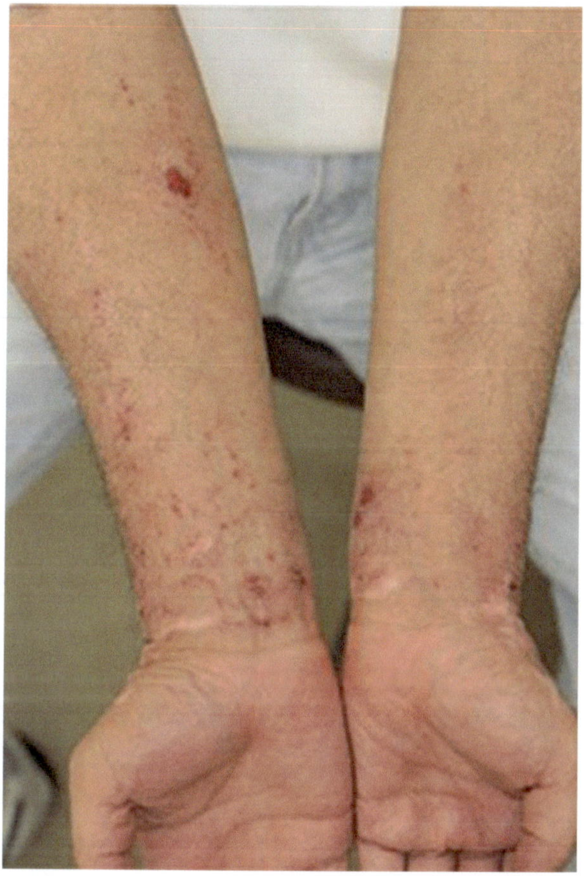

Fig. 17.2 Serous or crusted papules and erosions of forearm after scratching with intensity

intensity at the same area of the skin brings on symptoms such as serous or crusted papules and erosions (Fig. 2). Then the skin becomes thick and subsequently lichenified or pruritus after scratching over the years (Figs. 3 and 4). These manifestations are common in AD as well as in dry skin regardless of the age (Fig. 5 [5, 6]). In adult (adolescence/adulthood) phase, eruptions become marked in the upper body, including the face (Figs. 1, 6 and 7), and they are diverse.

There are many causes of symptoms of adult AD patients which are side effect of long-term use of topical corticosteroids [7], psychological stress [8], or some occupational environments including working at a restaurant, hair salon, hospital, etc. [9]. Hand eczema (Fig. 8) is also a common symptom for them, and it is intractable. It is caused by constantly exposing to various antigens and washing hands many times.

Furthermore, long-term inappropriate treatment without identifying and eliminating the individual risk factor like various antigens for AD patients frequently leads to the severe condition like erythroderma (Fig. 9).

Fig. 17.3 Prurigo

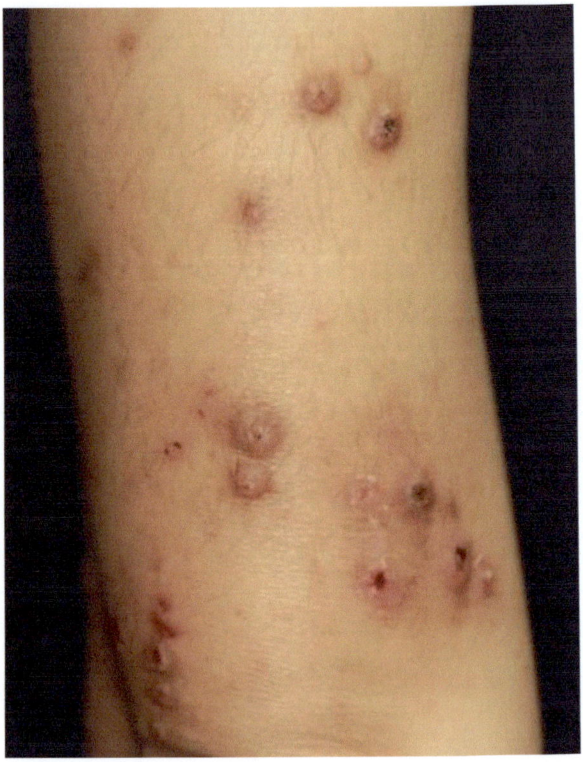

17.3 Manifestations Characteristic of AD

17.3.1 Prurigo (Fig. 3)

Prurigo is an intractable condition of unknown etiology in which there are independent itchy papules or solid nodular eruptions. It is induced by diabetes mellitus, chronic renal failure, internal malignancies, or atopic condition and is aggravated by repeated itching and scratching. There are various studies about its etiology. Hashimoto et al. established prurigo model mouse, and they present that the condition is a basophil-dependent allergic inflammation [11].

17.3.2 Lichenification (Fig. 4)

Lichenification is a chronic skin disorder which is a thickened skin condition with accentuated skin markings like an elephant, usually the result of constant scratching and rubbing. It presents elevated sulcus cutis, clear crista cutis, and dryness of area cutanea.

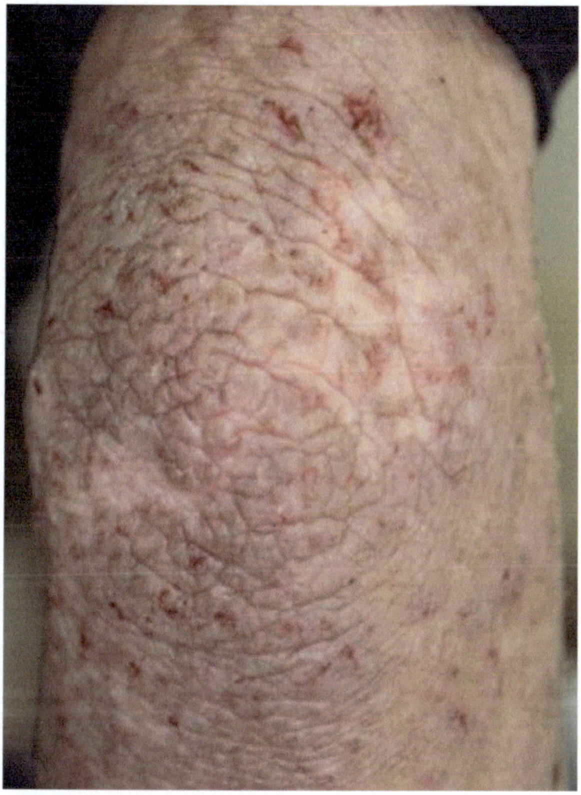

Fig. 17.4 Lichenification

17.3.3 Dry Skin (Fig. 5)

This is the common feature of atopic dermatitis among all ages. Increase of transepidermal water loss (TEWL) and decrease of water holding capacity (WHC) cause skin dryness in AD [5]. Sweating is thought to be a major source of water in the stratum corneum. And the functional abnormality of the stratum corneum in AD patients might impair the evaluation of WHC, even in cases of sufficient sweat volume [6].

17.3.4 Scratch Marks with White Dermographism (Fig. 6)

In adult (adolescence/adulthood) phase, atopic eczema is found commonly in the upper chest. This is the photograph of "white dermography" on the upper chest region. Patients of AD often develop the symptom when they scratch their skin lightly. It is characterized by blood vessel constriction, and the white scratch mark appears for over an hour.

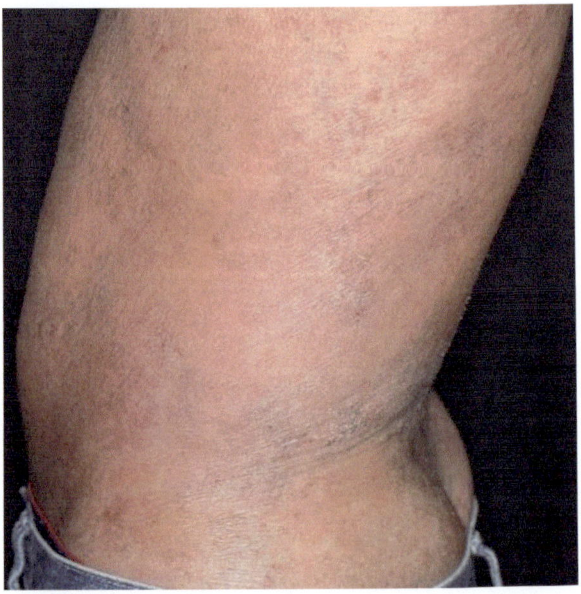

Fig. 17.5 Dry skin

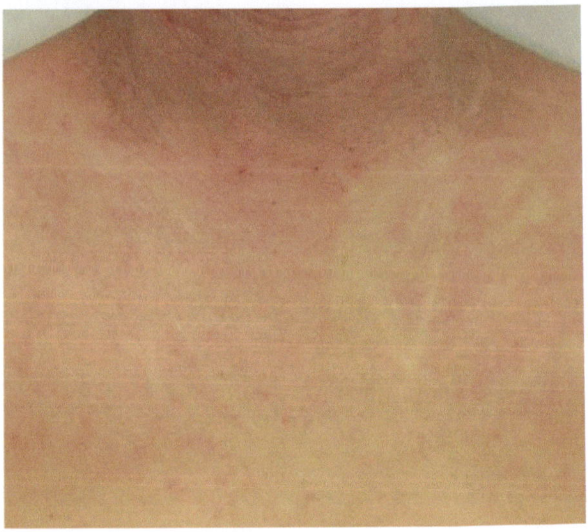

Fig. 17.6 Scratch marks with white dermography

17.3.5 Dirty Neck (Fig. 7)

Dirty neck is a protracted condition with various manifestations such as reticulate pigmentation, erythema, papules, and scratch marks. The main manifestation is reticulate pigmentation; skin atrophy, depigmentation, and telangiectasia appear in its development to a completely poikiloderma-like lesion. It is also called ripple pigmentation of the neck or poikiloderma-like skin changes and is attributable to chronic inflammation and prolonged using topical corticosteroid for treatment [12].

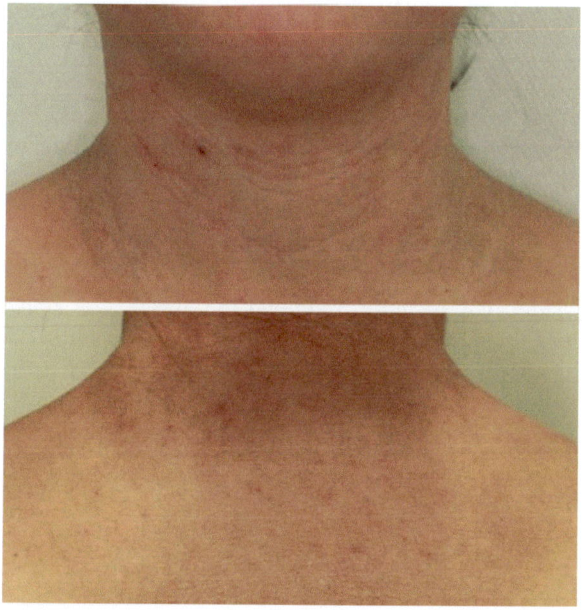

Fig. 17.7 Dirty neck

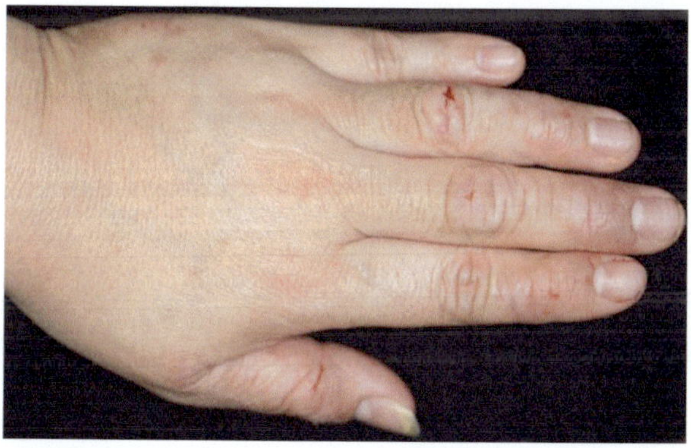

Fig. 17.8 Hand eczema

17.3.6 Hand Eczema (Fig. 8)

Hand eczema is characterized by xerosis, fissures, lichenification, etc. The nails are often coarse pitting and ridging.

It is an intractable and common symptom for AD patients whose skin barrier function is impaired. We constantly touch various antigens or irritants such as foods, pet animals, and chemical cleanser etc. And the people who work at a restaurant, hospital, or hair salon wash their hands many times. For AD patients whose skin barrier function is impaired, hand eczema is common and intractable. In addition, AD patients who work with papers and metals and take care of their baby or child often show severe hand eczema [10].

17.3.7 Erythroderma (Fig. 9)

Erythroderma is an inflammatory skin condition in which erythema and scaling affect nearly the entire body surface. It is induced by prolonged inappropriate or no treatment and is sometimes triggered by infection.

17.3.8 Dennie-Morgan Fold (Fig. 10)

Many folds increase in around the eyelid after skin inflammation persists for a long time. Dennie-Morgan fold is a deep fold in the lower eyelid.

It is a specific symptom for AD, and then certain paper suggests that the symptom is one of the criteria to diagnose AD [13, 14].

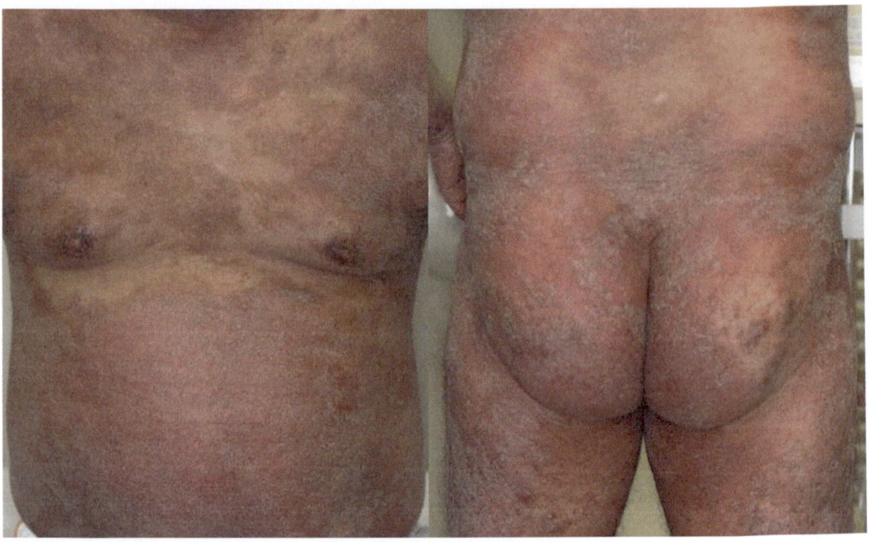

Fig. 17.9 Erythroderma

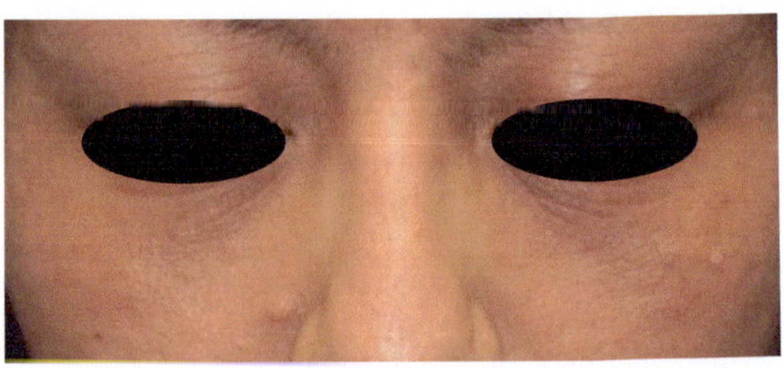

Fig. 17.10 Dennie-Morgan fold

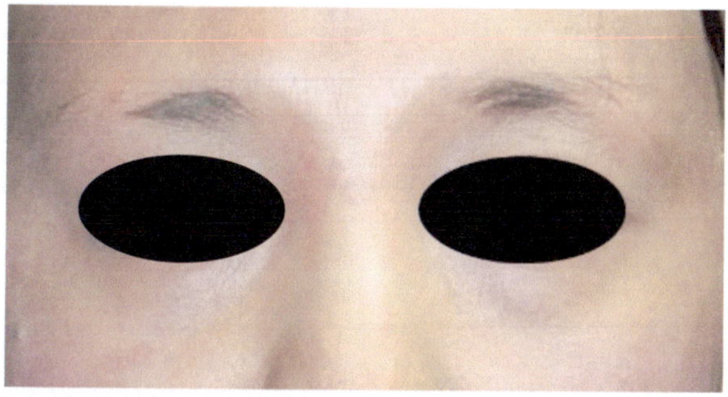

Fig. 17.11 Hertoghe's sign

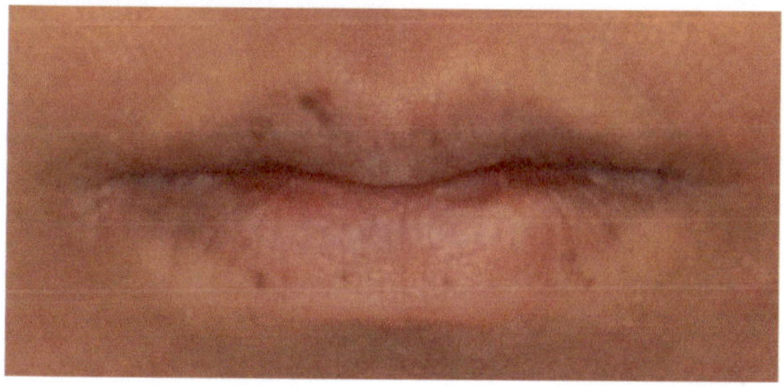

Fig. 17.12 Labial melanosis

17.3.9 Hertoghe's Sign (Fig. 11)

Hertoghe's sign is the sinning or loss of the outer third of the eyebrows and is caused by repeated rubbing or scratching of the skin around the eyes. It is also known as the famous symptom of hypothyroidism.

17.3.10 Labial Melanosis (Fig. 12)

Labial melanosis is seen in many AD patients. Repeated inflammation of their lips is considered a major cause of this symptom. There is another theory that some pigmented and depigmented areas appear after acute cheilitis. It is contributory to the diagnosis of AD.

17.3.11 Lichen Amyloidosis (Fig. 13)

Lichen amyloidosis is a chronic pruritic skin disorder characterized by amyloid deposition in the skin. Clinically, it is characterized by isolated, intensely pruritic, hyperkeratotic papules that may coalesce into plaques. It is often found on the anterior legs, back, forearms, and thighs. Pathologically, amyloid deposition is found in the papillary dermis and hyperkeratosis and acanthosis of the epidermis.

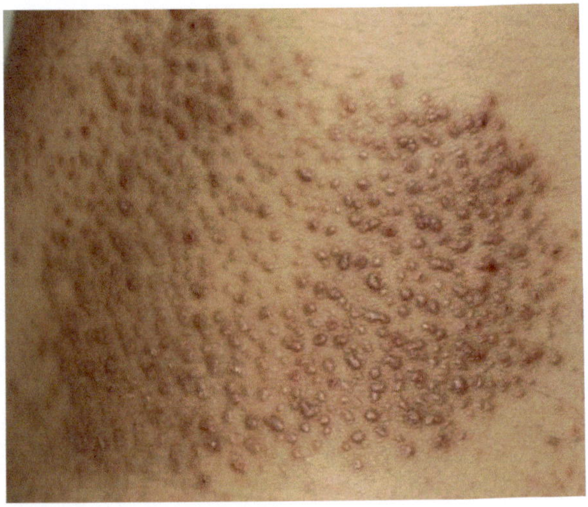

Fig. 17.13 Lichen amyloidosis

A working hypothesis is that the epidermal trauma induced by long-term scratching and rubbing seen in associated chronic diseases results in keratinocyte degradation and formation of amyloid [15].

17.3.12 Ichthyosis

Ichthyosis is severely dry, scaly, or flaky skin. It is like scales on fish, and ichthyosis means "fish" in ancient Greece. Mutations in the gene encoding filaggrin (FLG) were identified as the underlying cause of ichthyosis vulgaris and also shown to predispose to AD [16]. FLG is a main source of natural moisturizing factor (NMF)-associated skin barrier function. Loss-of-function mutations in the gene encoding filaggrin induce a decline in skin barrier function. Hasebe et al. reported that about 30% of patients of AD in Japan have mutations in the gene encoding FLG [17].

17.3.13 Hyperlinearity in Atopic Dermatitis, on the Palm

Patients with atopic dermatitis characteristically have increased numbers and depth of skin lines (hyperlinearity) on the palms and wrist with little erythema. Genetic epidemiological studies have shown that FLG null mutations are significantly associated with palmar hyperlinearity [18–21], keratosis pilaris, fine scaling, and dry skin, each of which may be feature of ichthyosis vulgaris.

17.3.14 Hair Loss (Fig. 14)

Hair loss or thin hair especially in the temporal region of the head is also common among patients with AD. Skin dryness of head or repeated scratching can cause

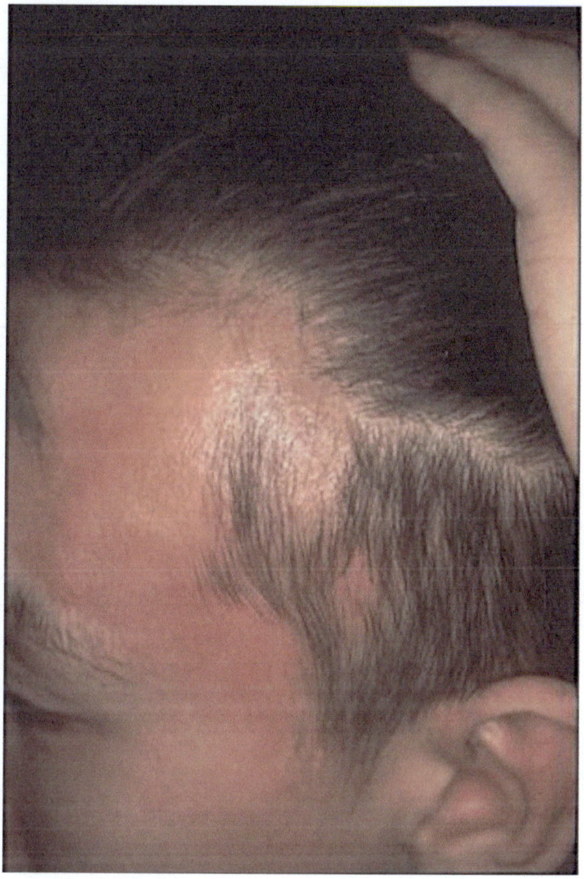

Fig. 17.14 Hair loss

hair loss. It usually improves when the dermatitis of the head skin is cured. Some of the patients have alopecia areata or alopecia totalis.

17.4 Complications

Dry skin, repeated rubbing, and deteriorating of eruption induce a decrease in skin barrier function or skin immune activity. Then various infectious diseases frequently occur in patients with AD. There is colonization of *Staphylococcus aureus* in almost lesions in patient with AD. Increased bacterial mass causes bacterial infection and symptoms such as impetigo, impetiginous erythema (Fig. 15), erysipelas, and cellulitis. Viral infections also often occur. Herpes simplex virus infection in AD patients is easy to become severe, and it is called kaposi's varicelliform eruption (Fig. 16). Common site of infection is the face and sometimes spreads to their limbs or trunk. Eruptions are many small, round vesicles with erosion, crust, and pain. It accompanies a fever or swollen lymph nodes.

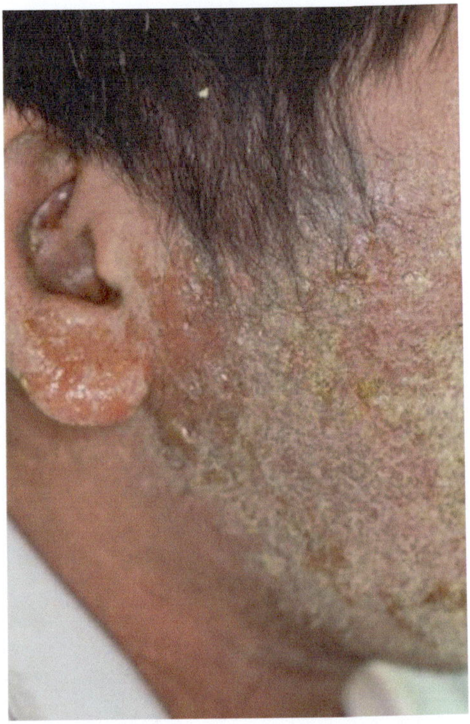

Fig. 17.15 Impetiginous erythema

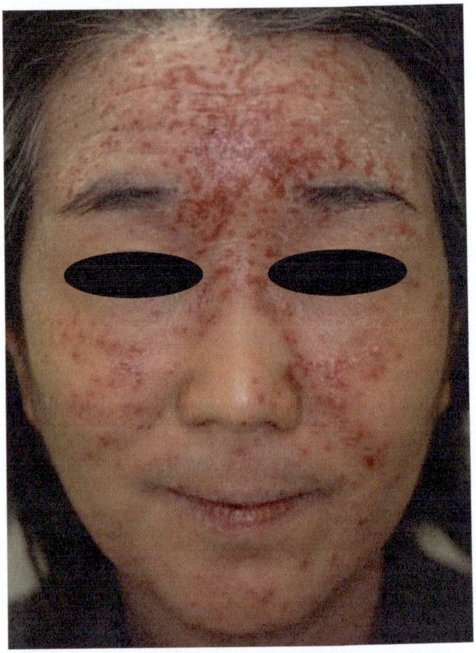

Fig. 17.16 Kaposi's varicelliform eruption

Ocular disease, such as keratoconjunctivitis, keratoconus, cataract, and retinal detachment, frequently develops when skin symptoms in the face are severe.

References

1. Hanifin JM, Rajka G. Diagnostic features of atopic dermatitis. Acta Derm Venereol. 1980;92:44–7.
2. The Japanese Dermatological Association. Definition and diagnostic criteria for atopic dermatitis. Jpn J Dermatol. 1994;104:1210. (in Japanese)
3. Saeki H, Nakahara T, Tanaka A, et al. Clinical practice guidelines for the management of atopic dermatitis 2016. J Dermatol. 2016;43:1117–45.
4. Lewis WH, Marion BS, et al. Evolution of atopic dermatitis. Arch Derm Syphilol. 1935;32:451–63.
5. Werner Y, Lindberg M. Transepidermal water loss in dry and clinically normal skin in patients with atopic dermatitis. Acta Derm Venereol. 1985;65(2):102–5.
6. Takahashi A, Tani S, Murota H, et al. Histamine modulates sweating and affects clinical manifestations of atopic dermatitis. Kerger Curr Probl Dermatol. 2016;51:50–6.
7. Hajar T, Leshem YA, Hanifin JM, et al. A systematic review of topical corticosteroid withdrawal ("steroid addiction") in patients with atopic dermatitis and other dermatoses. J Am Acad Dermatol. 2015;72(3):541–9.
8. Oh SH, Bae BG, Park CO, et al. Association of stress with symptoms of atopic dermatitis. Acta Derm Venereol. 2010;90:582–8.
9. Nilsson EJ, Knutsson A. Atopic dermatitis, nickel sensitivity and xerosis as risk factors for hand eczema in women. Contact Dermatitis. 1995;33:401–6.
10. Arase N, Murakami Y, Takahashi A, et al. Analysis of work productivity and activity impairment (WPAI), quality of life (QOL) and healthcare costs for Japanese patients with hand eczema. J Environ Dermatol Cutan Allergol. 2013;7(2):87–92.
11. Hashimoto T, Satoh T, Yokozeki H. Protective role of STAT6 in basophil-dependent prurigo-like allergic skin inflammation. J Immunol. 2015;194(10):4631–40.
12. Mukai H, Nishioka K, Kamimura K, et al. Poikiloderma-like lesions on the neck in atopic dermatitis: a histopathological study. J Dermatol. 1990;17(2):85–91.
13. Schram ME, Leeflang MM, DEN Ottolander JP, et al. Validation and refinement of the Millennium Criteria for atopic dermatitis. J Dermatol. 2011;38(9):850–8.
14. Uehara M. Infraorbital fold in atopic dermatitis. Arch Dermatol. 1981;117(10):627–9.
15. Wong CK, Lin CS. Friction amyloidosis. Int J Dermatol. 1988;27(5):302–7.
16. Smith FJD, Irvine AD, Terron-Kwiatkowski A, et al. Loss-of-function mutations in the gene encoding filaggrin cause ichthyosis vulgaris. Nat Genet. 2006;38:337–42.
17. Nemoto-Hasebe I, Akiyama M, Nomura T, Sandilands A, et al. FLG mutation p.Lys4021X in the C-terminal imperfect filaggrin repeat in Japanese patients with atopic eczema. Br J Dermatol. 2009;161(6):1387–90.
18. Novak N, Baurecht H, Schafer T, et al. Loss-of-function mutations in the filaggrin gene and allergic contact sensitization to nickel. J Invest Dermatol. 2008;128:1430–5.
19. Sergeant A, Campbell LE, Hull PR, et al. Heterozygous null alleles in filaggrin contribute to clinical dry skin in young adults and the elderly. J Invest Dermatol. 2009;129:1042–5.
20. Brown SJ, Relton CL, Liao H, et al. Filaggrin null mutations and childhood atopic eczema: a population-based case–control study. J Allergy Clin Immunol. 2008;121:940–6.
21. Brown SJ, Relton CL, Liao H, et al. Filaggrin haploinsufficiency is highly penetrant and is associated with increased severity of eczema: further delineation of the skin phenotype in a prospective epidemiological study of 792 school children. Br J Dermatol. 2009;161(4):884–9.

Senile Atopic Dermatitis

18

Ryoji Tanei

Abstract

Atopic dermatitis (AD) in the elderly represents a newly defined subgroup of AD. Elderly patients with AD show some characteristic clinical manifestations. Skin manifestations of elderly AD basically match those of adolescent/adult AD, but a lack of involvement of the folds of the elbows and knees is more common than the classic sign of localized lichenification in those folds. Elderly patients with immunoglobulin (Ig)E-allergic AD show high rates of positivity for specific IgE antibodies against house dust mites. In immunohistopathology, IgE-mediated allergic inflammation with IgE+ mast cells and IgE+ dendritic cells (i.e., Langerhans cells and inflammatory dendritic cells) in association with environmental allergens (e.g., house dust mites) may exist in the lichenified eczema of IgE-allergic elderly AD. The prevalence of elderly AD, which shows a tendency toward a male predominance, is approximately 1–3% among elderly populations in industrialized countries. In clinical practice, most elderly patients with AD obtain amelioration of skin manifestations once suitable management is implemented, but most elderly patients with AD still reach the end of life with AD. AD should now be considered as a lifelong allergic condition in some populations.

Keywords

Clinical manifestations • Elderly • Immunohistopathology • Immunoglobulin E
Prognosis

The original version of this chapter was revised. An erratum to this chapter can be found at https://doi.org/10.1007/978-981-10-5541-6_30

R. Tanei, M.D., Ph.D.
Department of Dermatology, Tokyo Metropolitan Geriatric Hospital and Institute of Gerontology, 35-2 Sakaecho, Itabashi, Tokyo 173-0015, Japan
e-mail: rtanei@aol.com; rtanei@tmghig.jp

I. Katayama et al. (eds.), *Evolution of Atopic Dermatitis in the 21st Century*,
https://doi.org/10.1007/978-981-10-5541-6_18

18.1 Introduction

Atopic dermatitis (AD) is a chronic inflammatory skin disease associated with a pathogenesis involving allergic inflammation and skin barrier defects. Prior to the 1960s–1970s, AD was basically considered a pediatric disease with good prognosis. This condition was known as classic child AD, as the onset of AD commonly begins in early infancy or childhood and resolution of AD typically occurs with increasing age until puberty. Although cases of prolonged AD until young adult life (i.e., adult AD) were reported in the 1930s, Sulzberger, the pioneer of the "atopic" concept of AD, stated that AD in middle age was extremely rare, and no typical case of AD in a patient over 50 years old was observed in that era [1]. From the 1980s, cases of AD either persisting or first appearing in adolescence and adulthood increased in industrialized countries and were termed adult-type AD [2]. Cases of AD manifesting in later life (i.e., elderly AD, senile AD) have gradually been increasing with the aging of society [3, 4]. As a result, AD is now capable of being classified into four phases: infantile (age <2 years), childhood (age 2–12 years), adolescent/adult (age >12 years but <60 years), and senile (age ≥60 years) [5].

In this chapter, I focus on the clinical manifestations of this new subgroup of elderly AD [6–8].

18.2 Clinical Manifestations of Senile AD

Characteristics of the clinical manifestations of elderly AD with regard to the following contents are summarized in Table 18.1.

18.2.1 Clinical Type

In general, at least two types of AD have been identified: an immunoglobulin (Ig) E-allergic type associated with high levels of serum total IgE (more than approximately 200 or 400 IU/L, according to the standards of the individual facility) and IgE-mediated sensitization to environmental allergens (positive results of allergen-specific IgE in skin prick test and/or serum evaluations) and a non-IgE-allergic type with normal levels of serum total IgE and a lack of sensitization to environmental allergens [9, 10]. Similar to other age groups, both IgE-allergic and non-IgE-allergic types of AD exist in elderly AD, if the diagnosis of AD is based upon standardized diagnostic criteria [6]. In addition, as is the case with infantile AD [11], an indeterminate-allergic type also exists in elderly AD with normal levels of serum total IgE and positivity for allergen-specific IgEs or with high levels of serum total IgE and non-detectable allergen-specific IgEs, as an intermediate, vague state between IgE-allergic and non-IgE-allergic types. In our clinical study ($n = 60$), the frequencies of IgE-allergic type, indeterminate-allergic type, and non-IgE-allergic type in elderly AD were 63.3% ($n = 38$), 15.0% ($n = 9$), and 21.7% ($n = 13$), respectively [12].

Table 18.1 Clinical manifestations of senile atopic dermatitis

Clinical type	Three types have been categorized: IgE-allergic type, non-IgE-allergic type. and indeterminate-allergic type [8, 12]
Skin manifestations	Basically match those of adolescent/adult AD: Chronic eczema on the face and neck and exudative/lichenified eczematous dermatitis on the trunk and extremities Other stigmas of AD, e.g., atopic red face, Hertoghe's sign, Dennie-Morgan's infraorbital folds, dirty neck, etc., are observed Features of elderly AD that differ from adolescent/adult AD: The classic sign of localized lichenified eczema in the folds of the elbows and knees is uncommon Unaffected folds of the elbows and knees are common Reverse sign of lichenified eczema around unaffected elbow folds is frequently observed [3, 6, 8, 12]
IgE reactivity and cytokines	Mean serum total IgE levels of IgE-allergic elderly AD: approximately 2500–7000 IU/mL [4, 12] Major allergens for IgE-allergic elderly AD: HDMs (*Dermatophagoides* species) followed by pollens [4, 12] Dominance of Th2 cytokine profiles, i.e., IL-4, IL-5, and IL-13 in elderly patients with IgE-allergic elderly AD [4] Dominance of Th1 cytokine profiles, i.e., IL-2 and IFN-γ in elderly patients with low serum total IgE [4]
Histopathology and immunopathogenesis of skin lesions	Numerous IgE+ cells, i.e., MCs, CD11c+ inflammatory DCs, and CD1a+ epidermal DCs are found among inflammatory cells infiltrating in IgE-allergic elderly AD [22, 33] Existence of HDM allergens coincident with IgE+ DCs can be observed in the skin lesions of elderly patients with IgE-allergic AD and HDM sensitization [33] Only a few IgE+ MCs are found among inflammatory cells infiltrating in non-IgE-allergic elderly AD [22]
Diagnosis of elderly AD	A long follow-up (more than 6 months), analyses of diagnostic features of AD, and exclusion from other pruritic skin conditions are required
Epidemiology	The prevalence of elderly AD is approximately 1–3% among elderly individuals in industrialized countries [4, 43] Male predominance: particularly for IgE-allergic and indeterminate-allergic types [12]; the male-female ratio for elderly AD is approximately 2:1 [12], 1.75:1 [4]
Onset and clinical course	Three main patterns are apparent: senile onset (continuous type), senile recurrence with history of classic child AD (outgrowth-recurrence type), continuation and/or recurrence of adolescent/adult AD (both continuous and outgrowth-recurrence types) [3, 6, 8, 12]
Personal and family histories of disorders associated with AD	Associations with clinical phenotypes and asthmatic complications are seen in elderly patients with IgE-allergic AD with onset before 30 years old [12] Lower incidence of ichthyosis in elderly patients with IgE-allergic AD [12]
Complications of coexisting/underlying disorders and malignancy	Most elderly AD patients have some complications of nonallergic coexisting/underlying disorders Lower incidence of malignancy in elderly patients with IgE-allergic AD [8, 12]

(continued)

Table 18.1 (continued)

Management and prognosis	Majority of elderly AD patients show good prognosis after suitable management Powerful anti-inflammatory treatments like oral corticosteroids may be needed in moderate to severe cases Complete remission (outgrowth) rarely arises Most elderly AD patients reach the end of life with AD [12]

Table reproduced with permission from *Geriatrics Gerontology International* [8]
Abbreviations: *AD* atopic dermatitis, *CD* cluster of differentiation, *DCs* dendritic cells, *HDM* house dust mite, *IgE* immunoglobulin E, *IL* interleukin, *IFN-γ* interferon-γ, *MCs* mast cells, *Th* T-helper

18.2.2 Skin Manifestations

The characteristics of skin manifestations seen in elderly AD basically match those of adolescent/adult AD [2]. Chronic eczema on the face and neck and exudative/lichenified eczematous dermatitis on the trunk and extremities are observed as major symptoms in elderly AD. Other stigmata of AD such as refractory facial erythema (atopic red face), Hertoghe's sign (loss of the lateral eyebrows), Dennie-Morgan's infraorbital folds, and dirty neck are observed mainly in moderate to severe cases (Fig. 18.1a–f). Nummular-form eczema, prurigo-form papules and/or nodules, chronic hand and/or foot eczema, and erythrodermic rash may also be observed (Fig. 18.1g–k).

One feature of skin manifestations in elderly AD that might distinguish this form from adolescent/adult AD is the involvement of the folds of the elbows and knees. Localized lichenified eczema in the elbow and knee folds is a typical sign of classic childhood AD and adolescent/young adult AD [1, 5, 17], but is uncommon in elderly AD [3, 12]. In elderly AD, unaffected folds of the elbows and knees are common, and lichenified eczema surrounding the folds, particularly around the elbow folds, are frequently observed. In our clinical study of 38 patients with IgE-allergic elderly AD [12], lichenified eczema in the flexure and/or extensor sites of the upper and lower extremities were observed in 30 patients (78.9%) and 22 patients (57.9%), respectively. However, a lack of lichenified eczema in the folds of elbows and knees was observed in 29 patients (76.3%) and 28 patients (73.7%), respectively. The classic sign of localized lichenification in the elbow and knee folds was observed in only two patients (5.3%) and four patients (10.5%), respectively (Fig. 18.2a, d). Diffuse lichenified eczema in the flexure sites of the extremities, including the elbow and knee folds, was observed in seven patients (18.4%) and six patients (15.8%), respectively (Fig. 18.2b, e). On the other hand, the reverse sign of lichenified eczema around unaffected folds of the elbows and knees was observed in 15 patients (39.5%) and in 5 patients (13.2%), respectively (Fig. 18.2c, f). This feature of scarce involvement in the folds of the elbows and knees in elderly AD might be partly associated with age-related decrements in regional sweat function [8, 13], because sweating can be related to the development of skin lesions of AD at these sites [14], and a pathophysiology of AD as an irritant, a major source of skin moisture, and an allergen for immediate hypersensitivity reactions [14–16].

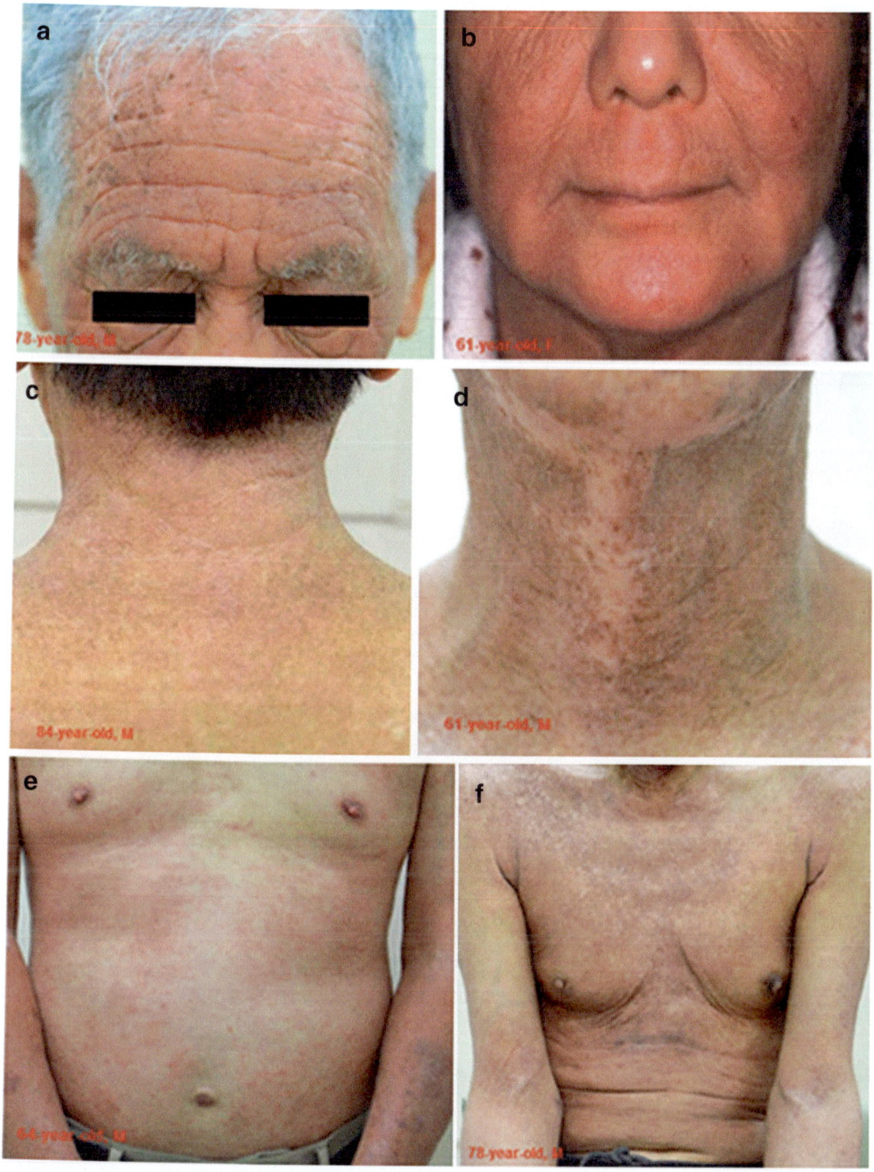

Fig. 18.1 Skin manifestations of elderly atopic dermatitis. (**a**) Lichenified eczema with post-inflammatory depigmentation, Hertoghe's sign (loss of lateral eyebrows), and Dennie-Morgan's infraorbital folds on the face. (**b**) Refractory eczematous erythema (atopic red face) on the face. Figure reproduced with permission from the *Japanese Journal of Allergology* [7]. (**c**) Lichenified eczema on the neck and upper back. Figure reproduced with permission from *Geriatrics & Gerontology International* [8]. (**d**) Lichenified eczema with post-inflammatory depigmentation on the neck (dirty neck). (**e**) Eczematous dermatitis with a diffuse exudative inflammation on the trunk. (**f**) Diffuse lichenified eczema on the trunk and localized lichenified eczema in the right elbow fold. (**g**) Nummular-form eczema on the back. (**h**) Prurigo-form papules on the left arm. (**i**) Lichenified hand eczema. (**j**) Lichenified foot eczema. (**k**) Lichenified eczema of erythroderma on the trunk

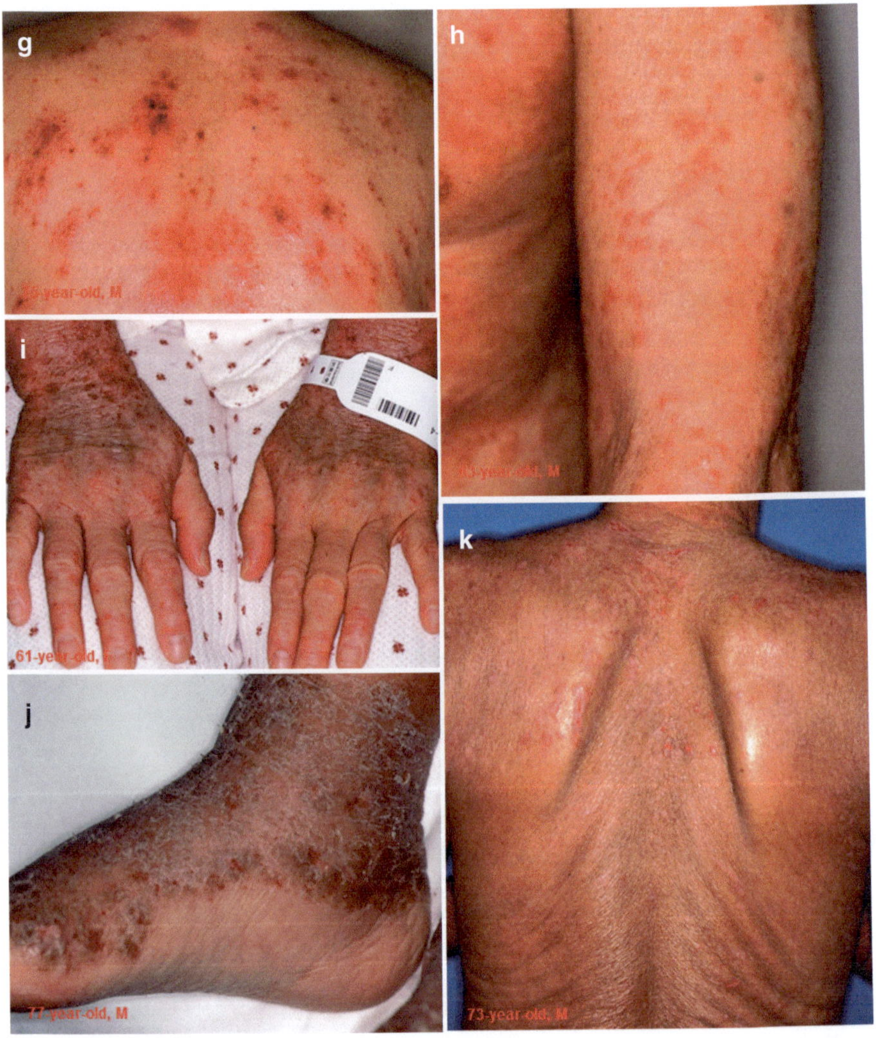

Fig. 18.1 (continued)

18.2.3 IgE Reactivity and Cytokines

The average level of serum total IgE in elderly patients with IgE-allergic AD has been reported as 2540 ± 2234 IU/mL in Poland [4] and 6975 ± 9908 IU/mL according to a previous study in our hospital [12]. The most common environmental allergens for IgE-allergic elderly AD are house dust mites (HDMs; e.g., *Dermatophagoides* species), followed by pollens (e.g., grass pollen and Japanese cedar). Positive rates were as follows: *D. pteronyssinus* (*Der p*), 72%; *D. farinae* (*Der f*), 70.9%; and grass pollen, 68.4% in the Polish study [4], and *Der f*, 83.8%, and Japanese cedar, 56.8% in the study of our patients [12]. Positive rates for foods, fungus, and animal dander were relatively lower in

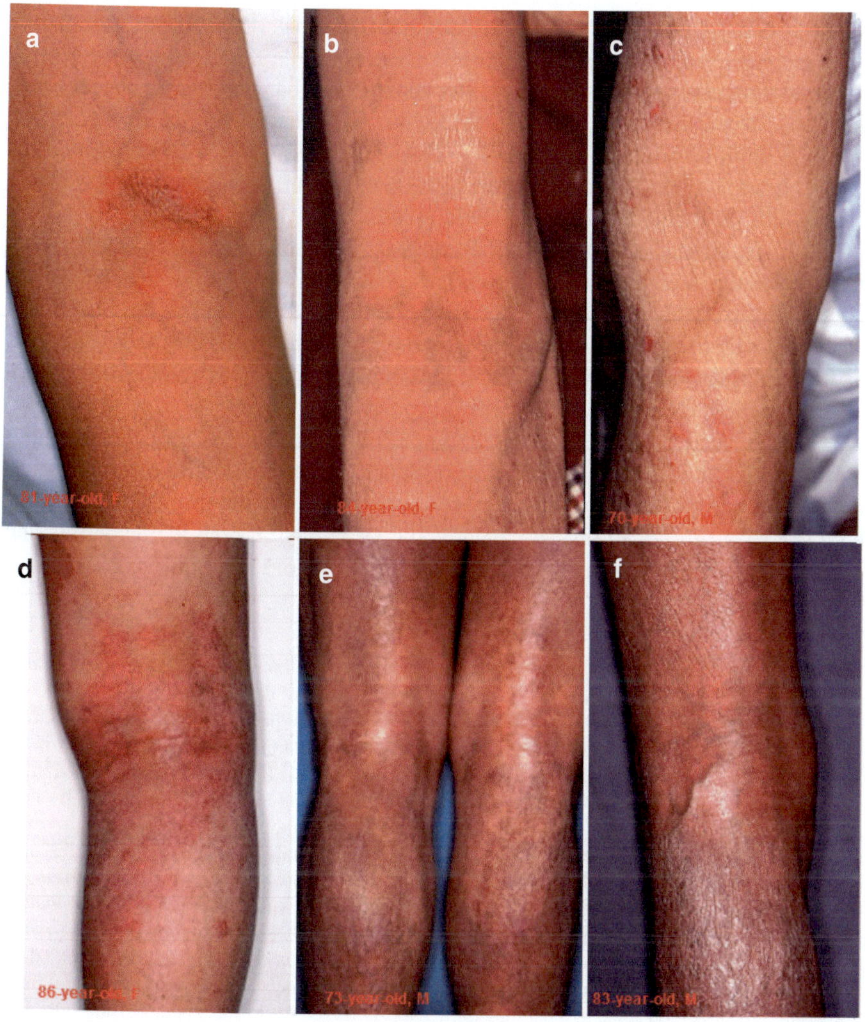

Fig. 18.2 Lichenification (lichenified eczema) in the antecubital and popliteal areas of elderly patients with atopic dermatitis. (**a**) Localized lichenified eczema in the elbow fold. (**b**) Diffuse lichenified eczema in the elbow fold and flexure site of the arm. (**c**) Lichenified eczema around the scarcely involved elbow fold. Figures reproduced with permission from the *Journal of Clinical Medicine* [12]. (**d**) Localized lichenified eczema in the knee fold. (**e**) Diffuse lichenified eczema in the knee folds and flexure site of the lower extremities. (**f**) Lichenified eczema around the scarcely involved knee fold

those studies. *Der f* also showed the highest average of titers for specific IgEs to environmental allergens in our patients [12].

Phenotypic analyses of peripheral blood cytokine concentrations in the Polish study [4] demonstrated the dominance of a T-helper (Th)2 cytokine profile, i.e., interleukin (IL)-4, IL-5, and IL-13, in elderly patients with IgE-allergic AD, and dominance of a Th1 cytokine profile, i.e., IL-2 and interferon-γ, in elderly patients with AD and low serum total IgE.

18.2.4 Histopathology and Immunopathogenesis of Skin Lesions

The pathogenesis of AD is complex. Recent research has provided a new concept for the immune pathomechanisms underlying AD, assigning roles to innate and adaptive immunity associated with Th1, Th2, Th17, Th22, and T-regulatory cells as well as innate lymphoid cells, macrophages, dendritic cells (DCs), mast cells (MCs), eosinophils, basophils, and keratinocytes [17–21].

On histopathological analysis, a chronic eczematous reaction with inflammatory infiltrating cells, mainly comprising cluster of differentiation (CD)4+ and CD8+ T cells, MCs, macrophages, and eosinophils, is observed in the lichenified eczema of elderly AD [22]. The composition of infiltrating cells is broadly the same as the compositions of nonatopic chronic dermatitides (e.g., asteatotic dermatitis), except for the increase in MCs [3, 22].

Among elderly patients with IgE-allergic AD, IgE-mediated allergic inflammation plays a critical role in the features of skin lesions. Immunohistochemical analysis of our previous study [22] showed IgE+ MCs in the upper dermis (Fig. 18.3a, b), IgE+ CD11c+ DCs (myeloid DCs; so-called atopic DCs [23]) in both the epidermis and upper dermis (Fig. 18.3c), and IgE+ CD1a+ DCs (myeloid DCs; mostly Langerhans

→

Fig. 18.3 Single immunohistochemical and double immunofluorescence staining with anti-immunoglobulin (Ig)E, anti-mast cell tryptase, and anti-cluster of differentiation (CD)11c monoclonal antibodies [22]. A lichenified skin lesion from an elderly patient with IgE-allergic atopic dermatitis (AD): (**a**–**c**). (**a**) Numerous IgE+ cells are seen in inflammatory infiltrating cells in the upper dermis. Original magnification: ×100. (**b**) Tryptase + mast cell infiltration is increased in the upper dermis. Original magnification: ×100. Note that, in (**a**) and (**b**), the majority of IgE+ cells and tryptase + mast cells in the upper dermis show the same morphology and localization (*arrows*). (**c**) Double-positive IgE+ CD11c+ cells (*yellow images*) accompanied by single-positive IgE+ cells (*red images*) and single-positive CD11c+ cells (*green images*) are observed in the epidermis and upper dermis. Original magnification: ×200. Figures reproduced with permission from the *Journal of the European Academy of Dermatology and Venereology* [22] and the *Japanese Journal of Allergology* [7]. A lichenified skin lesion from an elderly patient with non-IgE-allergic AD: (**d**–**f**). (**d**) Few IgE+ cells are present in inflammatory infiltrating cells in the upper dermis. Original magnification: ×100. (**e**) Tryptase + mast cell infiltration is increased in the upper dermis. Original magnification: ×100. (**f**) Only single CD11c+ cells (*green images*) are observed in the epidermis and upper dermis. Original magnification: ×200. Figures reproduced with permission from the *Japanese Journal of Allergology* [7]. An eczematous skin lesion from an elderly patient with non-atopic chronic eczema (asteatotic dermatitis): (**g**–**i**). (**g**) Few IgE+ cells are present in inflammatory infiltrating cells in the upper dermis. Original magnification: ×100. (**h**) Tryptase + mast cells are observed in the upper dermis. Original magnification: ×100. (**i**) Only single-positive CD11c+ cells (*green images*) are apparent in the upper dermis. Original magnification: ×200. Figures reproduced with permission from the *Journal of the European Academy of Dermatology and Venereology* [22] and the *Japanese Journal of Allergology* [7]. A skin lesion of vasculitis from an elderly patient with Churg-Strauss syndrome: (**j**–**l**). (**j**) Numerous IgE+ cells are observed in inflammatory infiltrating cells in the upper dermis. Original magnification: ×100. (**k**) Tryptase + mast cell infiltration is seen in the upper dermis. Original magnification: ×100. Note that, in specimens of (**j**) and (**k**), most IgE+ cells and tryptase + mast cells in the upper dermis show the same morphology and localization. (**l**) The majority of infiltrating stained cells in the epidermis and upper dermis represent single IgE+ cells (*red images*). No double-positive IgE+ CD11c+ cells (*yellow images*) are observed. Original magnification: ×200. Figures reproduced with permission from the *Japanese Journal of Allergology* [7]. Single immunohistochemical staining using serial paraffin sections (**a**, **b**, **d**, **e**, **g**,

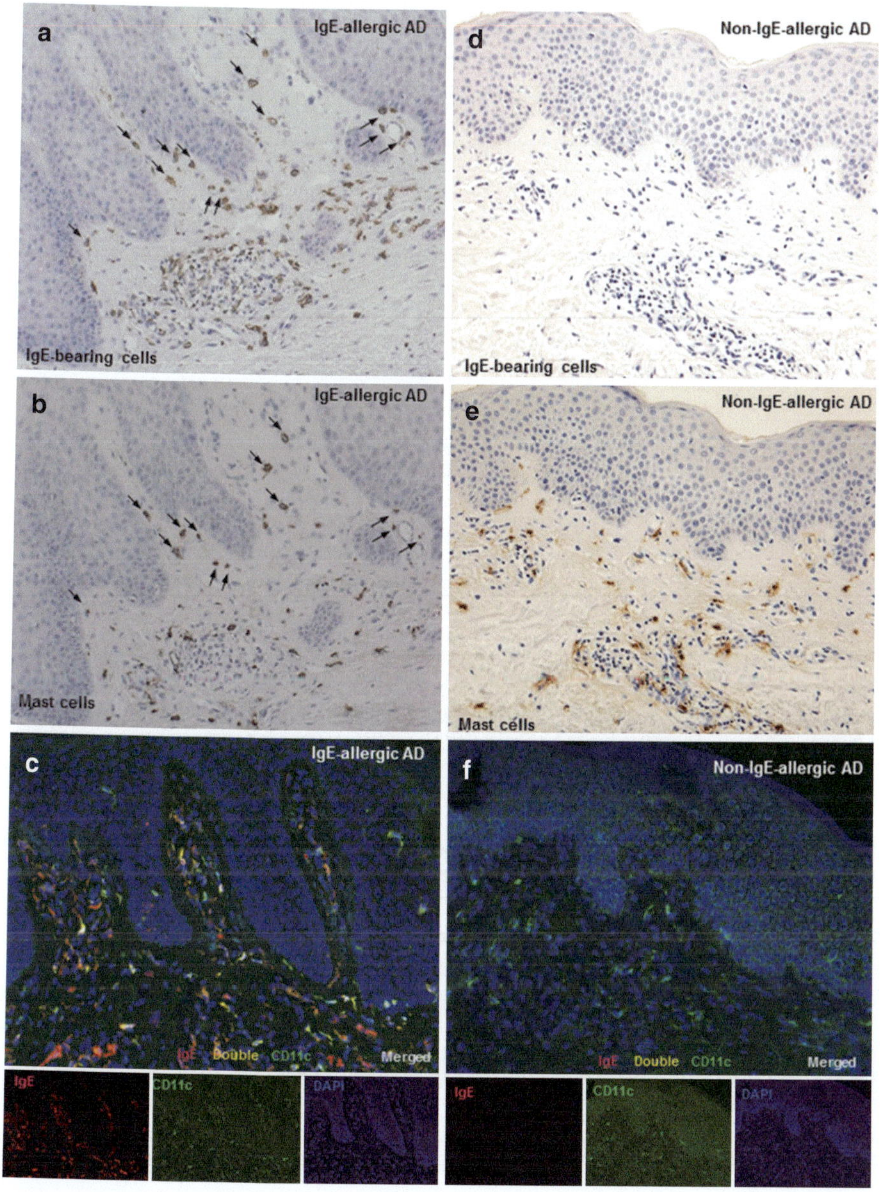

h, **j**, and **k**) and double immunofluorescence staining using frozen sections (**c**, **f**, **i**, and **l**). In the immunohistochemical staining, sets of figures (**a** and **b**, **d** and **e**, **g** and **h**, and **j** and **k**) represent serial sections. In the immunofluorescence staining, nuclei are labeled with 4′,6-diamidino-2-phenylindole (DAPI, *blue images*). Clinical findings: IgE-allergic AD, a 71-year-old man with an elevated serum total IgE level of 2413 IU/mL and specific IgEs for *Dermatophagoides farinae (Der f)* and Japanese cedar; non-IgE-allergic AD, a 63-year-old man with a serum total IgE level of 42 IU/mL and no detectable specific IgEs; asteatotic dermatitis, an 86-year-old man with a serum total IgE level of 16 IU/mL and no detectable specific IgEs; and Churg-Strauss syndrome, a 78-year-old man with an elevated serum total IgE level of 3007 IU/mL and weak positivity for specific IgEs for *Der f*

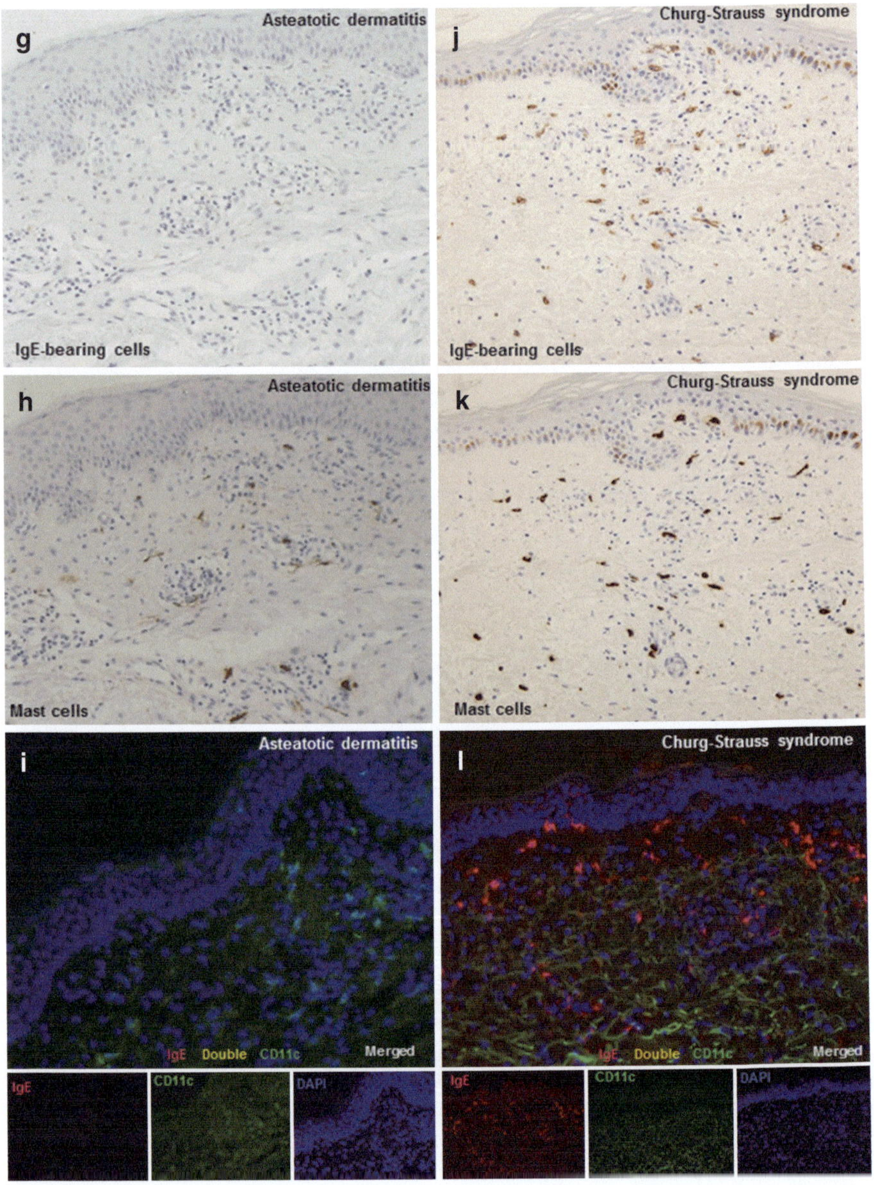

Fig. 18.3 (continued)

cells [24]) in the epidermis in the lichenified eczema of IgE-allergic elderly AD. IgE+ CD11c+ DCs are a type of inflammatory DC, and a group of IgE+ CD11c+ DCs with "CD1a+" could be termed as inflammatory dendritic epidermal cells when they infiltrate into the epidermis [17, 23, 25]. In contrast, although just a few IgE+ MCs were detected, no IgE+ CD11c+ cells or IgE+ CD1a+ cells were found in the lichenified eczema of non-IgE-allergic AD (Fig. 18.3d–f). As with the clinical condition of atopic allergy, immune histopathology of indeterminate-allergic AD showed a vague state between IgE-allergic and non-IgE-allergic AD. In control cases, only a few IgE+ MCs were observed in asteatotic dermatitis (Fig. 18.3g–i). In addition, although moderate IgE+ MCs and slight IgE+ CD1a+ DCs were observed, no IgE+ CD11c+ cells were found in the epidermis or upper dermis in noneczematous disorders with elevated serum total IgE levels (e.g., cholesterol embolism and Churg-Strauss syndrome) (Fig. 18.3j–l).

Complexes of IgE and high-affinity receptor (Fc epsilon receptor type I) on the cell surface of IgE+ MCs, IgE+ CD1a+ DCs, and IgE+ CD11c+ DCs can capture a large amounts of allergens [17, 22, 23], and IgE+ MCs may induce IgE-mediated immediate- and late-phase hypersensitivity reactions [26, 27], and the IgE+ CD1a+ DCs and IgE+ CD11c+ DCs might cause IgE-associated delayed-type hypersensitivity reactions as a result of the efficient presentation of allergens to naïve and/or specific memory T cells [28–30]. The possibility of eczematous skin reactions induced only by IgE-allergic sensitization has been reported using murine models [26]. The existence of HDM allergens in the dermis and epidermis coincident with DCs in naturally occurring AD lesions [31] and with IgE+ DCs in the site of atopy patch test for HDM [32] has been reported in adult patients with IgE-allergic AD and HDM sensitization. Indeed, the existence of HDM allergens (e.g., *Der f* 1) coincident with IgE+ CD11c+DCs in the upper dermis (Fig. 18.4a, b) and with IgE+ CD1a+ DCs (e.g., CD207+ Langerhans cells) in the epidermis (Fig. 18.5a–d) could be observed in the lichenified eczema of elderly patients with IgE-allergic AD and HDM sensitization in our immunohistological studies [33]. These findings suggest that not only IgE-mediated immediate- and late-phase hypersensitivities but also IgE-associated delayed-type hypersensitivity might contribute to the immunopathogenesis of skin manifestations of IgE-allergic elderly AD.

In non-IgE-allergic AD and indeterminate-allergic AD, microbial components (e.g., *Staphylococcus aureus* and resident fungi) [4, 34], metal antigens [10], and HDMs [35] might represent the main triggers for allergic skin inflammation in elderly AD, in which Th1 and/or Th17/Th22 responses presumably evolve [19, 36]. In addition, in indeterminate-allergic elderly AD, IgE-allergic inflammation to common environmental allergens with a moderate regulatory response [8] might also be associated with the development of skin manifestations.

18.2.5 Diagnosis of Elderly AD

At present, AD is considered as a clinical syndrome characterized by several phenotypes in association with heterogeneous genetic backgrounds and various environmental stimuli [9, 17, 20]. Diagnosis of elderly AD should conform to this concept, but some difficulties are encountered. Even now, single definitive clinical, histopathological, and laboratory diagnostic markers are lacking [37]. In addition, elderly individuals often show pruritic skin disorders, e.g., senile xerosis and asteatotic dermatitis, and commonly have other coexisting or underlying medical conditions, such as hypertension, cardiac/cerebral vascular diseases, and diabetes mellitus, which may induce itchy conditions caused directly by the medical conditions and/or as side effects of pharmacotherapy. In fact, most elderly patients with AD in our study [12] had coexisting/underlying disorders. These matters might complicate the diagnosis of elderly AD. A long follow-up (more than 6 months) of the clinical course, analyses of the diagnostic features of AD using standardized criteria, and exclusion of other pruritic skin conditions are thus required to diagnose elderly AD [6]. The main pruritic skin disorders necessitating differentiation from elderly AD are as follows: asteatotic dermatitis, nummular dermatitis, contact dermatitis, urticaria, chronic prurigo, idiopathic/secondary erythroderma [38, 39], papuloerythroderma [40], adverse drug reactions, scabies, and cutaneous T-cell lymphoma [41]. However, certain skin manifestations of the disorders, such asteatotic dermatitis, nummular dermatitis, urticaria, and chronic prurigo, may be involved in the clinical course of elderly AD and may precede its development [3, 6, 8].

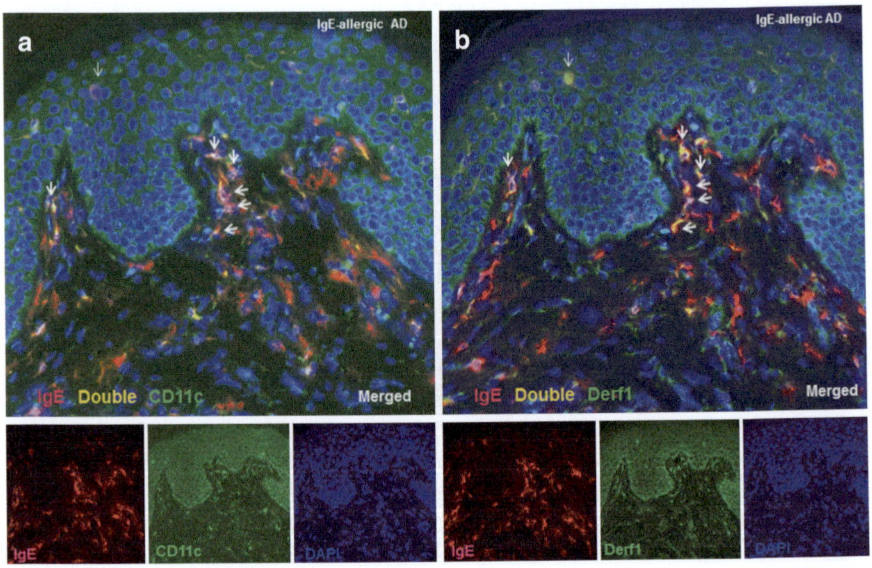

Fig. 18.4 Double immunofluorescence staining with anti-immunoglobulin (Ig)E and anti-cluster-of-differentiation (CD)11c monoclonal antibodies and anti-*Dermatophagoides-farinae (Der f)* 1 polyclonal antibodies. Figures (**a** and **b**) represent serial sections. (**a**) Double-positive IgE+ CD11c+ cells (*yellow images*) are observed in the upper dermis of lichenified eczema of an elderly patient with IgE-allergic atopic dermatitis (AD). Original magnification: ×200. (**b**) Double-positive IgE+ *Der f1*+ cells (*yellow images*) are also observed in the upper dermis of lichenified eczema. Original magnification: ×200. Note that, in specimens of (**a**) and (**b**), the majority of IgE+ CD11c+ cells and IgE+ *Der f1*+ cells in the papillary dermis show the same morphology and localization (*thick arrows*). However, coincidental presence of an IgE+ CD11c− cell and an IgE+ *Der f1*+ cell in the epidermis is also observed (*thin arrows*). Figures reproduced with permission from the *Dermatology Clinics & Research* [33]. Clinical findings: IgE-allergic AD, an 84-year-old man with an elevated serum total IgE level of 19,757 IU/mL and specific IgEs for *Dermatophagoides farinae* and other environmental allergens

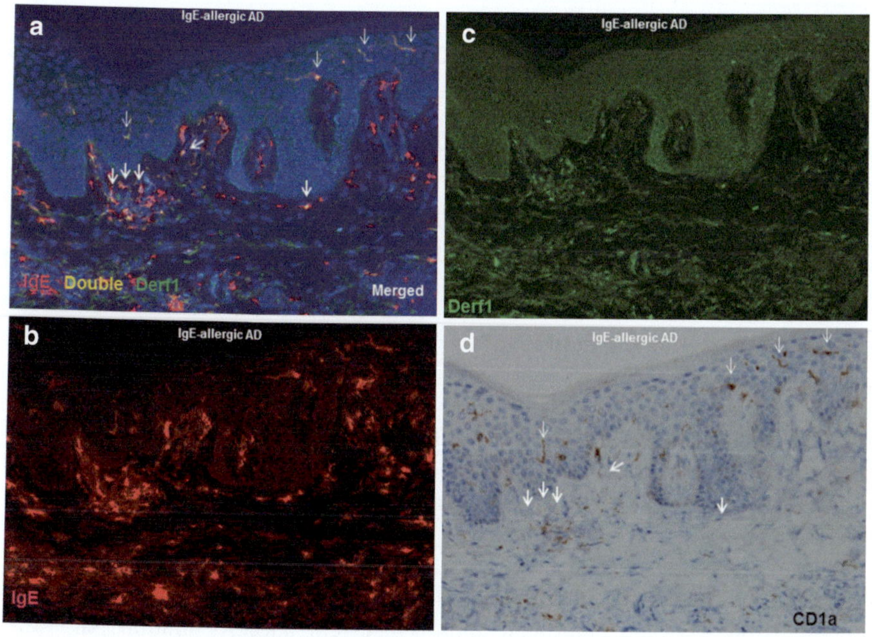

Fig. 18.5 Double immunofluorescence staining and an additional immunohistochemical staining with anti-immunoglobulin (Ig)E and anti-cluster-of-differentiation (CD)1a monoclonal antibodies and anti-*Dermatophagoides farinae (Der f) 1* polyclonal antibodies. Figures **a–c** and **d** represent double immunofluorescence sections and an immunohistochemical section, respectively. (**a**) Double-positive IgE+ *Der f1*+ cells (*yellow images*) are observed both in the epidermis and upper dermis of lichenified eczema of an elderly patient with IgE-allergic atopic dermatitis (AD). Original magnification: ×100. (**b**) Numerous IgE+ cells (*red images*) are seen in the epidermis and upper dermis of the lichenified eczema. Original magnification: ×100. (**c**) Scattered *Der f1*+ cells are observed both in the epidermis and upper dermis of the lichenified eczema. Original magnification: ×100. (**d**) The presence of epidermal CD1a+ dendritic cells coinciding with the morphology and localization of the IgE+ *Der f1*+ cells in figure (**a**) is confirmed in the epidermis of the lichenified eczema by additional immunohistochemical staining (*thin arrows*). Original magnification: ×100. Note that in (**a**) and (**d**), IgE+ *Der f1*+ cells not coinciding with the CD1a+ cells are also observed in the upper dermis (*thick arrows*). Additional immunohistochemical staining with anti-CD1a antibodies (**d**) was carried out after an image recording of double immunofluorescence staining (**a–c**). Figures reproduced with permission from the *Dermatology Clinics & Research* [33]. Clinical findings of the patients with elderly AD were the same as those described in Fig. 18.4

18.2.6 Epidemiology

An epidemiologic analysis in 2007–2008 reported that 3.39% of patients with AD in Japanese dermatology clinics were elderly (≥61 years, $N = 6733$) [42]. The prevalence of elderly AD was reported as 1.86% (≥60 years, $N = 6511$) in Poland [4] and 2.6% (≥60 years old, $N = 1494$) in Japan [43]. In both studies, a male predominance was found in the prevalence of elderly AD, with 2.9% in men and 1.1% in women in Poland

[4] and 3.0% in men and 1.9% in women in Japan [43]. The male-female ratio for elderly AD was approximately 2:1 in our study of 60 cases [12] and 1.75:1 in the study of 121 cases from Poland [4]. Male predominances in elderly AD were notable for the IgE-allergic and indeterminate-allergic types in our study [12]. These gender gaps in the development of elderly AD might reflect the influence of age-related changes to sex hormone levels on the immune system in the elderly, such as androgen deficiency in both sexes increasing the IL-4 production capacity of T cells and estrogen deficiency in elderly women increasing the interferon-γ production capacity of T cells [8, 44].

18.2.7 Onset and Clinical Course

From the perspective of geriatric dermatology, two clinical courses and three patterns of AD onset were mainly seen for elderly AD: senile onset (continuous type), senile recurrence with a history of classic child AD (outgrowth-recurrence type), and continuation and/or recurrence of adolescent/adult AD (both continuous and outgrowth-recurrence types with a history of infantile-, childhood-, adolescent-, or adult-onset AD) [12]. In our study of 60 cases of elderly AD [12], the incidences of senile-onset AD, senile recurrence with a history of classic child AD, and continued and/or recurrent adolescent/adult AD were 66.7%, 6.7%, and 26.7%, respectively. In addition, 13.3% of elderly patients with AD in total had a history of child AD. In the Polish study of 121 cases [4], the incidences of senile-onset AD, senile recurrence with a history of classic child AD, and adult-onset AD (another classification) were approximately 21%, 67%, and 12%, respectively. The discrepancies in the incidences of each type of elderly AD between Japan and Poland might be attributable to the differences in race, lifestyle, prevalence of child AD before the 1960s, and the medical record system in each country. Taking into consideration the obvious increase in AD among early- to middle-aged people from the 1980s [42], the frequencies of elderly patients with AD and with a history of infantile-, childhood-, adolescent-, or adult-onset AD may be speculated to increase in the near future in Japan and other industrialized countries.

18.2.8 Personal and Family Histories of Disorders Associated with AD

With regard to the personal history of allergic disorders associated with AD, incidences in elderly patients with IgE-allergic AD ($n = 38$), indeterminate-allergic AD ($n = 9$), and non-IgE-allergic AD ($n = 13$) in our study ($n = 60$) were as follows: bronchial asthma (BA), 36.8%, 44.4%, and 15.4%; allergic rhino-conjunctivitis (AR), 52.6%, 44.4%, and 38.5%; and urticaria, 21.1%, 22.2%, and 15.4%, respectively [12]. No significant differences were observed in incidences among the three types of elderly AD.

In terms of complications of BA, however, some interesting findings have been observed: in IgE-allergic elderly AD ($n = 38$), elderly patients with the outgrowth-recurrence type of early life-onset (until the young adult phase; <30 years old) AD

($n = 5$) showed a significantly higher incidence of childhood BA (60%; $n = 3$; $p < 0.05$) than those (0%; $n = 0$) with the continuous type of early life-onset AD ($n = 8$). In addition, elderly patients with continuous-type adolescent-/young-adult-onset AD ($n = 5$; 5 of the 8) had no history of childhood BA and adult/senile BA. These findings suggest that in early life-onset IgE-allergic elderly AD, at least two different phenotypes might exist: outgrowth-recurrence type with a history of childhood BA and continuous type from adolescent-/young-adult-onset AD without an asthmatic constitution. In the former, pathogenic dynamics similar to the so-called atopic (allergic) march [45] might be associated with the relapsing clinical course.

With regard to complications of nonallergic disorder, a significantly lower incidence of ichthyosis was observed in elderly patients with IgE-allergic AD (2.6%, $n = 1$) as compared with elderly patients with indeterminate-allergic AD (33.3%, $n = 3$; $p < 0.05$) or non-IgE-allergic AD (23.1%, $n = 3$; $p < 0.05$) in our study [12]. This result is supported by a previous study of adolescent/adult AD that presented a tendency toward a lower incidence of ichthyosis in IgE-allergic AD compared with non-IgE-allergic AD [46]. Meanwhile, ichthyosis-related gene mutation of filaggrin (FLG)—a protein with a key role in epidermal barrier function—is now considered the most widely reproducible genetic risk for AD. Several recent investigations [47–49] have suggested a strong association between FLG loss-of-function mutations and the development of AD in younger age groups (infancy to middle age) of IgE-allergic AD (approximately 30% of the AD population). Analyses of the FLG mutation in elderly patients with AD have not been widely undertaken. We analyzed FLG mutations (3321delA, Q1790X, Ser2554X, Ser2889X, Ser3296X, and Lys4022X) associated with the Japanese AD population [48, 49] in two elderly patients: a father-and-daughter pair, with IgE-allergic AD (one with continuous-type late adult-onset AD and another with continuous-type adolescent-onset AD) who had participated in the clinical study and lacked complicated ichthyosis, but could not detect any change to the risk [50]. In a previous study conducted using middle-aged to older adults (≥50 years old; mean age, 62.9 years; $N = 2057$) in the United Kingdom [51], FLG mutations (for R501X and/or 2282del4; highly significant risk factors in Caucasian populations) were significantly associated with a personal history of diagnosed eczema (probable AD, $p = 0.009$) and early onset before 20 years old ($p = 0.003$). However, FLG mutations were not associated with serum levels of total IgE or specific IgEs to HDM allergens among participants, and >80% of FLG mutation carriers had a history of neither BA nor atopic eczema in that study [51]. In view of these data, the FLG mutation may not represent a crucial genetic risk for the development of IgE-allergic elderly AD, particularly for the senile-onset type.

No significant difference in the family history of elderly patients with AD was evident among the three types. In cases of IgE-allergic AD, indeterminate-allergic AD, and non-IgE-allergic AD, incidences of family history were as follows: AD, 26.3%, 22.2%, and 38.5%; AR, 15.8%, 0%, and 7.7%; BA 15.8%, 11.1%, and 23.1%; and nonexistent, 50%, 33.3%, and 46.2%, respectively [12]. In our clinical study, we encountered a father-and-daughter pair with IgE-allergic elderly AD and found a major histocompatibility complex class II allele (i.e., human leukocyte antigen-DRB1*1501; a gene encoding an immunodominant epitope of HDMs) as a common genetic background for the development of AD [50].

18.2.9 Complications of Coexisting/Underlying Disorders and Malignancy

Most elderly patients with AD have some complications of nonallergic coexisting/underlying disorders (e.g., hypertension, heart disease, cerebrovascular disease, spinal disease, and diabetes mellitus). The incidence of complications of the disorders in elderly patients with AD does not show any marked divergence from trends for the incidence in the general population of elderly Japanese individuals [12]. In medical practice, however, the existence of these coexisting/underlying disorders may bring about difficulties in reaching a diagnosis of elderly AD and also place restrictions on treatment options, such as the use of oral corticosteroids and cyclosporine.

Meanwhile, the incidence of complicating malignancy in elderly patients with IgE-allergic AD might be lower than in the general elderly population. In our retrospective analysis [12], incidence of malignancy (2.6%; $n = 1$) among elderly patients with IgE-allergic AD ($n = 38$; 27 men, 11 women; ≥60 years old; mean age, 76.2 ± 8.7 years; mean duration of follow-up, 51.0 ± 46.1 months) was significantly lower than that (31.9%, $n = 23$; $p < 0.05$) in control subjects (elderly patients with benign epidermal cyst; $n = 72$; 47 men, 25 women; ≥60 years old; mean age, 74.7 ± 7.0 years; mean duration of follow-up, 57.7 ± 46.7 months) [8, 12]. Furthermore, elderly patients with IgE-allergic AD tended to show a lower incidence (0%; $n = 0$) of mortality from malignancy than control subjects (44.4%; $n = 4$), although the difference did not reach the level of significance due to the small number of cases (death was confirmed by our hospital in six patients with IgE-allergic elderly AD (mean age at death, 87.5 ± 7.9 years) and in nine control subjects (mean age at death, 81.1 ± 4.2 years)) [8, 12]. In addition, the chief cause of death among elderly Japanese (65–89 years old) is malignancy [12]. Although the limitations of retrospective analysis and a small sample size must be considered, these results suggest the hypothesis that the disease state in IgE-allergic elderly AD might involve immunological peculiarities acting against malignancy as a result of over-response against foreign substances, including self-antigens [17, 20], in which cancer antigens could be involved.

18.2.10 Management and Prognosis

In general, as with other age groups, management of elderly AD comprises treatment to maintain the skin barrier (e.g., moisturizer and emollients), anti-inflammatory measures (e.g., topical corticosteroids, topical tacrolimus, oral antihistamines, and oral anti-allergic agent), and the identification and avoidance of trigger factors (e.g., environmental allergens) [52]. Regular application of moisturizers and emollients in combination with topical corticosteroids and tacrolimus and oral antihistamines/

cytokine inhibitors has been the standard of treatment for elderly AD [6, 8]. In older patients, however, avoiding trigger factors in the environment and applying sufficient topical medication is difficult, because of potential decreases to activities of daily living with aging and lifestyle (e.g., isolated elderly individuals). Therefore, for moderate to severe cases and/or elderly cases with a lower ability to use topical treatments, powerful anti-inflammatory treatments like oral corticosteroid therapy (5–10 mg/day or 0.1–0.2 mg/kg body weight/day in prednisolone equivalents) may be used with standard treatments [12]. However, this requires appropriate monitoring and prevention of adverse events such as hypertension, peptic ulcer, cataract, osteoporosis, diabetes mellitus, and steroid purpura. As with other adjunctive treatments, narrowband ultraviolet B at a dosage of approximately 0.35–0.70 J/cm^2 per irradiation appears extremely effective for elderly AD [53]. Oral cyclosporine is also effective for the treatment of severe cases of elderly AD, but clinicians must pay attention to the increased risk of malignancy [54] and organ toxicity (e.g., renal dysfunction) in the elderly.

The majority of elderly AD patients would obtain amelioration of skin manifestations once they receive the aforementioned suitable managements in later life. In our clinical study ($n = 52$), with the principle use of standard treatments ($n = 25$) or combined therapy (standard treatments with oral corticosteroids, $n = 27$) for a duration of 6 months or more, the prognosis for elderly AD was as follows: clinical improvement was observed in 80.8% (IgE-allergic AD, 73.5%; indeterminate-allergic AD, 100%; and non-IgE-allergic AD, 90%) of cases, and clinical remission was obtained in 36.5% (IgE-allergic AD, 29.4%; indeterminate-allergic AD, 37.5%; and non-IgE-allergic AD, 60%) of cases. Clinical remission and clinical improvement were defined as follows: clinical remission is characterized by disappearance of skin lesions (≥6 months) in more than 95% of lesional areas observed with standard treatments or with combined therapy even after discontinuation of oral corticosteroids; clinical improvement is characterized by the same disappearance of skin lesions (<6 months) observed with standard treatments or the same disappearance of skin lesions (≥6 months) observed with combined therapy at a dosage of prednisolone ≤5 mg/day [8, 12].

However, complete remission (outgrowth, a condition without any need for treatment) was rarely achieved in elderly patients with AD. The majority of elderly patients who died had continued to receive treatments for AD until just before death [12]. Most elderly AD patients would thus reach the end of life with AD.

18.3 Future Directions

AD should now be considered as a lifelong allergic condition in some populations. In the near future, AD will become an ordinary disease of elderly people in an aging society. The natural lifetime courses of AD in accordance with the genetic background, environmental stimuli, and heterogeneous clinical phenotypes will become apparent. Risk classifications for the development of elderly AD in patients with or without a history of infantile-, childhood-, adolescent- and adult-onset AD will also eventually become apparent. For management, as in other age groups, new groups of therapeutics will also be used in elderly patients with AD, for example, antipruritic drugs [55], allergen-specific immunotherapy [56], and biologics [20, 21]. At that time, understanding the characteristic clinical manifestations of elderly AD will provide insights into relevant phenotyping and proper management, including the use of new therapeutics. Further investigation of larger cohorts of elderly patients with AD is warranted.

Acknowledgments The author thanks the *Japanese Journal of Allergology* (Japanese Society of Allergology) and *Geriatrics & Gerontology International* (Japan Geriatric Society and Wiley) for the permission to reuse a table, figures, and portions of text from original articles (Refs. 7, 8) in those journals.

References

1. Sulzberger MB, Goodman J. The relative importance of specific skin hypersensitivity in adult atopic dermatitis. JAMA. 1936;106:1000–3.
2. Nishioka K. Atopic eczema of adult type in Japan. Australas J Dermatol. 1996;37(Suppl):S7–9.
3. Tanei R, Katsuoka K. Clinical analyses of atopic dermatitis in the aged. J Dermatol. 2008;35:562–9.
4. Bozek A, Fisher A, Filipowska B, Mazur B, Jazab J. Clinical features and immunological markers of atopic dermatitis in elderly patients. Int Arch Allergy Immunol. 2012;157:372–8.
5. Bieber T, Bussmann C. Atopic dermatitis. In: Bolognia JL, Jorizzo JL, Schaffer JV, editors. Dermatology, vol. 1. 3rd ed. Amsterdam: Elsevier; 2012. p. 203–17.
6. Tanei R. Atopic dermatitis in the elderly. Inflamm Allergy Drug Targets. 2009;8:394–404.
7. Tanei R. Atopic dermatitis in the elderly. Jpn J Allergol. 2015;64:918–25. (in Japanese)
8. Tanei R, Hasegawa Y. Atopic dermatitis in older adults: a viewpoint from geriatric dermatology. Geriatr Gerontol Int. 2016;16(Suppl. 1):75–86.
9. Leung DYM, Boguniewicz M, Howell MD, Nomura I, Hamid QA. New insights into atopic dermatitis. J Clin Invest. 2004;113:651–7.
10. Tokura Y. Extrinsic and intrinsic types of atopic dermatitis. J Dermatol Sci. 2010;58:1–7.
11. Park JH, Choi YL, Namkung JH, Kim WS, Lee JH, Park HJ, et al. Characteristics of extrinsic and intrinsic atopic dermatitis in infancy: correlations with laboratory variables. Br J Dermatol. 2006;155:778–83.
12. Tanei R. Clinical characteristics, treatments, and prognosis of atopic eczema in the elderly. J Clin Med. 2015;4:979–97.
13. Smith CJ, Alexander LM, Kenney WL. Nonuniform, age-related decrements in regional sweating and skin blood flow. Am J Physiol Regul Integr Comp Physiol. 2013;305:R877–85.
14. Takahashi A, Murota H, Matsui S, Kijima A, Kitaba S, Lee JB, et al. Decreased sudomotor function is involved in the formation of atopic eczema in the cubital fossa. Allergol Int. 2013;62:473–8.
15. Shiohara T, Doi T, Hayakawa J. Defective sweating responses in atopic dermatitis. In: Shiohara T, editor. Pathogenesis and management of atopic dermatitis. Basel: Karger; 2011. p. 68–79.
16. Hide M, Tanaka T, Yamamura Y, Koro O, Yamamoto S. IgE-mediated hypersensitivity against human sweat antigen in patients with atopic dermatitis. Acta Derm Venereol. 2002;82:335–40.
17. Bieber T. Atopic dermatitis. N Engl J Med. 2008;358:1483–94.
18. Benedetto AD, Agnihothri R, McGirt LY, Bankova LG, Beck LA. Atopic dermatitis: a disease caused by innate immune defects? J Invest Dermatol. 2009;129:14–30.
19. Kabashima K. New concept of the pathogenesis of atopic dermatitis: interplay among the barrier, allergy, and pruritus as a trinity. J Dermatol Sci. 2013;70:3–11.

20. Eyerich K, Novak N. Immunology of atopic eczema: overcoming the Th1/Th2 paradigm. Allergy. 2013;68:974–82.
21. Werfel T, Allam JP, Biedermann T, Eyerich K, Gilles S, Guttman-Yassky E, et al. Cellular and molecular immunologic mechanisms in patients with atopic dermatitis. J Allergy Clin Immunol. 2016;138:336–49.
22. Tanei R, Hasegawa Y, Sawabe M. Abundant immunoglobulin E-positive cells in skin lesions support an allergic etiology of atopic dermatitis in the elderly. J Eur Acad Dermatol Venereol. 2013;27:952–60.
23. Guttman-Yassky E, Lowes MA, Fuentes-Duculan J, Whynot J, Novitskaya I, Cardinale I, et al. Major differences in inflammatory dendritic cells and their products distinguish atopic dermatitis from psoriasis. J Allergy Clin Immunol. 2007;119:1210–7.
24. Bruynzeel-Koomen C, van Wichen DF, Toonstra J, Berrens L, Bruynzeel PL. The presence of IgE molecules on epidermal Langerhans cells in patients with atopic dermatitis. Arch Dermatol Res. 1986;278:1993–205.
25. Hammad H, Plantinga M, Deswarte K, Pouliot P, Willart MAM, Kool M, et al. Inflammatory dendritic cells—not basophils—are necessary and sufficient for induction of Th2 immunity to inhaled house dust mite allergen. J Exp Med. 2010;207:2097–111.
26. Katayama I, Tanei R, Yokozeki H, Nishioka K, Dohi Y. Induction of eczematous skin reaction in experimentally induced hyperplastic skin of Balb/C mice by monoclonal anti-DNP IgE antibody: possible implication for skin lesion formation in atopic dermatitis. Int Arch Allergy Appl Immunol. 1990;93:148–54.
27. Okada M, Terui T, Honda M, Tanaka M, Chikama R, Tabata N, et al. Cutaneous late phase reaction in adult atopic dermatitis patients with high serum IgE antibody to *Dermatophagoides farinae*: correlation with IL-5 production by allergen-stimulated peripheral blood mononuclear cells. J Dermatol Sci. 2002;29:73–84.
28. Thepen T, Langeveld-Wildschut EG, Bihari IC, van Wichen DF, van Reijsen FC, Mudde GC, et al. Biphasic response against aeroallergen in atopic dermatitis showing a switch from an initial Th2 response to a Th1 response in situ: an immunocytochemical study. J Allergy Clin Immunol. 1996;97:828–37.
29. Bieber T. FcεRI-expressing antigen-presenting cells: new players in atopic game. Immunol Today. 1997;18:311–3.
30. Stingl G, Maurer D. IgE-mediated allergen presentation via Fc Epsilon RI on antigen-presenting cells. Int Arch Allergy Immunol. 1997;113:24–9.
31. Maeda K, Yamamoto K, Tanaka Y, Anan S, Yoshida H. House dust mite (HDM) antigen in naturally occurring lesions of atopic dermatitis (AD): the relationship between HDM antigen in the skin and HDM antigen-specific IgE antibody. J Dermatol Sci. 1992;3:73–7.
32. Tanaka Y, Tanaka M, Anan S, Yoshida H. Immunohistochemical studies on dust mite antigen in positive reaction site of patch test. Acta Derm Venereol (Stockh). 1989;144:93–6.
33. Tanei R, Hasegawa Y. Double-positive immunoglobulin E+ and Dermatophagoides farinae antigen+ dendritic cells are observed in skin Lesions of older adults with atopic dermatitis: an immunohistological study. Dermatol Clin Res. 2017;3(1):134–50.
34. Novak N, Allam JP, Bieber T. Allergic hyperreactivity to microbial components: a trigger factor of "intrinsic" atopic dermatitis? J Allergy Clin Immunol. 2003;112:215–6.
35. Kerschenlohr K, Decard S, Darsow U, Ollert M, Wollenberg A. Clinical and immunologic reactivity to aeroallergens in "intrinsic" atopic dermatitis patients. J Allergy Clin Immunol. 2003:111:195–7.
36. Suárez-Fariñas M, Dhingra N, Gittler J, Shemer A, Cardinale I, de Guzman SC, et al. Intrinsic atopic dermatitis shows similar Th2 and higher Th17 immune activation compared with extrinsic atopic dermatitis. J Allergy Clin Immunol. 2013;132:361–70.
37. Thijs JL, van Seggelen W, Bruijnzeel-Koomen C, de Bruin-Weller M, Hijnen D. New developments in biomarkers for atopic dermatitis. J Clin Med. 2015;4:479–87.
38. Asai T, Horiuchi Y. Senile erythroderma with serum hyper IgE. Int J Dermatol. 1989;28:255–8.
39. Nakano-Tahara M, Terao M, Nishioka M, Kitaba S, Murota H, Katayama I. T helper 2 polarization in senile erythroderma with elevated levels of TARC and IgE. Dermatology. 2015;230:62–9.

40. Camacho FM, García-Hernandez MJ, Muñoz-Pérez MA, Mazuecos J, Sotillo I. Ofuji papuloerythroderma in elderly woman with atopic erythroderma. J Eur Acad Dermatol Venereol. 2001;15:264–6.
41. Miyagaki T, Sugaya M. Erythrodermic cutaneous T-cell lymphoma: how to differentiate this rare disease from atopic dermatitis. J Dermatol Sci. 2011;64:1–6.
42. Furue M, Chiba T, Takeuchi S. Current status of atopic dermatitis in Japan. Asia Pac Allergy. 2011;1:64–72.
43. Muto T, Hsieh SD, Sakurai Y, Yoshinaga H, Suto H, Okumura K, et al. Epidemiology and health services research prevalence of atopic dermatitis in Japanese adults. Br J Dermatol. 2003;148:117–21.
44. Pietschmann P, Gollob E, Brosch S, Hahn P, Kudlacek S, Willheim M, et al. The effect of age and gender on cytokine production by human peripheral blood mononuclear cells and markers of bone metabolism. Exp Gerontol. 2003;38:1119–27.
45. Spergel JM, Poller AS. Atopic dermatitis and the atopic march. J Allergy Clin Immunol. 2003;112:S118–27.
46. Brenninkmeijer EEA, Spuls PI, Legierse CM, Lindeboom R, Smitt JHS, Bos JD. Clinical differences between atopic and atopiform dermatitis. J Am Acad Dermatol. 2008;58:407–14.
47. Irvine AD, McLean WH. Filaggrin mutation associated with skin and allergic diseases. N Engl J Med. 2011;365:1315–27.
48. Nomura T, Akiyama M, Sandilands A, Nemoto-Hasebe I, Sakai K, Nagasaki A, et al. Specific filaggrin mutations cause ichthyosis vulgaris and are significantly associated with atopic dermatitis in Japan. J Invest Dermatol. 2008;128:1436–41.
49. Enomoto H, Hirata K, Otuka K, Kawai T, Takahashi T, Hirota T, et al. Filaggrin null mutations are associated with atopic dermatitis and elevated levels of IgE in Japanese population: a family and case-control study. J Hum Genet. 2008;53:615–21.
50. Tanei R, Noguchi E. Elderly atopic dermatitis in a father and daughter associated with MHC class II allele HLA-DRB1*1501. Dermatol Clin Res. 2016;2(3):95–8. ISSN:2380-5609.
51. Rice NE, Patel BD, Lang IA, Kumari M, Frayling TM, Murray A, et al. Filaggrin gene mutations are associated with asthma and eczema in later life. J Allergy Clin Immunol. 2008;122:834–6.
52. Katayama I, Kohno Y, Akiyama K, Ikezawa Z, Kondo N, Tamaki K, et al. Japanese guideline for atopic dermatitis. Allergol Int. 2011;60:205–20.
53. Tanei R, Oda A, Hasegawa Y. Narrow-band ultraviolet B is a useful adjunctive treatment for atopic dermatitis in older adults: case reports. Dermatol Clin Res. 2016;2(3):112–7.
54. Nakamura S, Takeda K, Hashimoto Y, Mizumoto T, Ishida-Yamamoto A, Iizuka H. Primary cutaneous CD30+ lymphoproliferative disorder in an atopic dermatitis patient on cyclosporine therapy. Indian J Dermatol Venereol Leprol. 2011;77:253.
55. Furue M, Kadono T. New therapies for controlling atopic itch. J Dermatol. 2015;42:847–50.
56. Novak N, Bieber T, Hoffmann M, Fölster-Holst R, Homey B, Werfel T, et al. Efficacy and safety of subcutaneous allergen-specific immunotherapy with depigmented polymerized mite extract in atopic dermatitis. J Allergy Clin Immunol. 2012;130:925–31.

Differential Diagnosis of Atopic Dermatitis

19

Ichiro Katayama

Abstract

Regarding the treatment of atopic dermatitis (hereafter referred to "AD"), diagnostic criteria proposed by the Japanese Dermatological Association [1] and therapeutic guidelines established by the Japanese Society of Allergology [2] have been published. These guidelines enable us to conduct standard therapy for mild to severe pediatric and adult AD. Therapeutic methodology based on EBM will likely be established in the twenty-first century. Using these criteria, all diseases that meet the three requirements of itching, characteristic rashes and distribution, and chronic/recurrent progression will be diagnosed as atopic dermatitis irrespective of the severity of symptoms [1]. From this point of view, in this chapter, we summarize the differential diagnosis of AD (Table 19.1), which is required for assessing daily treatment. Important differential diagnoses listed in diagnostic criteria proposed by the Japanese Dermatological Association are as follows: contact dermatitis, seborrheic dermatitis, prurigo simplex, scabies, miliaria, ichthyosis, xerotic eczema, hand dermatitis (non-atopic), cutaneous lymphoma, psoriasis, immune deficiency diseases, collagen diseases (systemic lupus erythematosus and dermatomyositis), and Netherton syndrome. However, skin diseases or manifestations which should be differentiated from AD are different among infantile, childhood, and adult atopic dermatitis (Table 19.1). Misdiagnosis occasionally results in unfavorable prognosis, especially for cutaneous lymphoma, dermatomyositis, or infectious diseases. Therefore, careful observation and evaluation of skin manifestations is required to make a correct diagnosis of AD.

Keywords

Atopic Dermatitis • Differential Diagnosis • Vitiligo • Cedar Pollen Dermatitis • IgE

I. Katayama
Department of Dermatology, Course of Integrated Medicine, Graduate School of Medicine, Osaka University, 2-2 Yamada-Oka, Suita, Osaka 565-0871, Japan
e-mail: katayama@derma.med.osaka-u.ac.jp

I. Katayama et al. (eds.), *Evolution of Atopic Dermatitis in the 21st Century*,
https://doi.org/10.1007/978-981-10-5541-6_19

19.1 Introduction

Regarding the treatment of atopic dermatitis (hereafter referred to "AD"), diagnostic criteria proposed by the Japanese Dermatological Association [1] and therapeutic guidelines established by the Japanese Society of Allergology [2] have been published. These guidelines enable us to conduct standard therapy for mild to severe pediatric and adult AD. Therapeutic methodology based on EBM will likely be established in the twenty-first century. Using these criteria, all diseases that meet the three requirements of itching, characteristic rashes and distribution, and chronic/recurrent progression will be diagnosed as atopic dermatitis irrespective of the severity of symptoms [1]. From this point of view, in this chapter, we summarize the differential diagnosis of AD (Table 19.1), which is required for assessing daily

Table 19.1 Differential diagnosis of atopic dermatitis

Differential points	Infantile eczema	Childhood atopic dermatitis	Adult atopic dermatitis
Synonymous	Infantile seborrheic dermatitis	Prurigo Besnier	
	Infantile xerotic eczema		
Atopic diathesis	Unknown	Yes	Unknown
Clinical manifestations	Localized to the scalp and face	Generalized distribution	Onset at puberty, seborrheic area
		Flexor site of the extremities	Atopic red face, poikiloderma of the neck
		Dry skin	Erythrodermic change
Laboratory data	NP	Elevated IgE-RAST to food allergens	Elevated serum IgE, TARC
		Decreased IFN-γ production by umbilical blood	Elevated IgE-RAST to mite or pollen allergens
		Increased IL4/IL5 production by umbilical blood	Positive patch test to metals, soaps, etc.
		Elevated phosphodiesterase in monocytes	
Differential diagnosis	Histiocytosis (Letterer-Siwe disease)	Hyper-IgE syndrome	Contact dermatitis
	Psoriasis	Mastocytosis	Xerotic eczema
	Contact dermatitis	Scabies	Seborrheic dermatitis
	Infantile xerotic eczema	Miliaria	Pityriasis versicolor
	Netherton syndrome	Ichthyosis	Hand eczema
	Wiskott-Aldrich syndrome	Strophulus	Chronic actinic dermatitis
		Juvenile dermatomyositis	Mycosis fungoides

treatment. Important differential diagnoses listed in diagnostic criteria proposed by the Japanese Dermatological Association are as follows: contact dermatitis, seborrheic dermatitis, prurigo simplex, scabies, miliaria, ichthyosis, xerotic eczema, hand dermatitis (nonatopic), cutaneous lymphoma, psoriasis, immune deficiency diseases, collagen diseases (systemic lupus erythematosus and dermatomyositis), and Netherton syndrome. However, skin diseases or manifestations which should be differentiated from AD are different among infantile, childhood, and adult atopic dermatitis (Table 19.1). Misdiagnosis occasionally results in unfavorable prognosis, especially for cutaneous lymphoma, dermatomyositis, or infectious diseases. Therefore, careful observation and evaluation of skin manifestations is required to make a correct diagnosis of AD.

19.2 Differential Diagnosis of Atopic Dermatitis

1. *Symptoms Associated with Sweat or Sebum*
   Infantile seborrheic eczema (Fig. 19.1, left top and bottom) is frequently observed on the head and face in infants. For diagnosis of AD, continuous observation of this eczema for longer than 2 months in infanthood or longer than 6 months in childhood is important [1, 2]. Observation of generalized eczema, fissured-ear base lichenification, randomly appearing dry skin, or association with atopic predisposition may be signs of transition to AD. In addition,

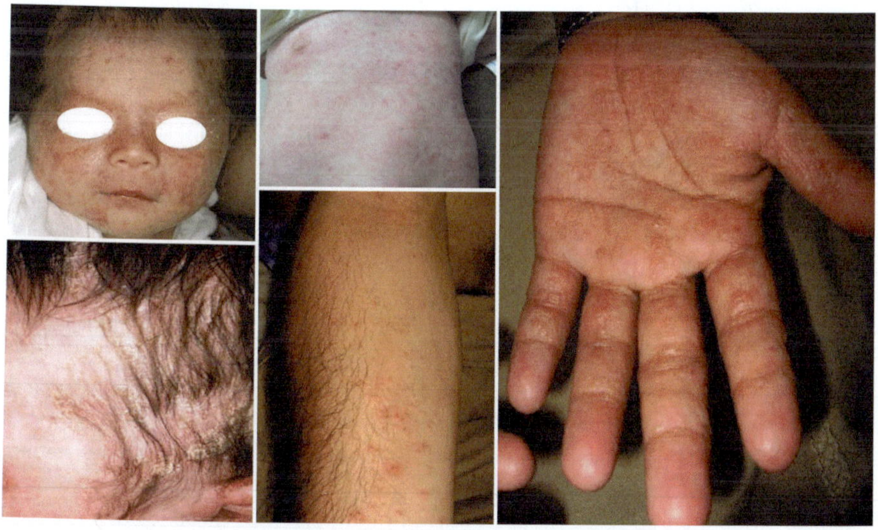

Fig. 19.1 Symptoms associated with sweat or sebum. Infantile seborrheic eczema (*left, top* and *bottom*) is frequently observed on the head and face in infants. Sweating is promoted, and serous papules or vesicles on the extremities or body trunk are occasionally observed (*center top* and *bottom*). Hand eczema is observed in relation to irritation by sand or sweating (*right*)

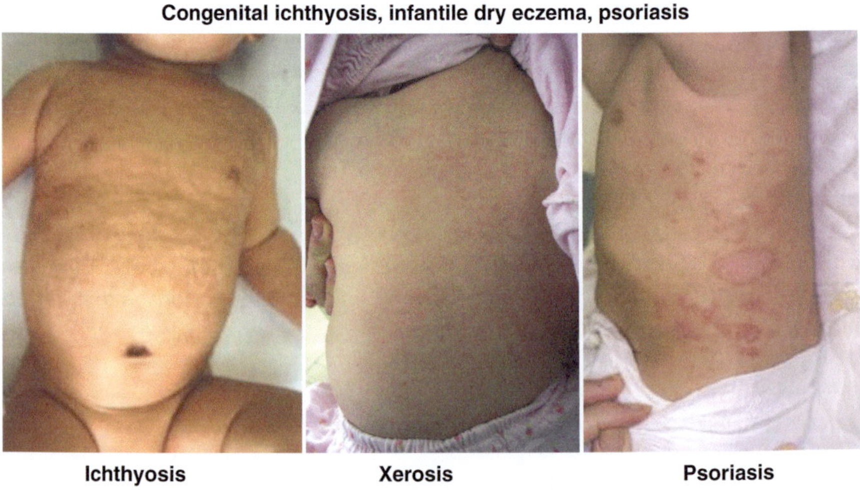

Fig. 19.2 Congenital ichthyosis, pediatric/infantile dry eczema. Fifteen percent of AD patients were reported to have ichthyosis vulgaris complications. In the winter season, scalelike cornified lesions are clearly observed (*left*). In winter, as children's skin is dry and pityroid dander is sometimes observed, these symptoms are referred to as simply dry skin (*center*) or pediatric dry eczema. In some cases, the symptom "pityriasis alba" may be observed. In psoriasis, circular keratotic erythema with white colored scales is observed. In infant patients, these lesions are frequently observed on the hip, and such lesions are referred to as "diaper psoriasis" (*right*)

in the summer season when sweating is promoted, serous papules or vesicles on the extremities or body trunk are occasionally observed (Fig. 19.1, center top and bottom) [3]. Hand eczema is observed in relation to irritation by sand or sweating (Fig. 19.1, right).

2. *Congenital Ichthyosis, Pediatric/Infantile Dry Eczema*
   Although Uehara et al. reported that 15% of observed AD patients were complicated with ichthyosis vulgaris [4], there are also some single cases. In the winter season, scalelike cornified lesions are clearly observed (Fig. 19.2, left). Expression of ceramide 10 and filaggrin 11 decreases in skin with atopic dermatitis, particularly in lesions, and is considered as a primary cause of barrier dysfunction [5, 6].

   This is also considered as a secondary phenomenon associated with inflammation and as a cause of atopic dermatitis. Patients with the above symptoms should be carefully treated because steroids have no effects on dry skin and instead disrupt skin barrier function [7, 8]. In winter, as children's skin is dry and pityroid dander is sometimes observed, these symptoms are referred to simply as dry skin (Fig. 19.2, center) or pediatric dry eczema. In some cases, the symptom of "pityriasis alba" may be observed. In psoriasis, circular keratotic erythema with white colored scales is observed. In infant patients, these lesions are frequently observed on the hip and sometimes such lesions are referred to as "diaper psoriasis" (Fig. 19.2, right).

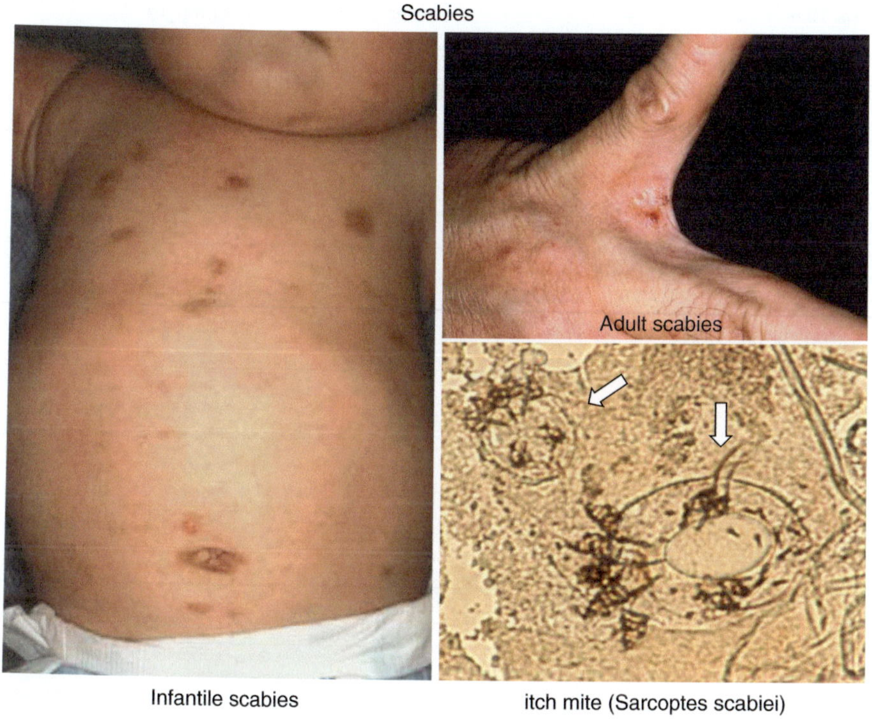

Fig. 19.3 Scabies. Scabies is transmitted from the care stuff at elderly hospitals in many cases but also may be transmitted from pets such as dogs or cats (canine scabies). Symptoms are mainly pruritic lesions, in which exacerbation or delay of healing are observed in response to topical steroid application

3. *Scabies*
   Scabies is transmitted from the care stuff at elderly hospitals in many cases but also may be transmitted from pets such as dogs or cats (canine scabies). Symptoms are mainly pruritic lesions, in which exacerbation or delay of healing are observed in response to topical steroid application (Fig. 19.3). This disease causes family infection. It should be noted that in some dog, cat, or pediatric patient cases, no skin eruptions are observed on the predisposition site. Diagnosis is confirmed by microscopic tests to visually confirm the scabies worm white arrows or its eggs. Treatment should be guided by specialists.
4. *Mast Cell Disease*
   Mast cell disease is also called "urticaria pigmentosa," in which sporadically occurring brownish pigment macules or papules are observed, mainly on the body trunk. Large numbers of mast cells are observed on the upper cutis, and urticarial lesions are shaped on pigment macules (Darier's sign) by scrabbling. In some cases, histiocytosis X should be excluded because of positive CD1a staining [9].

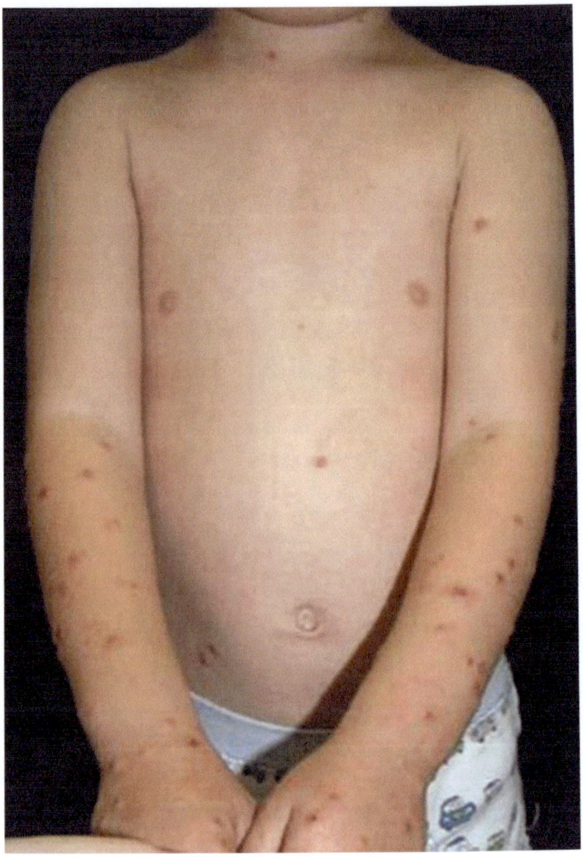

Fig. 19.4 Pediatric strophulus. In pediatric strophulus, large numbers of erythemas similar to urticaria occur after insect bite by mosquito, blackfly, etc., and sometimes shift to solid prurigo (known as strophulus). These symptoms frequently occur on all four limbs in the summer season

5. *Pediatric Strophulus (Acute Prurigo)*
   In pediatric strophulus, large numbers of erythemas similar to urticaria occur after insect bite by mosquito, blackfly, etc., and sometimes shift to solid prurigo (known as strophulus) (Fig. 19.4). These symptoms frequently occur on all four limbs in the summer season. Eczema on intertriginous areas usually found in AD patients is not observed in this case. The symptoms are relieved by topical steroid application and oral administration of antihistamine drugs.
6. *Contact Dermatitis, Photocontact Dermatitis*
   Contact dermatitis or photocontact dermatitis is sometimes observed in response to moisturizing agents, topical drugs, soaps, shampoos, etc. These symptoms may appear similar to refractory lesions of AD but rapidly disappear by discontinuation of causative agents and topical steroid application (Fig. 19.5, left). In cases where the causative agents are unknown, the effects of topical steroids will gradually decrease and symptoms will become

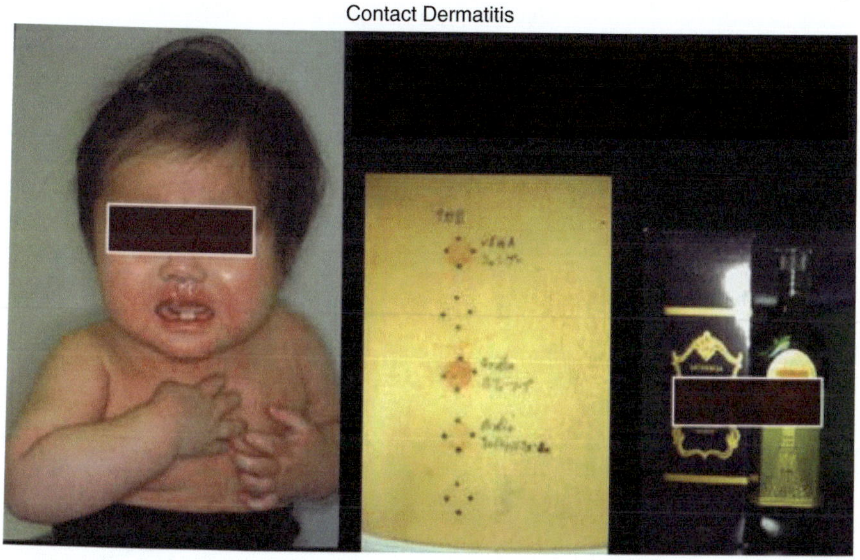

Fig. 19.5 Contact dermatitis, photocontact dermatitis. Contact dermatitis or photocontact dermatitis sometimes resembles refractory lesions of AD but rapidly disappears by discontinuation of the causative agents and topical steroid application (*left*). Diagnosis should be made by patch tests (contact dermatitis) or photopatch tests (photocontact dermatitis). An example of a positive response in a patch test is shown in *center*, with the suspected soap and shampoo in *right*

refractory. Diagnosis should be made by patch tests (contact dermatitis) or photopatch tests (photocontact dermatitis). An example of positive response in the patch test is shown in Fig. 19.5, center, with the suspected soap and shampoo in Fig. 19.5, right.

7. *Connective Tissue Disease*
   Childhood dermatomyositis is especially important in this disease. Erythemas on the face or body trunk or keratotic erythemas on the backside of joints are usually observed. In some cases, itching accompanies these erythemas with elevation of the serum IgE level [10, 11]. The patient shown in Fig. 19.6, left and right, was diagnosed with AD in childhood, and the picture in the center of Fig. 19.6 shows the clinical picture taken at the period of adolescence after growth. In this picture, calcareous depositions are observed.
8. *Histiocytic Disorders*
   Erythemas or papules associated with bleeding or other characteristic events are observed on the face, head, and body trunk (Fig. 19.7, upper, Langerhans cell histiocytosis). Pathological tests should be carried out to make a differential diagnosis. In this disease, CD1a is positive and Birbeck granules are observed by electronic microscopy (Fig. 19.7, lower pictures). In severe cases, chemotherapy should be conducted.

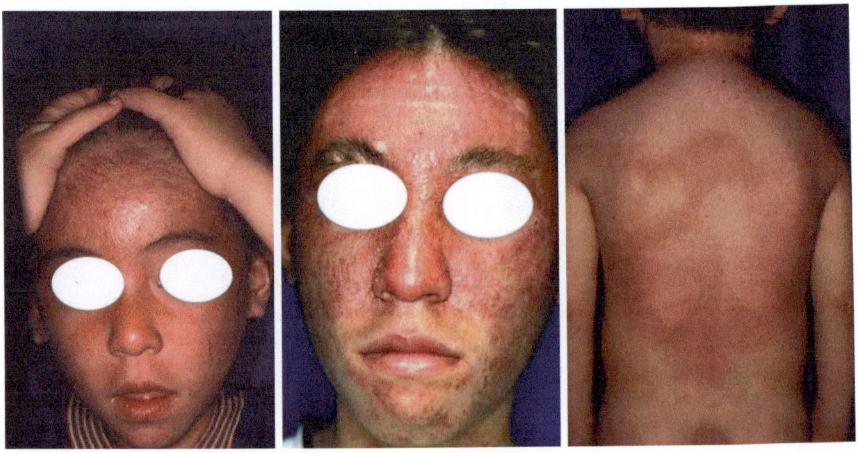

Fig. 19.6 Connective tissue disease. Childhood dermatomyositis is especially important in this disease. Erythemas on the face or body trunk or keratotic erythemas on the backside of joints are usually observed; in some cases, itching is accompanied by these erythemas, with elevation of the serum IgE level. The patient was diagnosed with AD in childhood, and the picture in the *center* of figure shows the clinical picture taken at the period of adolescence after growth. In this picture, calcareous depositions are observed

9. *Immune Deficiency Disease*
   In some cases of severe combined immune deficiency (SCID), erythemas or papules with dry pityroid dander are observed over the entire body. In Wiskott-Aldrich syndrome, eczema lesions similar to AD are observed. Netherton syndrome is characterized by ichthyosis, atopic diathesis, eczematous skin lesions with bamboo hairs, and SPINK5 gene mutation [12]. Hyper-IgE syndrome is a hereditary immune deficiency syndrome characterized by atopic dermatitis-like skin lesions, cold abscesses and pulmonary cysts with increased serum IgE and associated with STAT3, TYK2, or DOCK8 gene mutation [13].
10. *GVHD (Graft Versus Host Disease)*
    According to the pathology of GVHD, apoptotic cells observed on the epidermis and the disappearance of Langerhans cells are characteristic of this disease (Fig. 19.8). AD-like clinical manifestations are observed in chronic GVHD even though the donor has no predisposition to atopic dermatitis [14].
11. *Dermatitis Caused by Japanese Cedar Pollen*
    During the season when Japanese cedar pollen is released, typically from February to March in Japan, itchy urticaria and scaly dermatitis are observed on the face, especially around periorbital and nostril areas or the neck in some patients (Fig. 19.9, left). In AD patients, this is also important as one of the seasonally exacerbated factors [15, 16]. Patients with a history of aggravation of dermatitis exhibit positive delayed-onset scratch-patch tests to cry J1 (Fig. 19.9, right).

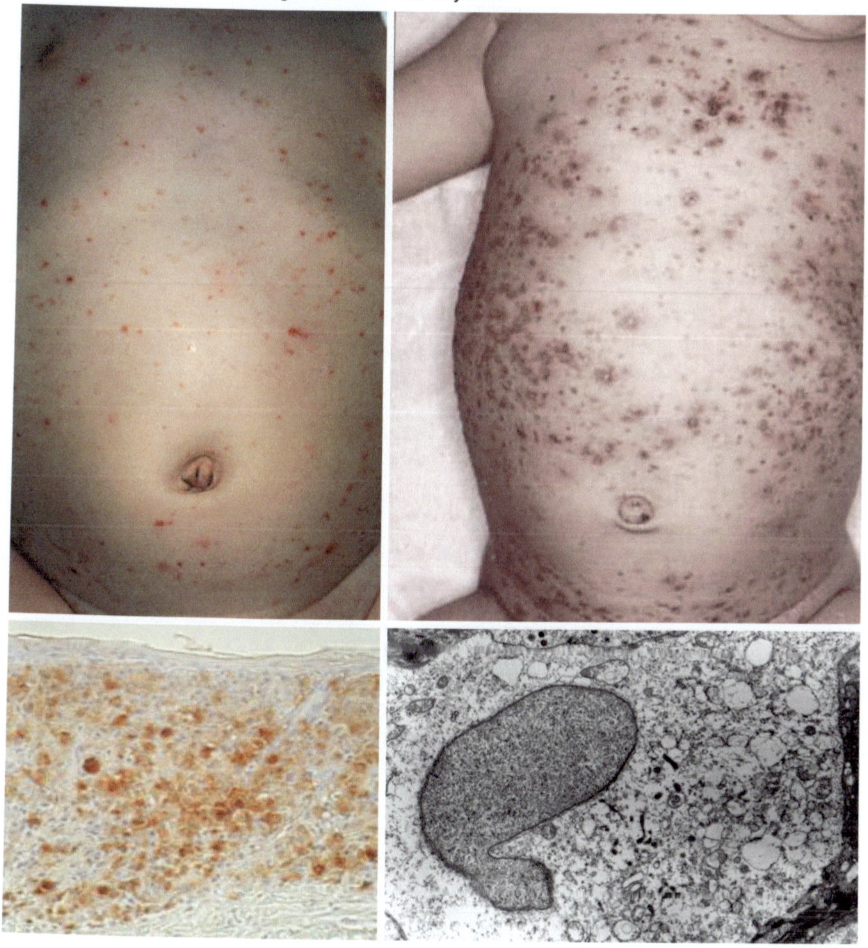

Fig. 19.7 Histiocytic disorders. Erythemas or papules associated with bleeding or other characteristic events are observed on the face, head, and body trunk (*upper*). Pathological tests should be carried out to make a differential diagnosis. In this disease, CD1a is positive and Birbeck granules are observed by electronic microscopy (*lower pictures*)

12. *Cutaneous T-Cell Lymphoma*
    It is important to differentiate mycosis fungoides from AD. In adult cases of AD, pruritic erythematous plaques or dirty poikilodermic lesions are occasionally observed with topical glucocorticoid resistance (Fig. 19.10, left and upper right). Histopathological evaluation (Fig. 19.10, lower left) using immunohistochemical analysis is recommended for differential diagnosis [17, 18].

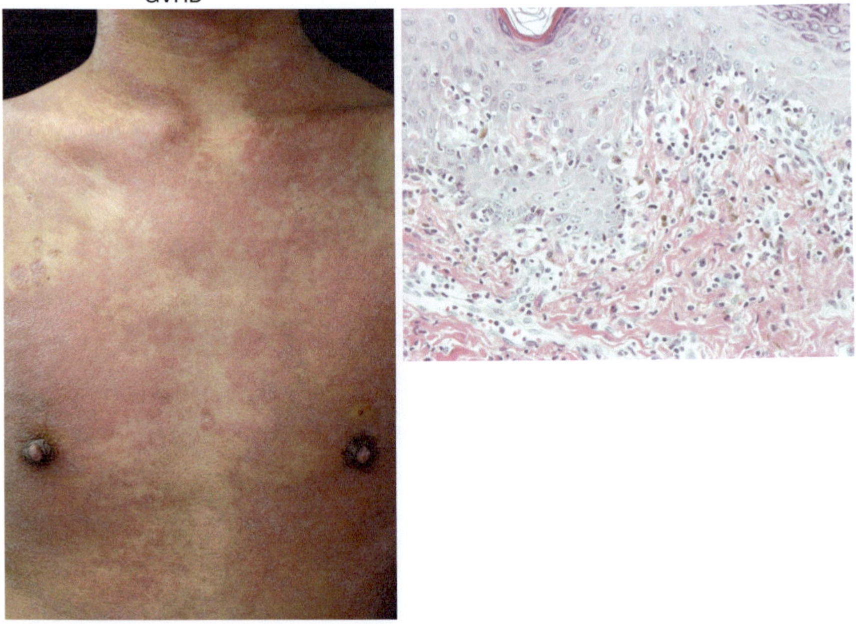

Fig. 19.8 GVHD (graft versus host disease). According to the pathology of GVHD, apoptotic cells observed on the epidermis and the disappearance of Langerhans cells are characteristic of this disease. AD-like clinical manifestations are observed in chronic GVHD even if the donor has no atopic dermatitis predisposition

19.3 Complicated AD Disease: Skin Infections

It is well known that the following infections are strongly associated with AD. Careful attention should be paid, especially in cases where immunosuppressive ointment is applied. It is reported that the defensive capability of skin is decreased in AD, and this is thought to be one of the reasons for the high frequency of complicated infections.

(a) *Contagious impetigo (Impetigo caused by Staphylococcus aureus or hemolytic streptococcus)*: Contagious impetigo caused by *Staphylococcus aureus* is often observed in pediatric skin infections. In cases of impetigo caused by hemolytic streptococcus, as symptoms of inflammation are relatively strong and erosions or ulcers are also severe, differentiation from Kaposi varicelliform eruption is important. In some cases, glomerular nephritis may be associated; thus, early diagnosis and administration of antibiotics are necessary (Fig. 19.11, upper left).
(b) *Body ringworm, cutaneous candidiasis*: In body ringworm, scaling erythematous macules with clear boundaries on all four limbs are characteristic. In cases where erythemas occur on genitocrural regions, diagnosis is easy, but

Cedar pollen dermatitis

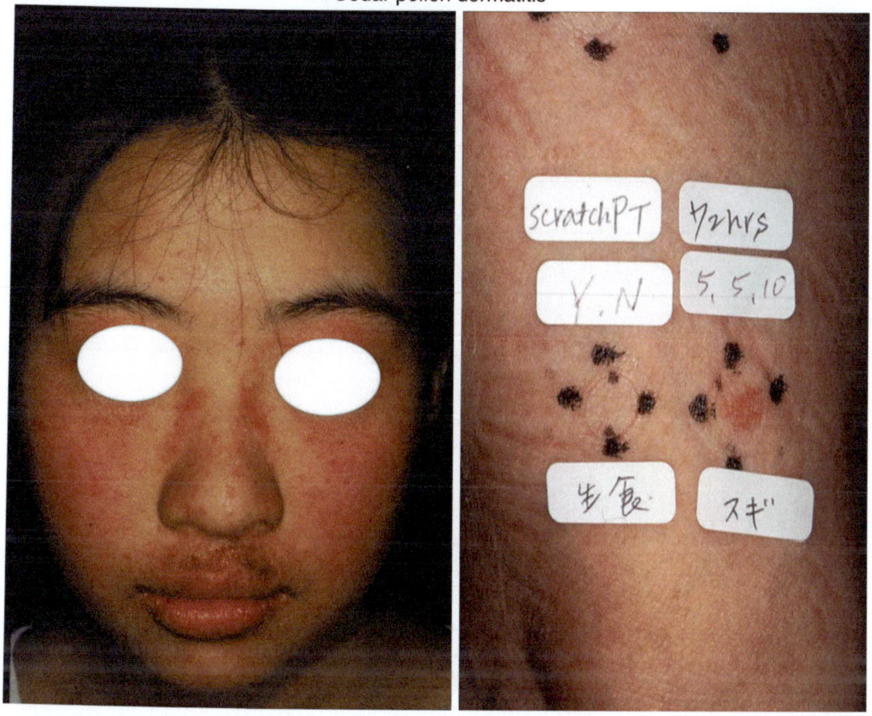

Fig. 19.9 Dermatitis caused by Japanese cedar pollen. During the season when Japanese cedar pollen is released, typically from February to March in Japan, itchy urticarial and scaly dermatitis are observed on the face, especially around periorbital and nostril areas or the neck in some patients (*left*). In AD patients, this is also important as one of the seasonally exacerbated factors. Patients with a history of aggravation of dermatitis exhibit positive delayed-onset scratch-patch tests to cry J1 (*right*)

some cases where erythemas occur on the body trunk may be missed. Topical steroids exacerbate these symptoms. Diagnosis should be confirmed by microscopic testing to confirm trichophyton or by cultivation. Cutaneous candidiasis is frequently observed on the external genitals, in which red plaques combined with vesicles or small pustules are observed (Fig. 19.11, bottom left).

(c) *Kaposi varicelliform eruption (Eczema herpeticum)*: This disease is caused by the initial infection of the herpes simplex virus. In this disease, small center-umbilicated vesicles are observed (Fig. 19.11, upper right). These vesicles are widely spread in an eczema-lesion-like pattern, with fever and enlargement of lymph nodes. Administration of antiviral agents or immunoglobulin and management of transfusion are necessary for treatment [19, 20].

(d) *Molluscum contagiosum*: This disease is caused by the molluscum contagiosum virus, which frequently infects patients in places such as swimming pools. Treatment is by removal of the molluscum before it spreads.

Cutaneous T cell lymphoma

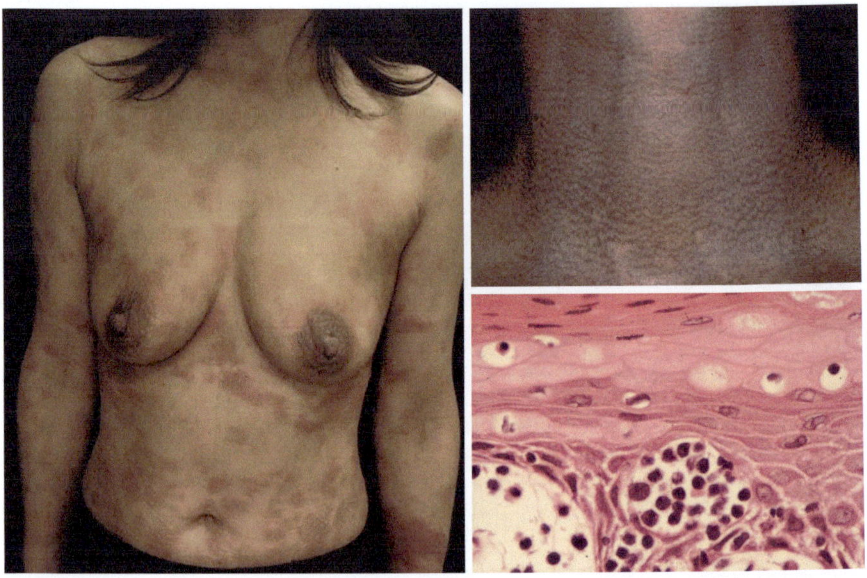

Fig. 19.10 Cutaneous T-cell lymphoma. It is important to differentiate mycosis fungoides from AD. In adult cases of AD, pruritic erythematous plaques or dirty poikilodermic lesions are occasionally observed with topical glucocorticoid resistance (*left* and *upper right*). Histopathological evaluation (*lower left*) using immunohistochemical analysis is recommended for the differential diagnosis of cutaneous T-cell lymphoma [17, 18]

19.4 Complications of Atopic Dermatitis: Autoimmune Diseases

(a) *Alopecia*: Patients with either vitiligo or AA, especially alopecia totalis or alopecia universalis, have a significantly increased risk for AD [21], opposite from our clinical observations [manuscript in preparation]. In AD, sparse alopecia is occasionally observed on the temporal area of the scalp as atopic alopecia (Fig. 19.11, left bottom center).

(b) *Vitiligo*: Vitiligo patches in patients with AD may be induced when the autoimmune background resembles that of autoimmune vitiligo and Sutton's nevus, both of which may be governed by Th17 cells [22] (Fig. 19.11, lower left). Fifty-six percent of patients with a history of atopic dermatitis had hypopigmented skin in the form of guttate psoriasis and patches. Kierland et al. reported that vitiligo was observed more frequently in patients with atopic dermatitis [23]. Although it is not fully understood how vitiligo arises on atopic skin, the incidence of vitiligo in atopy seems to be higher than that of vitiligo. As reported by Jin et al., *NALP1*-gene mutation is frequently observed in autoimmune vitiligo and is accompanied by several autoimmune disorders, including diabetes

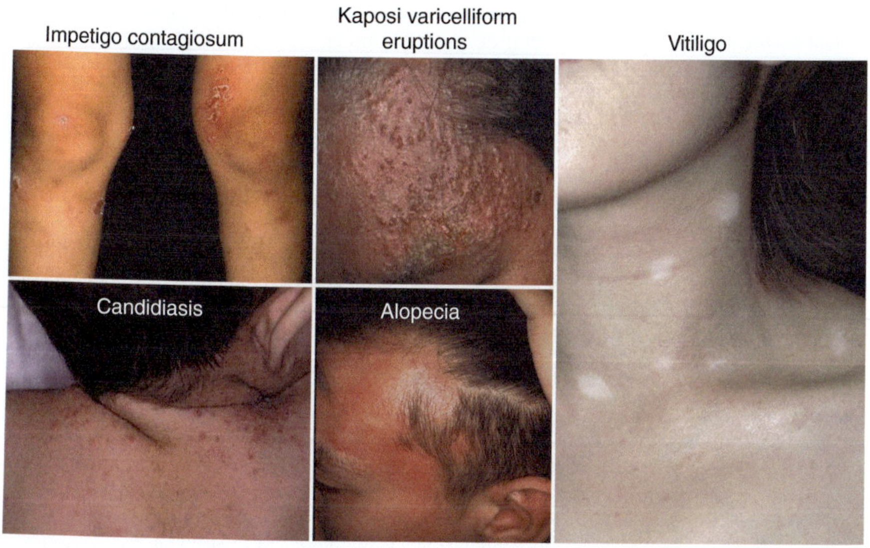

Fig. 19.11 Complicated AD disease: skin infections and autoimmune diseases. Contagious impetigo caused by *Staphylococcus aureus* is occasionally observed in pediatric skin infections (*upper left*). Cutaneous candidiasis is frequently observed on skin fold regions, especially on the external genitals, in which red plaques combined with vesicles or small pustules are observed (*bottom left*). Kaposi varicelliform eruption (eczema herpeticum) is caused by the initial infection of herpes simplex virus. In this disease, center-umbilicated small vesicles are observed (*upper right*). In AD, sparse alopecia is occasionally observed on the temporal area of the scalp as atopic alopecia (*left bottom center*). Vitiligo patches in patients with AD may be induced when the autoimmune background resembles that of autoimmune vitiligo and Sutton's nevus, both of which may be controlled by Th17 cells (*lower left*)

mellitus, Hashimoto's thyroiditis, Addison's disease, or skin diseases such as psoriasis vulgaris or alopecia areata [24].

(c) *Sjögren's syndrome*: We have recently reported four adult cases of AD complicated by Sjögren's syndrome (SS). The patients fulfilled the diagnostic criteria for AD and SS. All cases exhibited persistent itchy dry skin and eczematous lesions complicated with sicca symptoms including dry eyes and dry mouth with moderate joint pain. In the present cases, impaired sweat response in AD is attributable to abnormal sudomotor function, which is accelerated and modulated when complicated by SS, resulting in dry skin [25].

References

1. Saeki H, Furue M, Furukawa F et al.; Committee for Guidelines for the Management of Atopic Dermatitis of Japanese Dermatological Association. Guidelines for management of atopic dermatitis. J Dermatol 2009;36:563–577.
2. Katayama I, Kohno Y, Akiyama K, et al. Japanese Guideline for Atopic Dermatitis 2014. Japanese Society of Allergology. Allergol Int. 2014;63:377–98.

3. Takahashi A, Tani S, Murota H, Katayama I. Histamine modulates sweating and affects clinical manifestations of atopic dermatitis. Curr Probl Dermatol. 2016;51:50–6.
4. Uehara M, Hayashi S. Hyperlinear palms: association with ichthyosis and atopic dermatitis. Arch Dermatol. 1981;117:490–1.
5. Imokawa G, Abe A, Jin K, et al. Decreased level of ceramides in stratum corneum of atopic dermatitis: an etiologic factor in atopic dry skin? J Invest Dermatol. 1991;96:523–6.
6. Sugiura A, Nomura T, Mizuno A, et al. Reevaluation of the non-lesional dry skin in atopic dermatitis by acute barrier disruption: an abnormal permeability barrier homeostasis with defective processing to generate ceramide. Arch Dermatol Res. 2014;306:427–40.
7. Kao JS, Fluhr JW, Man MQ, et al. Short-term glucocorticoid treatment compromises both permeability barrier homeostasis and stratum corneum integrity: inhibition of epidermal lipid synthesis accounts for functional abnormalities. J Invest Dermatol. 2003;120:456–64.
8. Danby SG, Chittock J, Brown KA, et al. The effect of tacrolimus compared with betamethasone valerate on the skin barrier in volunteers with quiescent atopic dermatitis. Br J Dermatol. 2014;170:914–21.
9. Arase N, Wataya-Kaneda M, Oiso N, et al. CD1a-positive familial cutaneous mastocytosis without germ-line or somatic mutations in c-kit. Br J Dermatol. 2013;169:201–4.
10. Ishida T, Ohashi M, Matsumoto Y, et al. Connection of atopic disease in Japanese patients with juvenile dermatomyositis based on serum IgE levels. Clin Rheumatol. 1993;12:41–8.
11. Okiyama N, Kohsaka H, Ueda N, et al. Seborrheic area erythema as a common skin manifestation in Japanese patients with dermatomyositis. Dermatology. 2008;217:374–7.
12. Briot A, Deraison C, Lacroix MB, et al. Kallikrein 5 induces atopic dermatitis-like lesions through PAR2-mediated thymic stromal lymphopoietin expression in Netherton syndrome. J Exp Med. 2009;206:1135–47.
13. Hagl B, Heinz V, Schlesinger A, et al. Key findings to expedite the diagnosis of hyper-IgE syndromes in infants and young children. Pediatr Allergy Immunol. 2016;27:177–84.
14. Wei J, Zhang Y, Xu H, Jin J, Zhang J. Atopic dermatitis-like presentation of graft-versus-host disease: a novel form of chronic cutaneous graft-versus-host disease. J Am Acad Dermatol. 2013;69:34–9.
15. Yokozeki H, Takayama K, Katayama I, Nishioka K. Japanese cedar pollen as an exacerbation factor in atopic dermatitis: results of atopy patch testing and histological examination. Acta Derm Venereol. 2006;86:148–51.
16. Murakami Y, Matsui S, Kijima A, et al. Cedar pollen aggravates atopic dermatitis in childhood monozygotic twin patients with allergic rhino conjunctivitis. Allergol Int. 2011;60:397–400.
17. Tuzova M, Richmond J, Wolpowitz D, et al. CCR4+T cell recruitment to the skin in mycosis fungoides: potential contributions by thymic stromal lymphopoietin and interleukin-16. Leuk Lymphoma. 2015;56:440–9.
18. Hanafusa T, Matsui S, Murota H, et al. Increased frequency of skin-infiltrating FoxP3+ regulatory T cells as a diagnostic indicator of severe atopic dermatitis from cutaneous T cell lymphoma. Clin Exp Immunol. 2013;172:507–12.
19. Wollenberg A. Eczema herpeticum. Chem Immunol Allergy. 2012;96:89–95.
20. Wollenberg A, Seba A, Antal AS. Immunological and molecular targets of atopic dermatitis treatment. Br J Dermatol. 2014;170(Suppl 1):7–11.
21. Mohan GC, Silverberg JI. Association of vitiligo and alopecia areata with atopic dermatitis: a systematic review and meta-analysis. JAMA Dermatol. 2015;151:522–8.
22. Tanemura A, Yajima T, Nakano M, et al. Seven cases of vitiligo complicated by atopic dermatitis: suggestive new spectrum of autoimmune vitiligo. Eur J Dermatol. 2012;22:279–80.
23. Fregert S, Moller H, Rorsman H. Observations on vitiligo in a patient with atopic dermatitis. Acta Derm Venereol. 1959;39:225–9.
24. Jin Y, Mailoux CM, Gowan K, Riccardi SL, LaBerge G, Bennett DC, Fain PR, Sprits RA. NALP1 in vitiligo-associated multiple autoimmune disease. N Engl J Med. 2007;356:1216–25.
25. Kitaba S, Matsui S, Iimuro E, et al. Four cases of atopic dermatitis complicated by Sjögren's syndrome: link between dry skin and autoimmune anhidrosis. Allergol Int. 2011;60:387–91.

Part VII

Diagnosis

Diagnosis and Japanese Guideline 20

Hidehisa Saeki

Abstract

Based on the definition and diagnostic criteria for atopic dermatitis (AD) by the Japanese Dermatological Association (JDA), patients meeting three basic items – (1) pruritus, (2) typical morphology and distribution of the eczema, and (3) chronic or chronically relapsing course – are regarded as having AD. Eruption is symmetrically distributed and frequently develops on the forehead, periorbital area, perioral area, lips, periauricular area, neck, joint areas of limbs, and trunk. Its distribution is characterized by age. The clinical practice guidelines for the management of AD 2016 by the JDA were prepared as a regular revision for all children to adults with all severity of AD, involving internationally published novel findings on AD in 2016. Treatment measures for AD basically consist of drug therapy, skin care with emollients for physiological abnormalities in the skin, and investigations/elimination of exacerbating factors based on its pathogenesis. Drugs that potently reduce AD-related inflammation and of which the efficacy and safety have been scientifically examined include topical corticosteroids and tacrolimus. It is important to promptly and accurately reduce inflammation related to AD, and treatments are based on how topical corticosteroids and tacrolimus should be selected/combined for this purpose.

Keywords

Atopic dermatitis • Diagnostic criteria • Japanese guideline • Tacrolimus • Topical corticosteroids

H. Saeki, M.D.
Department of Dermatology, Nippon Medical School, 1-1-5, Sendagi, Bunkyo-ku, Tokyo 113-8603, Japan
e-mail: h-saeki@nms.ac.jp

I. Katayama et al. (eds.), *Evolution of Atopic Dermatitis in the 21st Century*,
https://doi.org/10.1007/978-981-10-5541-6_20

20.1 Diagnosis

20.1.1 Diagnostic Criteria

20.1.1.1 Diagnostic Criteria by the Japanese Dermatological Association (JDA)

Based on the "Definition and Diagnostic Criteria for Atopic Dermatitis (AD)" (revised in 2008) prepared by the JDA in 1994, patients meeting three basic items – (1) pruritus, (2) typical morphology and distribution of the eczema, and (3) chronic or chronically relapsing course (usually coexistence of old and new lesions) – are regarded as having AD regardless of the severity of symptoms. An English translation of these diagnostic criteria was published in 1995 and revised in 2009 (Table 20.1) [1, 2].

Eruption is symmetrically distributed and frequently develops on the forehead, periorbital area, perioral area, lips, periauricular area, neck, joint areas of limbs, and trunk. Its distribution is characterized by age. During infancy, eruption initially appears in the scalp and face, often expanding to the trunk and limbs. It appears in AD-specific sites during childhood, such as the neck and the flexural surfaces of the arms and legs. During adolescence/adulthood, it becomes marked in the upper body, including the face. AD-suspected patients are regarded as having acute or chronic eczema, and diagnoses are made based on their age and courses.

In a revision published in 2009, cutaneous lymphoma, psoriasis, immunodeficiency diseases (such as hyper-immunoglobulin E (IgE) syndrome and Wiskott-Aldrich syndrome), collagen disease (systemic lupus erythematosus and dermatomyositis), and Netherton's syndrome were newly added as disorders to be ruled out (Table 20.1) [2]. Therefore, it is essential to differentiate these disorders and be familiar with the complications of AD.

20.1.1.2 Diagnostic Criteria by Hanifin and Rajka

The diagnostic criteria defined by Hanifin and Rajka in 1980 are frequently used worldwide [3]. One of the differences between Hanifin and Rajka's criteria and the JDA criteria is that a personal or family history of atopic diseases (asthma, allergic rhinitis/conjunctivitis, and AD) is defined as a basic feature in the former and as a diagnostic aid in the latter. However, atopic diathesis is clearly addressed in the definition of AD by the JDA (Table 20.1).

The 23 minor features listed in the Hanifin and Rajka's criteria are characteristic for AD and often observed in this disease. However, their frequencies of development vary, and discrete expressions are used for some of the features; therefore they are excluded from the diagnostic criteria by the JDA, although some of them are referred to as diagnostic aids, clinical types, or significant complications (Table 20.1). Subsequently, an "abridged edition of Hanifin and Rajka's diagnostic criteria" was published in 2003 [4].

Table 20.1 Definition and diagnostic criteria for atopic dermatitis by the Japanese Dermatological Association

Definition
Atopic dermatitis is a pruritic, eczematous dermatitis; its symptoms chronically fluctuate with remissions and relapses. Most individuals with atopic dermatitis have atopic diathesis
Atopic diathesis: (1) personal or family history (asthma, allergic rhinitis and/or conjunctivitis, and atopic dermatitis) and/or (2) predisposition to overproduction of immunoglobulin E (IgE) antibodies
Diagnostic criteria for atopic dermatitis
1. Pruritus
2. Typical morphology and distribution:
(1) Eczematous dermatitis
• Acute lesions: erythema, exudation, papules, vesiculopapules, scales, and crusts
• Chronic lesions: infiltrated erythema, lichenification, prurigo, scales, and crusts
(2) Distribution
• Symmetrical
Predilection sites: forehead, periorbital area, perioral area, lips, periauricular area, neck, joint areas of limbs, and trunk
• Age-related characteristics
Infantile phase: starts on the scalp and face, often spreads to the trunk and extremities
Childhood phase: neck and the flexural surfaces of the arms and legs
Adolescent and adult phase: tendency to be severe on the upper half of the body (face, neck, anterior chest, and back)
3. Chronic or chronically relapsing course (usually coexistence of old and new lesions):
• More than 2 months in infancy
• More than 6 months in childhood, adolescence, and adulthood
Definitive diagnosis of atopic dermatitis requires the presence of all three features without any consideration of severity. Other cases should be evaluated on the basis of the age and clinical course with the tentative diagnosis of acute or chronic, nonspecific eczema
Differential diagnosis (association may occur)
Contact dermatitis, seborrheic dermatitis, prurigo simplex, scabies, miliaria, ichthyosis, xerotic eczema, hand dermatitis (non-atopic), cutaneous lymphoma, psoriasis, immunodeficiency diseases, collagen diseases (SLE, dermatomyositis), and Netherton's syndrome
Diagnostic aids
Family history (bronchial asthma, allergic rhinitis and/or conjunctivitis, atopic dermatitis), personal history (bronchial asthma, allergic rhinitis, and/or conjunctivitis), follicular papules (gooseskin), elevated serum IgE level
Clinical types (not applicable to the infantile phase)
Flexural surface type; extensor surface type; dry form in childhood; head, face, neck, upper chest, and back type; prurigo type; erythroderma type; combinations of various types are common
Significant complications
Ocular complication (cataract and/or retinal detachment), especially in patients with severe facial lesions; Kaposi's varicelliform eruption; molluscum contagiosum; and impetigo contagiosa

Cited from ref. [2]

20.1.1.3 Nationwide Investigation by Inquiry/Questionnaire

A questionnaire for AD diagnosis was developed in 1994 by the UK Working Party, and it has been used worldwide [5]. Its Japanese translation version has proven to be useful [6]. Furthermore, based on the questionnaire developed by the International Study of Asthma and Allergies in Childhood (ISAAC), global epidemiological surveys about eczema, including AD, have been conducted periodically (http://isaac.auckland.ac.nz/Index.html) [7]. Its Japanese translation version is used for epidemiological surveys [8].

20.1.2 Severity Classification

20.1.2.1 Severity Classification for the Whole Body

The classification of the severity of AD prepared by the Atopic Dermatitis Severity Classification-Reviewing Committee of the JDA is available for clinical studies because its statistical reliability and usefulness have been verified (Fig. 20.1) [2, 9]. For the severity classification, three elements of eruption (erythema/acute papules, exudation/crusts, and chronic papules/nodules/lichenification) are evaluated in the most severely affected part of each of the five body sites (head/neck, anterior trunk, posterior trunk, upper limbs, and lower limbs). The areas of eruption on the five body sites are also evaluated, and both scores are totalized (Fig. 20.1) (maximum

This severity classification can be adopted only for the cases that are definitely diagnosed as atopic dermatitis.

Three elements of eruption are evaluated in the most severely affected part of each of the five body regions (15 times in total).

The areas of eruption on the five body regions are also evaluated (5 times in total). Both scores are totalized (20 times in total).

For evaluation of severity of eruption on each region, the severest part is selected for each element.

Evaluation of the area of eruption should be done considering all three elements for all five body regions.

The highest possible score is 60 points.

	Head / Neck	Anterior Trunk	Posterior Trunk	Upper Limbs	Lower Limbs	Total
Erythema / Acute papules						
Exudation / Crusts						
Chronic papules / Nodules / Lichenification						
Area of eruption						

Total Score ______

Evaluation method

I. Evaluation criteria for three elements of eruption

0=absent, 1=mild, 2=moderate, 3=severe

*Explanation of three elements of eruption

Erythema: All the redness, flushing and edema are included, Acute papules: Papules not affected by scratching.

Exudation / Crusts: Erosion by scratching is included.

Chronic papules: Papules affected by scratching. Nodules / Lichenification: Eruption in which chronic papules progressed further.

II. Evaluation criteria for area of eruption

0=no eruption, 1=<1/3, 2=1/3~2/3, 3=>2/3

Fig. 20.1 Severity classification of atopic dermatitis by the Japanese Dermatological Association (Cited from ref. [2])

score, 60). As a simple method reviewed by this committee, a method to divide the whole body into the same five sites and calculate the sum of the global assessment scores of these sites is also presented (Fig. 20.2) (maximum score, 20) [2, 10].

In addition, as another simple method, the severity index has also been proposed by the Research Group of the Ministry of Health, Labour and Welfare (Table 20.2) [11]. Internationally, the Severity Scoring of Atopic Dermatitis (SCORAD) (maximum score, 103) [12] established by the European Task Force on Atopic Dermatitis or the Eczema Area and Severity Index (EASI) (maximum score, 72) [13] in the USA is widely used.

Severity in each region (Evaluated globally by considering both degrees and areas of eruption).
(Evaluation of area of eruption should be done considering all the eight elements; erythema, papules, erosion, crusts, excoriation, lichenification, pruriginous nodules, depilation)

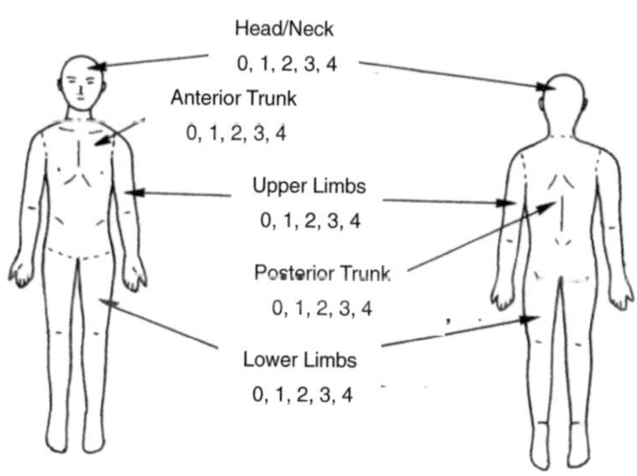

Evaluation method
The entire body is divided into five regions as illustrated in the figure. Severity is evaluated globally for each region (0=absent, 1=mild, 2=moderate, 3=severe, 4=very severe), and their total is calculated. The highest possible score is 20 points.

Fig. 20.2 Severity classification of atopic dermatitis by the Japanese Dermatological Association (simple method) (Cited from ref. [2])

Table 20.2 Severity index

There are several criteria proposed for severity assessment of atopic dermatitis at present that require proficiency in assessment. Accordingly, the following severity levels are defined as indices for treatment.
Mild: Only mild rashes are observed irrespective of the area Moderate: Rashes with severe inflammation are observed in less than 10% of the body surface area Severe: Rashes with severe inflammation are observed ≥10% to <30% of the body surface area Most severe: Rashes with severe inflammation are observed ≥30% of the body surface area
Mild rash: Lesions are seen chiefly with mild erythema, dry skin, or desquamation Rashes with severe inflammation: Lesion with erythema, papule, erosion, infiltration, lichenification, etc.

Cited from ref. [11]

20.1.2.2 Severity Classification Considering Clinical Course

As a severity classification considering the clinical course, the system of grading of the severity of AD published by Rajka and Langeland is frequently used [14]. Additionally, in the abovementioned ISAAC questionnaire, the question "In the last 12 months, how often, on average, have you (has your child) been kept awake at night by this itchy rash?" diagnoses patients as severe when they answer "1 or more nights per week" [7].

20.1.2.3 Evaluation of Pruritus

The visual analogue scale (VAS) is useful for evaluating pruritus [15]. In this scale, 1 point is marked on a 10-cm axis in accordance with the degree of pruritus, and the distance (mm) from the left end to the marked point is evaluated as the pruritus scale score, regarding the left end "no itch" as zero and the right end "the worst imaginable itch" as 100. As described in SCORAD (evaluated by the scale of 0–10 in SCORAD), VAS can also be used for sleep loss.

20.1.2.4 Evaluation of Quality of Life (QOL)

The Skindex-16 and Dermatology Life Quality Index (DLQI) have been statistically analyzed [16, 17]. Their Japanese versions were published and have been applied to the treatment of various skin diseases including AD [18, 19].

20.1.2.5 Severity of Eruption

The primary treatment, application of topical corticosteroid, should be determined based on "the severity of each eruption" (Tables 20.3 and 20.4) [20]. Briefly, potent

Table 20.3 Severity of eruption and topical corticosteroid application

Severity	Eruption	Topical corticosteroid application
Severe	Primarily severe swelling/edema/infiltration or erythema with lichenification, multiple papules, severe scales, crusts, vesicles, erosion, multiple excoriations, and pruriginous nodules	The use of very strong or strong-class topical corticosteroids is the first-line treatment Strongest-class topical corticosteroids are also available for refractory pruriginous nodules if sufficient effects are not achieved by applying very strong-class topical corticosteroids
Moderate	Primarily moderate erythema, scales, a few papules, and excoriations	The use of strong- or medium-class topical corticosteroids is the first-line treatment
Mild	Primarily dryness, mild erythema, and scales	The use of medium- or weak-class topical corticosteroids is the first-line treatment
Slight	Primarily dryness with negligible inflammation	Topical application of medicines other than corticosteroids (emollients)

Cited from ref. [20]

Table 20.4 Rank of topical corticosteroids

Strongest	
0.05%	Clobetasol propionate
0.05%	Diflorasone diacetate
Very strong	
0.1%	Mometasone furoate
0.05%	Betamethasone butyrate propionate
0.05%	Fluocinonide
0.064%	Betamethasone dipropionate
0.05%	Difluprednate
0.1%	Amcinonide
0.1%	Diflucortolone valerate
0.1%	Hydrocortisone butyrate propionate
Strong	
0.3%	Deprodone propionate
0.1%	Dexamethasone propionate
0.12%	Dexamethasone valerate
0.1%	Halcinonide
0.12%	Betamethasone valerate
0.025%	Fluocinolone acetonide
Medium	
0.3%	Prednisolone valerate acetate
0.1%	Triamcinolone acetonide
0.1%	Alclometasone dipropionate
0.05%	Clobetasone butyrate
0.1%	Hydrocortisone butyrate
0.1%	Dexamethasone
Weak	
0.5%	Prednisolone

As of September, 2015. Cited from ref. [20]

topical therapy is selected to treat severe eruption even when its extent is narrow. However, it is not required for patients with mild eruption even when its area is extensive. Therefore, "the severity of each eruption" is the most important factor to consider when selecting topical therapy, and a severity assessment must be performed by physicians with dermatological skills in order to evaluate severity and predict the treatment response.

20.1.2.6 Examinations for Diagnosis and Severity Assessment

Serum IgE Level

Total serum IgE levels are high in approximately 80% of patients with AD. This parameter is useful for making diagnoses. In adults, a total serum IgE level of 200 IU/mL or greater is regarded as high (differs among examination organizations). In infants, the upper limit of its normal range is lower at a younger age. The total serum IgE level reflects the long-term severity and activity of AD, but not its short-term changes. The IgE antibody may be produced in patients with AD in response to several allergens, such as mites, house dust, pollen, fungi, and foods. Most patients show positive reactions on serum-allergen-specific IgE antibodies and skin prick tests.

Peripheral Blood Eosinophil Counts, Serum Lactate Dehydrogenase (LDH) Levels, and Thymus and Activation-Regulated Chemokine (TARC, CCL17) Levels
The parameters of the short-term severity and activity of AD include peripheral blood eosinophil counts, serum LDH levels, and TARC levels [21]. According to the literature, serum TARC levels were useful as a marker of the disease activity of AD. The literature analysis indicated that serum TARC levels more sensitively reflected the activity of AD than serum IgE levels, LDH levels, and peripheral blood eosinophil counts in children and adults with this disease [22, 23]. It may also be possible to review patient education and treatments by using serum TARC levels as a parameter. Serum TARC levels are higher in younger children, and its reference range differs among ages.

20.2 Japanese Guideline

20.2.1 Introduction

The guidelines for therapy for AD by the JDA were first prepared in 2000 and basically designed for dermatologist who treats patients in primary care to advanced specialty-required phases in the treatment of AD [24]. Thereafter, they were revised in 2003 and 2004. In 2008, guidelines for the management of AD in which diagnostic criteria for AD, severity classification, and treatment guidelines were integrated were prepared, partially revised, and translated into English in 2009 [2].

The clinical practice guidelines for the management of AD 2016 were prepared as a regular revision for all children to adults with all severity of AD, involving internationally published novel findings on AD in 2016 [20]. In this revision, recommendations to review clinical research articles, evaluate the balance between the advantages and disadvantages of medical activities, and optimize medical activity-related patient outcomes with respect to several important points requiring decision-making in clinical practice were presented.

20.2.2 Definition

See Sect. 20.1.1.1 and Table 20.1.

20.2.3 Pathogenesis

The pathogenesis of AD can be explained from the perspectives of the skin barrier, allergic inflammation, and pruritus [25].

20.2.3.1 Skin Barrier

Skin barrier function is reduced in patients with AD; therefore, skin irritability to nonspecific stimuli is enhanced, frequently causing inflammation. A recent study reported that filaggrin gene mutations were involved in the pathogenesis of AD [26]. Filaggrin aggregates keratin fibers and, when decomposed, contributes to water retention in the cornified layer as a natural moisturizing factor.

20.2.3.2 Allergic Inflammation

A reduction in skin barrier function leads to antigen (allergen) invasiveness in the skin. Allergens, such as mites and pollen, function as protein antigens and induce T-helper (Th)2-type immune responses that are mediated by the proteases contained in them. Th2-type immune responses then induce the production of IgE.

20.2.3.3 Pruritus

The effects of histamine H1 receptor antagonists (antihistamines) on AD-related pruritus vary among patients, and the presence of a mediator other than histamine has been suggested. A recent study reported that IL-31, a cytokine produced by Th2 cells, induced pruritus [27].

20.2.4 Course and Prognosis

Although AD shows a chronic course, remission may be achieved when symptoms are continuously controlled by appropriate treatments. According to the literature, age-related remission was achieved in a specific proportion of patients with AD. The remission rate was higher in patients with milder symptoms.

20.2.5 Diagnosis

See Sect. 20.1.

20.2.6 Treatments

20.2.6.1 Goal of Treatment

The goal of treatment is to reach and maintain a state in which symptoms are absent or mild without being disturbed in daily activities by the disease and drug therapy is not required. Even when this level is not reached, the objective is to maintain a state in which symptoms are mild without rapid exacerbations that affect daily activities.

20.2.6.2 Treatment Measures

Treatment measures for AD basically consist of drug therapy, skin care for physiological abnormalities in the skin, and investigations/elimination of exacerbating factors based on its pathogenesis. These measures are important and are adequately combined for individual patients based on the grade of symptoms and background.

20.2.6.3 Drug Treatment

Topical Anti-inflammatory Drugs

Drugs that potently reduce AD-related inflammation and of which the efficacy and safety have been scientifically examined include topical corticosteroids and tacrolimus (a topical calcineurin inhibitor). It is important to promptly and accurately reduce inflammation related to AD, and treatments are based on how topical corticosteroids and tacrolimus should be selected/combined for this purpose.

Topical Corticosteroids

Previous studies indicated that the efficacy of topical corticosteroids was significantly greater than that of a placebo regardless of age, excluding a few articles. These drugs may reduce inflammation related to AD. A rank table of topical corticosteroids is shown in Table 20.4 [20]. It is important to adequately select drugs at a rank that matches the severity of each eruption using this rank as an index and use them at the required volume for the required period.

A volume (approximately 0.5 g) measuring 5 mm in diameter that is pushed out from a tube to an area between the tip and first joint of the second finger is appropriate for two palms of adults, that is, approximately 2% of the body surface area of adults (fingertip unit) [28]. As a rule, topical corticosteroids should be applied twice a day in cases of acute exacerbation. When inflammation is reduced, the number of applications should be decreased to once a day to induce remission.

In infants/children, as a rule, topical corticosteroids one rank lower than that presented in Table 20.3 should be used when the severity of eruption is evaluated as severe or moderate. In the area including the face and neck where the drug absorption rate is high, the appearance of local adverse reactions to topical corticosteroids such as skin atrophy and capillary dilatation must be particularly considered. Therefore, long-term continuous use should be avoided. As a rule, medium-class or lower topical corticosteroids should be used. Tacrolimus ointment is frequently indicated for the face, and its guidance-based administration should be positively considered.

Tacrolimus

Tacrolimus inhibits the activity of intracellular calcineurin. It reduces inflammation via an action mechanism that differs from that of corticosteroids. Tacrolimus ointment is available at the following concentrations: 0.1% for adults and 0.03% for children. The efficacy of this ointment (0.1% for adults) for the trunk and limbs may be similar to that of strong-class topical corticosteroids.

Based on the findings of a long term observational study involving adults, the upper limit of the volume of a 0.1% ointment per session (twice a day) for adults was established as 5 g to avoid an increase in its blood concentration and maintain its safety. In accordance with the physical status, the maximum volume of a 0.03% ointment per use was established as 1 g for children aged 2–5 years, 2–4 g for those aged 6–12 years, and a maximum of 5 g for those aged 13 years or older.

Irritative symptoms, such as a transient burning sensation and hot flushes, often appear at the site of application. However, these symptoms appear at the start of treatment, and most symptoms disappear with improvements in eruption. This should be explained to patients before the start of treatment. Evidence to show that the use of tacrolimus ointment does not increase the risk of skin cancer or lymphoma is increasing.

Proactive Therapy

Proactive therapy refers to a treatment method in which, after inducing remission by an acute-phase treatment for repeatedly relapsing eruption, topical corticosteroids or tacrolimus ointment is periodically applied to the skin (e.g., twice a week) in addition to skin care with moisturizers in order to maintain remission. Recently, proactive therapy has commonly been selected as a strategy for maintaining the remission of AD.

Oral Antihistamines

Histamine H1 receptor antagonists (antihistamines) are widely used to treat AD-related pruritus. However, their effects markedly differ among patients. In the treatment of AD, it is most important to reduce dermatitis by using topical anti-inflammatory drugs, such as corticosteroids and tacrolimus. The oral administration of antihistamines is recommended as adjuvant therapy. The use of nonsedative second-generation antihistamines is recommended for the following reasons: no differences have been reported in treatment responses, and the incidences of adverse reactions, such as sleepiness, malaise, and impaired performance, are low [29].

Cyclosporine

In 2008, the use of cyclosporine was approved for patients with severe adult AD who do not respond to conventional treatments, showing eruption with marked inflammation involving 30% or greater of the body surface area. The initial dose of this drug is 3 mg/kg/day. It should be increased or decreased in accordance with symptoms, but in such a manner that it does not exceed 5 mg/kg/day. Its administration should be completed in 8–12 weeks. It is important to promptly switch cyclosporine therapy to conventional topical treatment after the amelioration of symptoms. Intermittent administration involving a 2-week or much longer period of discontinuation should be performed if long-term administration is necessary.

Oral Corticosteroids

Although a double-blind randomized controlled study has not yet been conducted to investigate the effects of oral corticosteroids on AD, these drugs have sometimes been used to induce the remission of acute exacerbation or severe/the most severe conditions. Long-term oral corticosteroid therapy induces various serious systemic adverse reactions; therefore, long-term AD control with oral corticosteroids is not recommended.

Chinese Herbal Medicine

For patients with AD who do not respond to topical anti-inflammatory drugs, such as corticosteroids or tacrolimus, oral antihistamines, skin care, or strategies against triggering factors, combination therapy with traditional Chinese herbal medicines may be considered.

Consideration for Pregnancy/Lactating Women

Some patients discontinue drug therapy due to anxiety regarding its influence on fetuses, leading to the deterioration of symptoms. However, the required treatments should also be adequately performed during pregnancy/lactation. Standard topical corticosteroid therapy shows low-level absorption in systemic circulation, and neither congenital anomalies nor the influence on fetal growth has been raised as an issue.

20.2.6.4 Skin Care for Abnormalities in Skin Barrier Function

The water content of the stratum corneum is reduced in patients with AD, leading to dry skin and reduced skin barrier function [25]. The use of moisturizers for the dry skin reverses the reduction in the water content of the stratum corneum, thereby promoting skin barrier function recovery, preventing the recurrence of dermatitis/invasion of allergens, and inhibiting pruritus. Furthermore, the continuous application of moisturizers after the relief of dermatitis related to treatment with topical anti-inflammatory drugs is useful for maintaining remission.

20.2.6.5 Investigation of Triggering Factors and Avoidance

Daily/social life-related aggravating factors specific to individual patients exist in most cases. It is important to investigate such factors and establish strategies to avoid them.

Food

The involvement of food allergens has been suggested in patients with AD, especially in infants. However, an allergen-free diet is not useful for treating children and adults with AD in whom the involvement of food allergies is not clear. Elimination-diet therapy should be performed under the guidance of physicians after determining, prior to its initiation, whether it should be indicated based on an evaluation of the involvement of food allergies.

Environmental and Contact Antigens

In order to determine whether environmental allergens, such as mites, house dust, pollen, and animal hair aggravate eruption, a comprehensive evaluation is needed based on information, such as medical histories, environmental changes, and changes in eruption, but not on clinical symptoms or specific IgE antibody titers/prick test results alone. It is necessary to establish whether eruption subsides by avoiding contact with suspected substances, make a definitive diagnosis based on the results of patch tests, and avoid contact with causative substances.

Sweat

Although sweat has been identified as an AD-triggering factor, "sweating" must be differentiated from "sweat after sweating." It is not necessary to avoid sweating, but "sweat after sweating" may induce pruritus. Because taking a shower (with tap water) is effective for relieving symptoms in seasons with a high sweat rate [30], excess sweat after sweating should be washed away.

20.2.6.6 Psychosomatic Aspects

Skin symptoms affect psychosocial aspects, and psychosocial factors influence skin symptoms. A vicious circle has been shown to persist in many patients with protracted AD. Therefore, psychosomatic approach is necessary for providing medical services in many cases. The conditions of AD that require psychosomatic considerations have been classified into the following three groups: stress-related deterioration/protraction of AD, maladjustment caused by AD, and maladjustment to the treatment/management of AD. These three groups are not independent and are often mutually associated.

20.2.6.7 Complications

Bacterial/fungal/viral infections may concomitantly occur in patients with AD, and their conditions frequently become severe. Therefore, it is important to maintain the skin in a favorable state. Ocular diseases, such as eyelid dermatitis, keratoconjunctivitis, keratoconus, cataracts, and retinal detachment, frequently develop when skin symptoms in the face are severe. It is important to promote regular ophthalmological consultations, instruct patients not to rub/hit their eyes, and control eruption.

20.2.6.8 Other Therapies

Ultraviolet (UV) therapy is considered for nonresponders to treatments with topical anti-inflammatory drugs, antihistamines, or moisturizers as well as for patients with adverse reactions to conventional treatments. In Japan, irradiation systems for narrow-band UVB therapy with a peak of 311 nm have been installed in an increasing number of hospitals and clinics. This therapy may be applied further in the future because of its safety and needlessness of posttreatment light shielding.

20.2.6.9 Hospital Care

Hospital care is indicated for some severe patients in whom the area of eruption is extensive. Hospital care may make it possible to thoroughly perform intensive topical therapy with isolation from the daily environment, establish a healthcare professional-patient relationship of mutual trust, review triggering factors/application methods/skin care, and overcome these problems in the early phase.

20.2.6.10 Education

In patients with AD, insufficient understanding of their condition or treatment and anxiety often lead to inappropriate treatments. Previous studies indicated that several sessions of a multi-occupational patient population education program involving physicians and nurses markedly improved the QOL of patients and severity of eruption [31].

20.2.6.11 Adherence

In medical care for AD, a chronic disease, it is important for patients and their parents to understand their condition/the significance of treatments, positively participate in the selection of therapeutic strategies, accomplish treatments according to these strategies, and improve the will to continue treatments, that is, adherence to

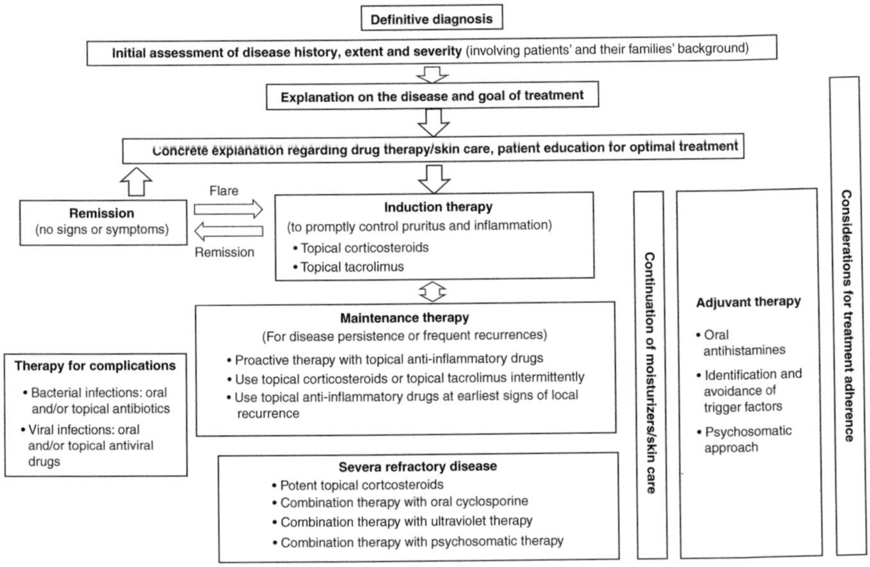

Fig. 20.3 Algorithm for treatment of atopic dermatitis (Cited from ref. [20])

treatments. Treatment adherence-associated factors include patient-/disease-/treatment-/healthcare professional-related and socioeconomic factors.

As factors related to healthcare professionals, their relationships with patients, explanations of the disease and treatment methods, and continuous information provision/support contribute to improvements in adherence. It is important to explain the necessity of drug therapy/skin care to patients and motivate them.

20.2.6.12 Treatment Procedures

Treatment procedures for AD are shown in Fig. 20.3 [20]. After making an accurate diagnosis and evaluating its severity, appropriate treatment methods should be combined in accordance with the state of eruption. In the initial consultation, it is important to explain the condition of AD and treatment methods to patients and have a common understanding with them.

References

1. Tagami H. Japanese Dermatological Association Criteria for the diagnosis of atopic dermatitis. J Dermatol. 1995;22:966–7.
2. Saeki H, Furue M, Furukawa F, et al. Guidelines for management of atopic dermatitis. J Dermatol. 2009;36:563–77.
3. Hanifin JM, Rajka G. Diagnostic features of atopic eczema. Acta Dermatol Venereol Suppl (Stockh). 1980;92:44–7.
4. Eichenfield LF, Hanifin JM, Luger TA, et al. Consensus conference on pediatric atopic dermatitis. J Am Acad Dermatol. 2003;49:1088–95.

5. Williams HC, Burney PGJ, Pembroke AC, et al. The UK Working Party's Diagnostic criteria for atopic dermatitis. III. Independent hospital validation. Br J Dermatol. 1994;131:406–16.
6. Saeki H, Iizuka H, Mori Y, et al. Community validation of the U.K. diagnostic criteria for atopic dermatitis in Japanese elementary schoolchildren. J Dermatol Sci. 2007;47:227–31.
7. Williams H, Robertson C, Stewart A, et al. Worldwide variations in the prevalence of symptoms of atopic eczema in the international study of asthma and allergies in childhood. J Allergy Clin Immunol. 1999;103:125–38.
8. Nishima S, Odajima H. Prevalence of childhood allergic diseases in Japan using international study of asthma and allergies in childhood (ISAAC) phase I protocol. Jpn J Pediatr Allergy Clin Immunol. 2002;16:207–20. (in Japanese with English abstract)
9. Aoki T. The second report from the Advisory Committee for Atopic Dermatitis Severity Classification. Jpn J Dermatol. 2001;111:2023–33. (in Japanese)
10. Yoshida H. Interim report from the Advisory Committee for Atopic Dermatitis Severity Classification. Jpn J Dermatol. 1998;108:1491–6. (in Japanese)
11. Katayama I, Kohno Y, Akiyama K, et al. Japanese guideline for atopic dermatitis 2014. Allergol Int. 2014;63:377–98.
12. European Task Force on Atopic Dermatitis. Severity scoring of atopic dermatitis: the SCORAD index. Dermatology. 1993;186:23–31.
13. Hanifin JM, Thurston M, Omoto M, et al. The eczema area and severity index (EASI): assessment of reliability in atopic dermatitis. Exp Dermatol. 2001;10:11–8.
14. Rajka G, Langeland T. Grading of the severity of atopic dermatitis. Acta Derm Venereol Suppl (Stockh). 1989;144:13–4.
15. Furue M, Ebata T, Ikoma A, et al. Verbalizing extremes of the visual analogue scale for pruritus: a consensus statement. Acta Derm Venereol. 2013;93:214–5.
16. Chren MM, Lasek RJ, Sahay AP, et al. Measurement properties of Skindex-16: a brief quality-of-life measure for patients with skin diseases. J Cutan Med Surg. 2001;5:105–10.
17. Finlay AY, Khan GK. Dermatology Life Quality Index (DLQI)—a simple practical measure for routine clinical use. Clin Exp Dermatol. 1994;19:210–6.
18. Higaki Y, Kawamoto K, Kamo T, et al. The Japanese version of Skindex-16: a brief quality-of-life measure for patients with skin diseases. J Dermatol. 2002;29:693–8.
19. Takahashi N, Suzukamo Y, Nakamura M, et al. Japanese version of the Dermatology Life Quality Index: validity and reliability in patients with acne. Health Qual Life Outcomes. 2006;4:46.
20. Saeki H, Nakahara T, Tanaka A, et al. Clinical practice guidelines for the management of atopic dermatitis 2016. J Dermatol. 2016;43:1117–45.
21. Saeki H, Tamaki K. Thymus and activation regulated chemokine (TARC)/CCL17 and skin diseases. J Dermatol Sci. 2006;43:75–84.
22. Tamaki K, Saeki H, Kadono T, et al. Serum TARC/CCL17 levels as a disease marker of atopic dermatitis. Jpn J Dermatol. 2006;116:27–39. (In Japanese with English abstract)
23. Fujisawa T, Nagao M, Noma Y, et al. Clinical utility of serum TARC/CCL17 for monitoring clinical course of atopic dermatitis in children. Jpn J Pediatr Allergy Clin Immunol. 2005;19:744–57. (In Japanese with English abstract)
24. Kawashima M, Takigawa M, Nakagawa H, et al. Guidelines for therapy for atopic dermatitis. Jpn J Dermatol. 2000;110:1099–104. (In Japanese with English abstract)
25. Kabashima K. New concept of the pathogenesis of atopic dermatitis: interplay among the barrier, allergy, and pruritus as a trinity. J Dermatol Sci. 2013;70:3–11.
26. Palmer CN, Irvine AD, Terron-Kwiatkowski A, et al. Common loss-of-function variants of the epidermal barrier protein filaggrin are a major predisposing factor for atopic dermatitis. Nat Genet. 2006;38:441–6.
27. Dillon SR, Sprecher C, Hammond A, et al. Interleukin 31, a cytokine produced by activated T cells, induces dermatitis in mice. Nat Immunol. 2004;5:752–60.
28. Long CC, Finlay AY. The finger-tip unit - a new practical measure. Clin Exp Dermatol. 1991;16:444–7.

29. Yanai K, Zhang D, Tashiro M, et al. Positron emission tomography evaluation of sedative properties of antihistamines. Expert Opin Drug Saf. 2011;10:613–22.
30. Murota H, Takahashi A, Nishioka M, et al. Showering reduces atopic dermatitis in elementary school students. Eur J Dermatol. 2010;20:410–1.
31. Staab D, Diepgen TL, Fartasch M, et al. Age related, structured educational programmes for the management of atopic dermatitis in children and adolescents: multicentre, randomised controlled trial. BMJ. 2006;332:933–8.

Part VIII

Management

Management: Drug Therapy—Ointment 21

Takahiro Satoh

Abstract

Atopic dermatitis (AD) is an allergic inflammatory skin disease etiologically associated with disrupted skin barrier function. Topical treatment is a fundamental approach for the management of AD. This includes various kinds of emollients/moisturizers as skin care and anti-inflammatory drugs, such as corticosteroids and tacrolimus. Improvement of barrier function could lead to reduced risk for the development and/or exacerbation of AD and reduces the chance for epicutaneous sensitization against environmental allergens, which may induce systemic allergy. Anti-inflammatory drugs are used for controlling flare-up of skin inflammation during the course of the disease. Proactive therapy, comprising continuous or periodical use and gradual tapering of anti-inflammatory drugs with emollients/moisturizers even when clinical symptoms improve, has been found to be useful for obtaining long-term remission. Patient adherence to external application is essential for reaching successful treatment outcomes with topical drugs.

Keywords

Barrier function • Corticosteroids • Proactive therapy • Tacrolimus

T. Satoh
Department of Dermatology, National Defense Medical College,
3-2 Namiki, Tokorozawa 359-8513, Japan
e-mail: tasaderm@ndmc.ac.jp

I. Katayama et al. (eds.), *Evolution of Atopic Dermatitis in the 21st Century*,
https://doi.org/10.1007/978-981-10-5541-6_21

21.1 Introduction

Atopic dermatitis (AD) is a chronic eczematous skin disease. Patients are commonly complicated by repeated exacerbation and remission. Skin inflammation is closely associated with dry skin and barrier dysfunction. Topical therapies are the principal therapeutic approaches for AD. Basically, these consist of two components: emollients/moisturizers and topical anti-inflammatory drugs.

21.2 Emollients/Moisturizers

Rectification of dry skin and disrupted barrier function by emollients/moisturizers is a fundamental treatment for AD. Continuous use of moisturizers has been found to be effective for maintaining remission of AD [1]. In addition, a recent study conducted in Japan elegantly demonstrated that daily application of moisturizer to neonates prevented the development of AD [2].

The pharmaceutical effects of emollients/moisturizers appear to be determined by the composition of agents and constituents. Physicians should also consider the skin condition of the patient, weather (temperature and humidity), and patient preferences.

Olive oil and camellia oil are simple agents for increasing water content in the stratum corneum by inhibiting water evaporation through occlusion of skin surface. Petrolatum is also commonly used in emollients. A thick layer of petrolatum has been found to not only increase skin hydration but also improve transepidermal water loss (TEWL) [3]. Classical topical agents, such as hydrophilic ointment (cream) and zinc oxide ointment (10, 20%), are also useful.

Moisturizing agents actively keeping water include 10–20% urea cream and 0.3% heparinoid ointment/cream/lotion (Hirudoid®). A recent study demonstrated that topical urea application normalized skin barrier function and promoted antimicrobial peptide generation [4]. Many other types of moisturizers that include glycerin, hydrolyzed collagen, chondroitin sulfate, ceramides, free fatty acids, squalene, and/or cholesterol are available as clinically exclusive cosmetics, OCT (over-the-counter) products, or general cosmetics/products.

21.3 Topical Anti-inflammatory Drugs

Topical corticosteroids and an immunosuppressant, tacrolimus, represent a highly recommended therapeutic option as a topical therapy for AD. Since repeated exacerbation of symptoms is common, topical anti-inflammatory drugs are generally used to obtain remission at the time of flare (reactive therapy). Recently, an alternative method, proactive therapy, has been recommended for patients with repeatedly relapsing eruptions [5, 6]. Anti-inflammatory drugs are used for obtaining remission of exacerbated lesions, followed by periodical application instead of cessation of topical drugs, even when skin inflammation is clinically improved; this could lead to the maintenance of long-term remission. Serum TRAC levels have been reported as a useful marker for determining the dose, application frequency, and/or time of cessation of anti-inflammatory drugs [5]. Concomitant use of emollients/moisturizers with anti-inflammatory drugs during proactive therapy is recommended. A randomized, investigator-blinded study demonstrated that proactive therapy, but not reactive therapy, with corticosteroids in children with AD prevented sensitization against aeroallergens in addition to decreased clinical severity and serum TARC levels [6]. Apparently, physicians should take care of adverse reactions.

In contrast to topical corticosteroids and tacrolimus, nonsteroidal anti-inflammatory drugs (NSAIDs) have minimal or no effect on eczematous skin inflammations. Considering the risk of contact dermatitis, NSAIDS are not ideal for treating AD. Reliable evidence for the clinical effects of topical Chinese herbal medicines is not yet available. Physicians should also pay attention to the risk of contact dermatitis from topical Chinese herbal medicines.

21.3.1 Corticosteroids

In Japan, topical corticosteroids are classified into five ranks (strongest, very strong, strong, medium, and weak) [5]. Physicians need to select an adequate rank of corticosteroids depending on skin severity, age, and anatomical sites. In neonates and infants, drugs more than one rank lower than in adults are recommended. The face, neck, and groin are known to be sites that are highly absorbent of corticosteroids [7]. Drugs lower than medium class should thus generally be used.

The fingertip unit (FTU) [8] is useful for estimating the adequate volume of topical corticosteroid, with ointment from a tube on the second finger between the fingertip and first joint (approximately 0.5 g) corresponding to a two-hand area (approximately 2% of the body surface area).

In principle, topical corticosteroids are initially applied twice a day, in the morning and evening. When acutely exacerbated lesions improve, the frequency of application can be gradually reduced to frequencies such as once a day or three times a week.

Systemic adverse reactions, such as adrenal insufficiency, and local adverse reactions, such as skin atrophy, telangiectasia, acne, and infections commonly from fungus, need to be carefully monitored by dermatologists. A large amount and/or long-term application of corticosteroids to periorbital regions increases the risk of glaucoma.

21.3.2 Topical Tacrolimus

Tacrolimus is a calcineurin inhibitor that down-modulates immune responses. In Japan, 0.1 and 0.03% ointments are available for adults and children, respectively. These do not induce skin atrophy and telangiectasia, which are common adverse reactions in corticosteroids. Absorption of tacrolimus is influenced by skin barrier function. Because of its high molecular weight (822.03), tacrolimus is not easily absorbed through the normal skin. When skin inflammation improves and the disrupted barrier function recovers through the use of tacrolimus, no further absorption can occur, avoiding unwanted and excess absorption. Topical tacrolimus is thus useful for treating regions that can easily absorb corticosteroids, such as the face and neck, and is suitable for AD patients with severe adverse responses due to long-term corticosteroid use. A recent study demonstrated that application of corticosteroids for 4 weeks increased transepidermal water loss (TEWL), indicating reduced skin barrier function. In contrast, topical tacrolimus reduced TEWL and improved skin hydration [9]. Topical tacrolimus may be preferable to topical corticosteroids in AD patients for long-term application, particularly as proactive therapy.

Adverse reactions often include burning sensation or hot flushing; these are mostly transient and gradually disappear along with the improvement of skin inflammation. Tacrolimus should not be applied to erosive and ulcerative lesions. Occlusive dressing techniques should also not be used. As with corticosteroids, patients should be aware of increased risk of bacterial, fungal, and viral infections. Topical tacrolimus may be useful for treating rosacea but also causes rosacea-like eruptions that are occasionally accompanied by granulomatous reaction and increased *Demodex* in hair follicles [10, 11].

Conclusions

Dry skin and skin inflammation in AD are principally managed by topical therapies. In addition to the pharmacological actions of topical drugs, patient adherence to external application in daily life is an important factor for achieving successful outcomes compared with oral drugs.

References

1. Szczepanowska J, Reich A, Szepietowski JC. Emollients improve treatment results with topical corticosteroids in childhood atopic dermatitis: a randomized comparative study. Pediatr Allergy Immunol. 2008;19(7):614–8. doi:10.1111/j.1399-3038.2007.00706.x.
2. Horimukai K, Morita K, Narita M, Kondo M, Kitazawa H, Nozaki M, et al. Application of moisturizer to neonates prevents development of atopic dermatitis. J Allergy Clin Immunol. 2014;134(4):824–830. e6. doi:10.1016/j.jaci.2014.07.060.
3. Loden M. The increase in skin hydration after application of emollients with different amounts of lipids. Acta Derm Venereol. 1992;72(5):327–30.
4. Grether-Beck S, Felsner I, Brenden H, Kohne Z, Majora M, Marini A, et al. Urea uptake enhances barrier function and antimicrobial defense in humans by regulating epidermal gene expression. J Invest Dermatol. 2012;132(6):1561–72. doi:10.1038/jid.2012.42.
5. Saeki H, Nakahara T, Tanaka A, Kabashima K, Sugaya M, Murota H, et al. Clinical practice guidelines for the Management of Atopic Dermatitis 2016. J Dermatol. 2016;43:1117–45. doi:10.1111/1346-8138.13392.
6. Fukuie T, Hirakawa S, Narita M, Nomura I, Matsumoto K, Tokura Y, et al. Potential preventive effects of proactive therapy on sensitization in moderate to severe childhood atopic dermatitis: a randomized, investigator-blinded, controlled study. J Dermatol. 2016;43:1283–92. doi:10.1111/1346-8138.13408.
7. Feldmann RJ, Maibach HI. Regional variation in percutaneous penetration of 14C cortisol in man. J Invest Dermatol. 1967;48(2):181–3.

8. Long CC, Finlay AY, Averill RW. The rule of hand: 4 hand areas = 2 FTU = 1 g. Arch Dermatol. 1992;128(8):1129–30.
9. Danby SG, Chittock J, Brown K, Albenali LH, Cork MJ. The effect of tacrolimus compared with betamethasone valerate on the skin barrier in volunteers with quiescent atopic dermatitis. Br J Dermatol. 2014;170(4):914–21. doi:10.1111/bjd.12778.
10. Antille C, Saurat JH, Lubbe J. Induction of rosaceiform dermatitis during treatment of facial inflammatory dermatoses with tacrolimus ointment. Arch Dermatol. 2004;140(4):457–60. doi:10.1001/archderm.140.4.457.
11. Fujiwara S, Okubo Y, Irisawa R, Tsuboi R. Rosaceiform dermatitis associated with topical tacrolimus treatment. J Am Acad Dermatol. 2010;62(6):1050–2. doi:10.1016/j.jaad.2009.01.029.

Drug Therapy: Systemic

22

Norito Katoh

Abstract

Systemic therapy is indicated for patients with severe atopic dermatitis (AD) who do not respond to adequate topical treatment or who cannot continue to receive topical therapy due to its side effects, such as skin atrophy. Before administering systemic immunosuppressive or immunomodulatory pharmaceuticals, clinicians should check whether the diagnosis of AD is correct, consider possible differential diagnoses, and examine whether the patient's adherence to topical treatments is sufficient. The currently available immunosuppressive and immunomodulatory drugs mainly produce their anti-inflammatory effects by suppressing the proliferation and functions of lymphocytes. However, since they can cause a range of adverse effects, strict monitoring before and during treatment is mandatory. Patient education regarding the possible adverse effects of treatment, the pathogenesis of AD, and the practical measures for treating AD is very important.

Keywords

Cyclosporine • Azathioprine • Mycophenolic acid • Methotrexate • Antihistamine

N. Katoh, M.D., Ph.D.
Department of Dermatology, Graduate School of Medical Science, Kyoto Prefectural University of Medicine, 465 Kajii-cho, Kawaramachi-Hirokoji, Kamigyo-ku, Kyoto 602-8566, Japan
e-mail: nkatoh@koto.kpu-m.ac.jp

I. Katayama et al. (eds.), *Evolution of Atopic Dermatitis in the 21st Century*,
https://doi.org/10.1007/978-981-10-5541-6_22

22.1 Introduction

Atopic dermatitis (AD) is a disease characterized by relapsing eczema and pruritus. Type 2 cytokines play critical roles in the pathogenesis of allergic inflammation in AD [1]. The current evidence-based strategies used to treat the condition consist of three primary measures: (1) the use of topical anti-inflammatory agents, such as topical corticosteroids and topical calcineurin inhibitors; (2) the application of emollients/moisturizers to treat cutaneous barrier dysfunction; and (3) the avoidance of exacerbating factors [2]. Most patients with AD can control their skin disease with these approaches. Systemic therapy is required in patients with severe AD who do not respond to these treatments. The systemic treatments for AD are subdivided into three categories: (1) immunosuppressive and immunomodulatory pharmaceuticals, (2) antihistamines, and (3) others. In this chapter, I briefly review the information about currently available systemic treatments for AD.

22.2 Immunosuppressive and Immunomodulatory Pharmaceuticals

22.2.1 Before the Start of Immunosuppressive and Immunomodulatory Pharmaceutical Treatment

Before judging that a patient's condition is refractory to treatment with topical corticosteroids and topical calcineurin inhibitors, clinicians should check whether the diagnosis of AD is correct and consider possible differential diagnoses including allergic contact dermatitis, seborrheic dermatitis, prurigo simplex, cutaneous mycosis, scabies, miliaria, ichthyosis, xerotic eczema, hand dermatitis (non-atopic), cutaneous lymphoma, psoriasis, immunodeficiency diseases (hyper-IgE syndrome and Wiskott-Aldrich syndrome), collagen diseases (systemic lupus erythematosus and dermatomyositis), and Netherton syndrome [2]. In addition, allergic contact dermatitis caused by topical medications is often misdiagnosed as refractory AD [3].

During the treatment of AD, if the expected effects are not obtained with topical corticosteroids and topical calcineurin inhibitors, it is important to confirm whether these drugs have been correctly applied. Physicians should educate patients and their caregivers about the appropriate amount of the prescribed drug to apply (e.g., a blob of ointment (0.5 g) measuring 5 mm in diameter that is pushed out from a tube onto the area between the tip and first joint of the second finger is appropriate for covering both palms of a British adult, i.e., approximately 2% of the body surface area of an adult (fingertip unit)) [2, 4, 5]. We should monitor patients' treatment adherence because poor treatment adherence often prevents patients from achieving disease control. Poor adherence can also be misinterpreted as a poor response to treatment, which might lead to the patient receiving more powerful and potentially dangerous systemic medications. In general, oral medication is associated with significantly better adherence than topical medication.

In patients with severe chronic eczema, hospitalization for a few weeks often leads to the patient's AD being brought under control with intensive topical therapy, and education aimed at increasing the patient's understanding of the mechanism responsible for their disease and improving their treatment adherence can also be provided [2, 6].

Before starting any immunosuppressive or immunomodulatory drug therapy for AD, a detailed clinical and laboratory examination of the patient is essential. In particular, underlying active infectious diseases including hepatitis B and C, HIV infections, and syphilis have to be ruled out. The organ function tests that should be performed before and during therapy depend on the drugs prescribed [7].

22.2.2 Cyclosporine

Cyclosporine, a cyclic non-ribosomal peptide composed of 11 amino acids, inhibits T-cell activation and proliferation by preventing the dephosphorylation of nuclear factor of activated T cells [8]. Cyclosporine inhibits the production of cytokines, such as interleukin (IL)-2, IL-3, and IL-6, by T cells, and, thus, has immunosuppressive effects.

In randomized placebo-controlled trials, cyclosporine has been shown to have significant beneficial effects on skin lesions and pruritus and, hence, to improve the quality of life of adult patients with severe AD [9, 10]. The efficacy of cyclosporine against severe childhood AD has also been demonstrated in clinical studies [11, 12]. A meta-analysis assessing the effectiveness of systemic cyclosporine in patients with severe AD showed that cyclosporine consistently decreased the severity of AD and was similarly effective in children and adults [13]. It also revealed that 6–8 weeks of cyclosporine treatment had a relative effectiveness of 55% (95% confidence interval, 48–62%).

Cyclosporine has been approved as a first line systemic treatment for severe AD in children and adults in some European countries. In Japan, cyclosporine is licensed for use in patients with severe adult AD who do not respond to conventional treatments and exhibit eruptions and marked inflammation involving ≥30% of their body surface area. The initial dose of cyclosporine for adult patients with severe AD is 3 mg/kg per day in Japan, which should be increased or decreased in accordance with the patient's symptoms, but it should not exceed 5 mg/kg per day [2].

It is recommended that cyclosporine to be tapered and eventually discontinued after an improvement in the patient's AD has been achieved. In Japan, the package insert for cyclosporine warns physicians that the cyclosporine treatment period should be limited to ≤12 weeks in AD patients. Some clinical studies have examined relapse rates after the discontinuation of cyclosporine treatment in AD patients [12, 14, 15]. In these studies, the treatment protocol allowed the use of topical steroids after the discontinuation of cyclosporine. In one study, about 50% of patients relapsed within 2 weeks of the discontinuation of cyclosporine, and about 80% relapsed within 6 weeks [14]. In another study, 73% of the patients relapsed within 24 weeks [15]. In pediatric patients with AD, 86% of patients relapsed within

9 months [12]. Interestingly, Kim et al. compared the efficacy and relapse rate of cyclosporine treatment combined with topical therapy involving topical corticosteroids and topical calcineurin inhibitors with those of cyclosporine alone in moderate-to-severe AD patients [16]. The treatment success rate was significantly higher in the combination group. The combination group had a shorter median time to response, a lower cumulative dose, and a longer time to relapse than the monotherapy group [16].

Renal dysfunction and increased blood pressure are the most concerning adverse effects of cyclosporine and are particularly associated with long-term prescription. It is necessary to monitor patients' blood pressure, serum creatinine levels, complete blood counts, and blood biochemistry before and during cyclosporine therapy [7, 17]. Gastrointestinal symptoms and headache are the most commonly reported adverse events associated with cyclosporine treatment in pediatric patients with severe AD [13]. Adverse events appear to be more common in patients treated with higher doses [13]. Cyclosporine should not be combined with phototherapy because it increases the risk of nonmelanoma skin cancer [18].

22.2.3 Azathioprine

Azathioprine, an imidazolyl derivative of 6-mercaptopurine, is converted to 6-mercaptopurine, which blocks the synthesis of RNA and DNA and, thus, inhibits the proliferation of T and B cells and suppresses the functions of natural killer cells [8]. It is widely used as immunosuppressant drug during solid organ transplants and as a treatment for rheumatic arthritis and inflammatory bowel disease [8]. Unlike cyclosporine, azathioprine takes several weeks to reach a steady-state level in the blood and is therefore slow to take effect [18]. Thiopurine methyltransferase (TPMT), one of the enzymes involved in the metabolism of 6-mercaptopurine into inactive compounds, is affected by genetic polymorphisms, and inherited changes in its activity can impact on patients' responses to azathioprine [8].

Regarding the efficacy of azathioprine against AD, some case series have indicated that azathioprine might be a useful treatment for recalcitrant pediatric, adolescent, and adult AD [19–24]. Two double-blind, randomized controlled trials have also demonstrated that treatment with azathioprine produced clinically relevant improvements in moderate-to-severe AD [25, 26]. In one study, 54 (86%) participants completed the study, 2 (3%) withdrew from the placebo group, and 7 (11%) withdrew from the azathioprine group. By week 12, azathioprine had brought about a 37% improvement in mean disease activity compared with the 20% improvement produced by the placebo [26]. In another study, 37 subjects were enrolled, and 16 were withdrawn (12 during azathioprine treatment and 4 during placebo treatment). After 3 months, the eruption score had fallen by 26% in the group treated with azathioprine, whereas it had only fallen by 3% in the placebo group [25].

The major adverse effects associated with azathioprine include gastrointestinal complaints, such as nausea, liver dysfunction, and leukopenia. Patients who exhibit reduced or no TPMT activity (about 10% and 0.3% of the population, respectively) are at higher risk of profound immunosuppression [27]. Reduced TPMT activity is also related to the risk of fatal myelosuppression [18]. Thus, patients' TMPT activity should be checked before the start of azathioprine treatment because the serious adverse effects of azathioprine treatment are dose-dependent [17]. Furthermore, an increased risk of nonmelanoma skin cancer has been detected in transplant recipients on long-term azathioprine treatment [18]. It is proposed that this is mediated via azathioprine-induced increases in photosensitivity, so all patients that receive such treatment should be advised about photoprotection [18].

22.2.4 Mycophenolic Acid

Mycophenolate mofetil is rapidly absorbed and hydrolyzed into the active compound mycophenolic acid [8]. Mycophenolic acid inhibits inosine monophosphate dehydrogenase, which is required for de novo purine synthesis, and has immunomodulatory effects on T and B cells [17]. Recently, enteric-coated mycophenolate sodium (EC-MPS) was developed as a way of decreasing the adverse gastrointestinal effects of mycophenolic acid treatment [18].

In an open-label pilot study, 1 g mycophenolate mofetil was administered orally twice daily for 4 weeks to ten adult patients with moderate-to-severe AD, which was followed by 500 mg twice daily from weeks 5 to 8 [28]. Treatment with mycophenolate markedly reduced the severity of AD within 4 weeks in all patients, and after 8 weeks, the mean ± SD SCORAD (SCORing Atopic Dermatitis) index had dropped from the pretreatment value of 49.2 ± 13.8 to 21.9 ± 26.5 ($P < 0.01$). In the latter study, most patients tolerated the treatment well, except one patient who developed herpes retinitis after 4 weeks. In a retrospective chart review of 20 adult patients with moderate-to-severe AD, the conditions of 17 patients improved within 4 weeks of the start of mycophenolate mofetil treatment [29]. Ten patients achieved disease remission and were subsequently able to discontinue mycophenolate mofetil. Two case series of pediatric AD patients also demonstrated positive responses to myco phenolate mofetil treatment [20, 30]. Haeck et al. performed an observer-blinded randomized controlled trial, in which the efficacy of EC-MPS was compared with cyclosporine as a maintenance treatment for adult patients with moderate-to-severe AD [31]. Although the clinical improvement achieved with EC-MPS was delayed in comparison with that induced by cyclosporine, both treatments were similarly effective as maintenance therapies in patients with AD. Interestingly, the disease activity of the patients in the cyclosporine study arm was significantly greater than that seen in the EC-MPS study arm after the withdrawal of medication, suggesting that EC-MPS might exhibit more prolonged treatment effects.

In studies of AD, mild headaches and nausea were the most commonly reported adverse effects of mycophenolic acid therapy [17, 28, 29, 31]. Treatment with mycophenolic acid also increases the risk of liver enzyme abnormalities and infections, such as herpes zoster, herpes simplex, or staphylococcal infections [28, 29, 31, 32]. Therefore, it is necessary to monitor patients' complete metabolic panels, liver enzyme levels, and complete blood counts before and during therapy with mycophenolic acid [17].

22.2.5 Methotrexate

Methotrexate is an analogue of folic acid, which inhibits purine and pyrimidine synthesis and, thus, suppresses cellular proliferation [8]. It is also considered to negatively affect T-cell function and is used to treat chronic inflammatory diseases, such as rheumatic arthritis and psoriasis.

A randomized controlled trial including 40 pediatric patients with severe AD, who ranged in age from 8 to 14, found that oral methotrexate (initial dose, 5 mg; maintenance dose, 7.5 mg weekly) and cyclosporine (2.5 mg/kg/day) exhibited similar efficacy during 12 weeks' treatment [33]. Mild and temporary adverse effects were reported in some patients in both groups. In another randomized controlled trial, the efficacy of methotrexate (dosage, 10–22.5 mg/week) was compared with that of azathioprine (dosage, 1.5–2.5 mg/kg/day) in adult patients with severe AD [34]. Both treatments displayed similar efficacy levels (42% versus 39% SCORAD reduction, respectively). Although no statistically significant differences in the number or severity of adverse events were detected, blood count abnormalities were more common in the azathioprine group. Therefore, it was indicated that methotrexate is an alternative first-line systemic treatment for severe AD [18, 35].

Gastrointestinal symptoms, such as nausea, and increases in liver enzyme levels were the main side effects observed in previous case series examining methotrexate therapy for AD [36–38]. Complete blood count monitoring is important during methotrexate treatment because of the risk of bone marrow suppression. Folic acid supplementation reduces the risk of hepatotoxicity, gastrointestinal symptoms, and bone marrow suppression [18]. In addition, teratogenicity has to be considered [7].

22.2.6 Corticosteroids

Corticosteroids affect the transcription of several mediators involved in the pathogenesis of inflammatory disorders, including AD, by binding to the regulatory elements of many genes via the glucocorticoid receptor [7].

Systemic corticosteroids have sometimes been used to induce remission after the acute exacerbation of AD or in severe/very severe AD. They are known to be effective and are commonly used in clinical practice [Simon]. However, long-term oral corticosteroid therapy induces various serious systemic adverse reactions, including diabetes, hypertension, gastric ulcers, osteoporosis, skin atrophy, glaucoma, Cushing's syndrome, and growth retardation [Simon]. Therefore, long-term AD control with oral corticosteroids is not recommended [2, 7, 35]. In a double-blind, placebo-controlled study of oral prednisolone (initial dose, 0.5–0.8 mg/kg/day) versus cyclosporine (2.7–4.0 mg/kg/day), 2 weeks' prednisolone treatment was not able to sufficiently control the symptoms of severe AD, and cyclosporine was more effective at maintaining remission [39].

22.2.7 Interferon Gamma

Th2 cytokines including IL-4, IL-5, and IL-13 are known to play important roles in the pathogenesis of AD [1, 40]. Interferon gamma (IFN-γ) inhibits IgE synthesis and the proliferation of Th2 cells [41, 42] and, thus, is considered to be effective against AD. A few studies have examined the efficacy of IFN-γ as a treatment for AD. The subcutaneous injection of IFN-γ produced a statistically significant improvement in the symptoms of severe AD compared with placebo injections [43, 44]. However, its "flu-like" side effects, which include fever, fatigue, and myalgia, and cost prevent its widespread use [Simon, Hanifin].

22.3 Antihistamines

Although histamine and the histamine H1 receptor (H1R) are considered to be representative mediators of pruritus, many other mediators might be involved in itching in AD [45]. Actually, antihistamines (H1R antagonists), especially the sedating type, have long been prescribed to AD patients in an attempt to reduce pruritus. However, histamines are not always involved in AD-related pruritus, and so antihistamines might not help all patients. As a consequence, neither the American nor European guidelines for the management of AD recommend the general use of antihistamines as part of AD treatment for pruritus [35, 46]. Due to their sedative properties, sedating antihistamines, such as hydroxyzine, are widely used to counteract eczema-induced sleep loss in children older than 2 years [17]. However, in a randomized, double-blind, placebo-controlled study, the addition of a non-sedating antihistamine, fexofenadine hydrochloride (60 mg BID), to a topical corticosteroid resulted in a significant reduction in AD-associated pruritus in adult patients [47]. Yamanaka et al. investigated the effects of an oral non-sedating antihistamine, olopatadine hydrochloride, and a placebo on the visual analog scale (VAS) scores for itching in 20 patients with moderate to severe AD and showed that the patients' VAS scores for itching were significantly reduced by olopatadine, but not the placebo. In addition, the drug did not affect sleep quality, according to simultaneously recorded electroencephalograms [48]. These results suggest that some AD patients might benefit from the use of non-sedating antihistamines when they are used in combination with topical corticosteroids. Clinical studies analyzing the factors correlated with the efficacy of non-sedating antihistamines in a large number of AD patients are required.

22.4 Others

22.4.1 Alitretinoin

Alitretinoin, 9-cis retinoic acid, is an antagonistic vitamin A derivative that binds to both retinoic acid receptors (RAR and RXR) [Simon]. A randomized, double-blind, placebo-controlled trial demonstrated that oral alitretinoin is an effective treatment for severe hand eczema and that its effects are dose-dependent [49]. Although alitretinoin was shown to be effective against all types of chronic hand eczema, hyperkeratotic and fingertip eczema exhibited the highest response rates and strongest responses compared with the placebo treatment [51]. Alitretinoin treatment is well tolerated, and its most common dose-dependent adverse effects include headaches, mucocutaneous events, hyperlipidemia, and decreased levels of free thyroxine and thyroid-stimulating hormone. Interestingly, the administration of oral alitretinoin at the standard dose of 30 mg daily significantly improved both the palmar lesions and the extra-palmar manifestations of AD in six adult patients [50]. Since all retinoids are teratogenic, alitretinoin is not indicated for pregnant women, and its use to treat women of childbearing age should be avoided unless strict contraceptive measures are employed [7].

22.5 Conclusion and Future Perspectives

During the treatment of psoriasis, another representative inflammatory skin disease, the blockade of a single cytokine with biologics, has been demonstrated to be very effective, and this technique is now widely used in clinical practice. So far, the effects of biologics on AD do not seem to bear comparison with those seen in psoriasis [Beck], mostly because of the heterogeneous characteristics of AD, the pathogenesis of which involves many types of cytokines.

Although immunosuppressive and immunomodulatory pharmaceuticals have been shown to be effective against severe AD in both pediatric and adult patients, their potential adverse effects limit their prescription in daily practice. Novel small molecules that are able to block the synthesis of several of the pro-inflammatory cytokines and chemokines involved in the pathogenesis of AD are required. Alternatively, personalized treatment using biologics that can block the most relevant cytokine in each AD patient might help to address current medical issues.

References

1. Werfel T, Allam JP, Biedermann T, Eyerich K, Gilles S, Guttman-Yassky E, et al. Cellular and molecular immunologic mechanisms in patients with atopic dermatitis. J Allergy Clin Immunol. 2016;138:336–49. doi:10.1016/j.jaci.2016.06.010.
2. Saeki H, Nakahara T, Tanaka A, Kabashima K, Sugaya M, Murota H, Committee for Clinical Practice Guidelines for the Management of Atopic Dermatitis of Japanese Dermatological Association, et al. Clinical practice Guidelines for the Management of Atopic Dermatitis 2016. J Dermatol. 2016;43:1117–45. doi:10.1111/1346-8138.13392.
3. Tamagawa-Mineoka R, Masuda K, Ueda S, Nakamura N, Hotta E, Hattori J, et al. Contact sensitivity in patients with recalcitrant atopic dermatitis. J Dermatol. 2015;42:720–2. doi:10.1111/1346-8138.12866.
4. Long CC, Finlay AY. The finger tip unit a new practical measure. Clin Exp Dermatol. 1991;16:444–7.
5. Long CC, Finlay AY, Averill RW. The rule of hand: 4 hand area = 2 FTU = 1 g. Arch Dermatol. 1992;128:1129–30.

6. Bieber T, Straeter B. Off-label prescriptions for atopic dermatitis in Europe. Allergy. 2015;70:6–11.
7. Simon D, Bieber T. Systemic therapy for atopic dermatitis. Allergy. 2014;69:46–55.
8. Smith GP, Chan ESL. Immunomodulating pharmaceuticals. In: Rich RR, Fleisher TA, Shearer WT, Schroeder H, Frew AJ, Weyand CM, editors. Clinical Immunology. 4th ed. Amsterdam: Elsevier; 2013. p. 1077–84.
9. Salek MS, Finlay AY, Luscombe DK, Allen BR, Berth-Jones J, Camp RD, et al. Cyclosporin greatly improves the quality of life of adults with severe atopic dermatitis. A randomized, double-blind, placebo-controlled trial. Br J Dermatol. 1993;129:422–30.
10. van Joost T, Heule F, Korstanje M, van den Broek MJ, Stenveld HJ, van Vloten WA. Cyclosporin in atopic dermatitis: a multicentre placebo-controlled study. Br J Dermatol. 1994;130:634–40.
11. Berth-Jones J, Finlay AY, Zaki I, Tan B, Goodyear H, Lewis-Jones S, et al. Cyclosporine in severe childhood atopic dermatitis: a multicenter study. J Am Acad Dermatol. 1996;34:1016–21.
12. Harper JI, Ahmed I, Barclay G, Lacour M, Hoeger P, Cork MJ, et al. Cyclosporin for severe childhood atopic dermatitis: short course versus continuous therapy. Br J Dermatol. 2000;142:52–8.
13. Schmitt J, Schmitt N, Meurer M. Cyclosporin in the treatment of patients with atopic eczema - a systematic review and meta-analysis. J Eur Acad Dermatol Venereol. 2007;21:606–19.
14. Granlund H, Erkko P, Sinisalo M, Reitamo S. Cyclosporin in atopic dermatitis: time to relapse and effect of intermittent therapy. Br J Dermatol. 1995;132:106–12.
15. Atakan N, Erdem C. The efficacy, tolerability and safety of a new oral formulation of Sandimmun®- Sandimmun Neoral® in severe refractory atopic dermatitis. J Eur Acad Dermatol Venereol. 1998;11:240–6.
16. Kim JE, Shin JM, Ko JY, Ro YS. Importance of concomitant topical therapy in moderate-to-severe atopic dermatitis treated with cyclosporine. Dermatol Ther. 2016;29:120–5. doi:10.1111/dth.12333.
17. Slater NA, Morrell DS. Systemic therapy of childhood atopic dermatitis. Clin Dermatol. 2015;33:289–99. doi:10.1016/j.clindermatol.2014.12.005.
18. Cookson H, Smith C. Systemic treatment of adult atopic dermatitis. Clin Med (Lond). 2012;12:172–6.
19. Caufield M, Tom WL. Oral azathioprine for recalcitrant pediatric atopic dermatitis: clinical response and thiopurine monitoring. J Am Acad Dermatol. 2013;68:29–35.
20. Waxweiler WT, Agans R, Morrell DS. Systemic treatment of pediatric atopic dermatitis with azathioprine and mycophenolate mofetil. Pediatr Dermatol. 2011;28:689–94.
21. Hon KL, Ching GK, Leung TF, Chow CM, Lee KK, Ng PC. Efficacy and tolerability at 3 and 6 months following use of azathioprine for recalcitrant atopic dermatitis in children and young adults. J Dermatolog Treat. 2009;20:141–5.
22. Buckley DA, Baldwin P, Rogers S. The use of azathioprine in severe adult atopic eczema. J Eur Acad Dermatol Venereol. 1998;11:137–40.
23. Kuanprasert N, Herbert O, Barnetson RS. Clinical improvement and significant reduction of total serum IgE in patients suffering from severe atopic dermatitis treated with oral azathioprine. Australas J Dermatol. 2002;43:125–7.
24. Hughes R, Collins P, Rogers S. Further experience of using azathioprine in the treatment of severe atopic dermatitis. Clin Exp Dermatol. 2008;33:710–1.
25. Berth-Jones J, Takwale A, Tan E, Barclay G, Agarwal S, Ahmed I, et al. Azathioprine in severe adult atopic dermatitis: a double-blind, placebo-controlled, crossover trial. Br J Dermatol. 2002;147:324–30.
26. Meggitt SJ, Gray JC, Reynolds NJ. Azathioprine dosed by thiopurine methyltransferase activity for moderate-to-severe atopic eczema: a double-blind, randomised controlled trial. Lancet. 2006;367:839–46.
27. Murphy LA, Atherton DJ. Azathioprine as a treatment for severe atopic eczema in children with a partial thiopurine methyl transferase (TPMT) deficiency. Pediatr Dermatol. 2003;20:531–4.
28. Grundmann-Kollmann M, Podda M, Ochsendorf F, Boehncke WH, Kaufmann R, Zollner TM. Mycophenolate mofetil is effective in the treatment of atopic dermatitis. Arch Dermatol. 2001;137:870–3.

29. Murray ML, Cohen JB. Mycophenolate mofetil therapy for moderate to severe atopic dermatitis. Clin Exp Dermatol. 2007;32:23–7.
30. Heller M, Shin HT, Orlow SJ, Schaffer JV. Mycophenolate mofetil for severe childhood atopic dermatitis: experience in 14 patients. Br J Dermatol. 2007;157:127–32.
31. Haeck IM, Knol MJ, Ten Berge O, van Velsen SG, de Bruin-Weller MS, Hantash B, et al. Liver enzyme abnormalities in patients with atopic dermatitis treated with mycophenolate mofetil. Arch Dermatol. 2006;142:109–10.
32. Hantash B, Fiorentino D. Liver enzyme abnormalities in patients with atopic dermatitis treated with mycophenolate mofetil. Arch Dermatol. 2006;142:109–10.
33. El-Khalawany MA, Hassan H, Shaaban D, Ghonaim N, Eassa B. Methotrexate versus cyclosporine in the treatment of severe atopic dermatitis in children: a multicenter experience from Egypt. Eur J Pediatr. 2013;172:351–6.
34. Schram ME, Roekevisch E, Leeflang MMG, Bos JD, Schmitt J, Spuls PI. A randomized trial of methotrexate versus azathioprine for severe atopic eczema. J Allergy Clin Immunol. 2011;128:353–9.
35. Sidbury R, Davis DM, Cohen DE, Cordoro KM, Berger TG, Bergman JN, et al. Guidelines of care for the management of atopic dermatitis. Section 3. Management and treatment with phototherapy and systemic agents. J Am Acad Dermatol. 2014;71:327–49.
36. Goujon C, Bérard F, Dahel K, Guillot I, Hennino A, Nosbaum A, et al. Methotrexate for the treatment of adult atopic dermatitis. Eur J Dermatol. 2006;16:155–8.
37. Lyakhovitsky A, Barzilai A, Heyman R, Baum S, Amichai B, Solomon M, et al. Low-dose methotrexate treatment for moderate-to-severe atopic dermatitis in adults. J Eur Acad Dermatol Venereol. 2010;24:434–9.
38. Weatherhead SC, Wahie S, Reynolds NJ, Meggitt SJ. An open-label, dose-ranging study of methotrexate for moderate-to severe adult atopic eczema. Br J Dermatol. 2007;156:346–51.
39. Schmitt J, Schäkel K, Fölster-Holst R, Bauer A, Oertel R, Augustin M, et al. Prednisolone versus cyclosporine for severe adult eczema. An investigator-initiated double-blind placebo-controlled multicentre trial. Br J Dermatol. 2010;162:661–8.
40. Beck LA, Thaçi D, Hamilton JD, Graham NM, Bieber T, Rocklin R, et al. Dupilumab treatment in adults with moderate-to-severe atopic dermatitis. N Engl J Med. 2014;371:130–9. doi:10.1056/NEJMoa1314768.
41. Jujo K, Renz H, Abe J, Gelfand EW, Leung DYM. Decreased interferon gamma and increased interleukin-4 production in atopic dermatitis promotes IgE synthesis. J Allergy Clin Immunol. 1992;90:323–31.
42. Gajewski TF, Fitch FW. Anti-proliferative effect of IFN-γ in immune regulation: IFN-γ inhibits the proliferation of TH2 but not TH1 murine helper T lymphocyte clones. J Immunol. 1988;140:4245–52.
43. Hanifin JM, Schneider LC, Leung DY, Ellis CN, Jaffe HS, Izu AE, et al. Recombinant interferon gamma therapy for atopic dermatitis. J Am Acad Dermatol. 1993;28:189–97.
44. Jang IG, Yang JK, Lee HJ, Yi JY, Kim HO, Kim CW, et al. Clinical improvement and immunohistochemical findings in severe atopic dermatitis treated with interferon gamma. J Am Acad Dermatol. 2000;42:1033–40.
45. Tominaga M, Takamori K. Itch and nerve fibers with special reference to atopic dermatitis: therapeutic implications. J Dermatol. 2014;41:205–12.
46. Ring J, Alomar A, Bieber T, Deleuran M, Fink-Wagner A, Gelmetti C, et al. Guidelines for treatment of atopic eczema (atopic dermatitis) part II. J Eur Acad Dermatol Venereol. 2012;26:1176–93.
47. Kawashima M, Tango T, Noguchi T, Inagi M, Nakagawa H, Harada S. Addition of fexofenadine to a topical corticosteroid reduces the pruritus associated with atopic dermatitis in a 1-week randomized, multicentre, double-blind, placebo-controlled, parallel-group study. Br J Dermatol. 2003;148:1212–21.
48. Yamanaka K, Motomura E, Noro Y, Umeda K, Morikawa T, Umeda-Togami K, et al. Olopatadine, a non-sedating H1 antihistamine, decreases the nocturnal scratching without affecting sleep quality in atopic dermatitis. Exp Dermatol. 2015;24:227–9.

49. Ruzicka T, Lynde CW, Jemec GBE, Diepgen T, Berth-Jones J, Coenraads PJ, et al. Efficacy and safety of oral alitretinoin (9-cis retinoic acid) in patients with severe chronic hand eczema refractory to topical corticosteroids: results of a randomized, double-blind, placebo-controlled, multicentre trial. Br J Dermatol. 2008;158:808–17.
50. Grahovac M, Molin S, Prinz JC, Ruzicka T, Wollenberg A. Treatment of atopic eczema with oral alitretinoin. Br J Dermatol. 2010;162:217–8.
51. Church MK, Maurer M. H1-antihistamines and itch in atopic dermatitis. Exp Dermatol. 2015;24:332–3.

Skin Care and Intervention

23

Yukihiro Ohya

Abstract

Atopic dermatitis (AD) is a chronic inflammatory skin disorder and also recognized as one of the allergic diseases that has increased within a half century when rapid environmental and lifestyle changes have occurred as a background. Most randomized controlled trials (RCTs) for high-risk infants with an intention of allergen elimination failed to prevent the onset of AD. Although some RCTs that administered probiotics during both prenatal and postnatal periods showed preventive effects on AD, a meta-analysis showed that probiotics were not effective as a viable treatment of established AD. Now, skin barrier dysfunction is recognized as a key initiator to progress AD, and the hypothesis that improving the properties of skin barrier early in life by applying emollients might prevent or delay the onset of AD was verified by two independent RCTs. One was a multicenter RCT carried out in the United States (USA) and United Kingdom (UK) applying emollients from birth to 6 months resulting in 50% reduction of the onset of AD. The other was a single-center RCT carried out in Japan applying an emollient from birth to 8 months resulting in 34% reduction of the onset. Skin care seems to be important not only for the prevention and treatment of AD but also for prevention of food allergy and other allergic diseases. In the future, larger-scale RCTs are expected to confirm preventive effect of skin care with emollients on AD and other allergic diseases in later life.

Keywords

Emollients • Food allergy • Prevention • RCT • Skin care

Y. Ohya
Division of Allergy, Department of Medical Subspecialties, National Center for Child Health and Development, 2-10-1, Okura, Setagayaku, Tokyo 157-8535, Japan
e-mail: ohya-y@ncchd.go.jp

I. Katayama et al. (eds.), *Evolution of Atopic Dermatitis in the 21st Century*,
https://doi.org/10.1007/978-981-10-5541-6_23

23.1 Preventive Intervention by Allergen Avoidance

Atopic dermatitis (AD) is a chronic inflammatory skin disorder and also recognized as one of the representative allergic disorders that has been increased worldwidely starting from industrialized countries in a half century. Rapid environmental and lifestyle changes caused by economic growth in advanced countries might have altered immunological diathesis from birth and increased prevalence of allergic diseases including AD.

As a general concept of allergy, onset of allergic diseases was thought to be preceded by allergen sensitization. An old randomized controlled trial (RCT) carried out three decades ago showed successful prevention of eczema and wheezing in the first year of life by multiple allergen avoidance measures from birth [1]; however, most of the larger-scale RCTs done later with an intention of eliminating environmental allergens could not reproduce successful outcomes [2–4].

Although a large proportion of patients with infantile AD are sensitized to any food allergen, maternal-specific food allergen avoidance during pregnancy and/or lactation failed to prevent not only the onset of offspring's AD but also their sensitization to the eliminated foods [5]. Furthermore, delayed introduction of solid food in infants who had eczema has turned out to be a risk factor of food allergy in later life [6–10].

Those clinical evidences indicate that allergen avoidance measures have been ineffective to prevent allergic diseases at least such as AD and food allergy.

23.2 Preventive Intervention by Probiotics

Probiotics are microorganisms with immune-modulative and beneficial functions on human beings when administered in adequate amounts of appropriate species. In 2001, a Finnish group published the first successful RCT of prenatally and postnatally administered probiotics to prevent AD resulting in the reduced onset of relative risk 0.51 (95% CI: 2.6–15.6) at 2 years of age [11]. They reported preventive effect of probiotics applied during pregnancy and infancy extended up to 4 years [12].

Additional interventions were carried out, and there are conflicting views, although a recently published meta-analysis showed prenatal administration of probiotics followed by postnatal administration was protective (OR, 0.61; $P < 0.001$) in contrast to only postnatal administration (OR, 0.95; $P < 0.82$) [13–15]. Another meta-analysis showed that probiotics were not effective as a viable treatment of established AD [16].

23.3 Preventive Strategy with Skin Care

Ecological studies have implied that epidermal barrier dysfunction caused by environmental and lifestyle changes in the modern world contributes to the development of AD [17, 18], and recent advances in basic cutaneous biology has suggested epidermal defects might be a key initiator of AD and possibly allergic sensitization

[19–21]. Now, skin barrier dysfunction is recognized as a key initiator to progress AD. These findings generate the hypothesis that improving the properties of skin barrier early in life by applying emollients might prevent or delay the onset of AD by providing skin with a source of exogenous lipids [22–24]. The result of an open-label trial performed in this century suggested the use of emollients on neonate from birth might protect against the onset of AD in infants and early childhood [25]. To verify the hypothesis that application of emollient from neonatal period is a safe and effective approach to the prevention of AD, two RCTs were carried out by two independent study groups [26, 27]: one was a dermatologist group working in the United States (USA) and United Kingdom (UK) and the other was a pediatric allergist and dermatologist group in Japan.

23.4 A Preventive RCT from the United States and United Kingdom [26]

The study design of the US and UK group was a multicenter, multinational, assessor-blind RCT of 6 months' duration of which intervention started within 3 weeks of birth. Participants of this study were infants at high risk of eczema, which was defined as having a parent or sibling who had physician-diagnosed AD, asthma, or allergic rhinitis.

Parents in the intervention group were offered a choice of three emollients of different viscosities (sunflower seed oil, Cetaphil cream in the United States/Doublebase gel in the United Kingdom, or Aquaphor healing ointment in the United States/liquid paraffin 50% in white soft paraffin in the United Kingdom). Parents were asked to apply the emollient to the baby's entire body surface, with the exception of the scalp, starting as soon as possible after birth and continuing until 6 months of age. Both the intervention and control groups were given an infant skin care advice booklet, which reflected current European guidelines [28].

Parents are advised to adhere the following five items: (1) to avoid soap and bubble bath; (2) to use a mild, fragrance-free synthetic cleanser designed specifically for babies; (3) to avoid bath oils and additives; (4) to use a mild, fragrance-free shampoo designed specifically for babies and avoid washing the suds over the baby's body; and (5) to avoid using baby wipes, where possible.

Recruitment took place in the United Kingdom and the United States between May 2010 and May 2011. In the United Kingdom, research nurses were based in three acute National Health Service hospital trusts (Nottingham University Hospitals, Derby Hospitals, and United Lincolnshire Hospitals) and one general practice surgery (the Surgery@Wheatbridge, Chesterfield). In the United States, the study was recruited in one hospital, Oregon Health & Science University Hospital and Clinics (Portland, Oregon).

The research nurse contacted parents by telephone at 10 days and 6 weeks, with a face-to-face visit at 12 weeks (usually at home in the United Kingdom and as a clinic visit in the United States). This was then followed by a further telephone call at 18 weeks, and the final contact was a clinic visit at 24 weeks for an assessment by the dermatologist or dermatology specialist nurse, who conducted a blinded assessment of the skin. In addition to these scheduled contact points, parents were encouraged to contact the research nurse if they had any concerns about the child's skin. If parents reported symptoms of eczema, then an unscheduled visit to the hospital to see the dermatologist was arranged so that the presence of eczema could be confirmed.

An independent outcome assessor who was blinded to treatment allocation performed the skin examinations and diagnosis of eczema. The statistician was blinded to treatment group until the analysis was complete.

Of the 295 eligible families, 124 (42%) accepted the initial invitation to participate and were randomized. Baseline characteristics including a loss-of-function mutation of filaggrin gene were similar between the two groups. By 6 months, nine participants in the intervention group and seven in the control group were lost to follow-up or withdrew in the intervention group (12.9% attrition).

All parents reported they found the emollient "acceptable," and none of the families withdrew because of the emollient. In the intervention group, the cream/gel formulation was the preferred emollient (67.2%), followed by oil (23.4%) and then ointment (9.4%). Approximately 85% of parents in the intervention group reported using emollients at least 5 days per week in the intervention group at 6 months.

Daily emollient use significantly reduced the cumulative incidence of AD at 6 months (43% in the control group vs. 22% in the emollient group). This corresponds to a relative risk reduction to 50% (relative risk, 0.50; 95% CI, 0.28–0.90; $P = 0.017$). This trial is a feasible study of large-scale RCT named the BEEP (Barrier Enhancement for Eczema Prevention) study which already finished the recruitment of 1395 participants to be followed up to 2 years of age to find out whether skin care advice using emollients can prevent eczema in newborn babies compared with skin care advice alone.

23.5 A Preventive RCT from Japan [27]

The study design of the Japanese study was an investigator-blinded, single-center RCT of which participants were born in the National Center for Child Health and Development (NCCHD) in Tokyo, Japan, from November 2010 through November 2013. Among women who visited the prenatal clinic of the NCCHD, 183 expectant mothers with family histories of AD (defined as a history of physician-diagnosed AD for at least one of the unborn baby's parents or siblings) were invited to participate in this trial. Informed consent was obtained from the parents before delivery. After birth, the study doctors and a dermatology specialist confirmed the eligibility of each neonate on the basis of the inclusion criteria (e.g., absence of treatment with corticosteroids) and exclusion criteria (e.g., abnormal skin disorders, such as ichthyosis), which had been registered with the University Hospital Medical Information Network Clinical Trials Registry (UMIN-CTR; UMIN000004544).

One hundred and eighteen neonates were enrolled and then randomly assigned to the intervention ($n = 59$) group or the control ($n = 59$) group. The intervention group started daily application of an emulsion-type emollient (2e [Douhet] emulsion) from the first week of life and continued for 32 weeks. Petroleum jelly was prescribed to all infants in both groups on request by the institutional review board because of the institutional treatment by default. All infants were examined by the same dermatologist blinded to the assignment of the groups at scheduled visits of 4, 12, 24, and 32 weeks of life. At each visit, the dermatologist examined the skin condition of the infant and recorded a diagnosis of AD, eczema, skin rash without pruritus, or healthy skin without any lesions.

The primary outcome measure was the cumulative incidence of AD, eczema, or both by temporal observation. The diagnostic criteria for infantile eczema, AD, or both (AD and eczema) were developed based on a modification of the UK Working Party's criteria and were applied by a dermatology specialist. Briefly, those criteria were a pruritic skin condition of at least 2 weeks' duration, a visible flexural dermatitis (on the cheeks and extensor surfaces), a history of dry skin, and a family history in a first-degree relative of the enrolled neonate. Secondary outcome measures were the presence of allergen-specific IgE, transepidermal water loss, stratum corneum hydration, stratum corneum pH, and skin colonization by *Staphylococcus aureus*.

Analyses of the primary and secondary outcomes were conducted according to the intention-to-treat principle and based on the full analysis set, which included all randomized participants. Two infants assigned to the control group were found to have accidently received and used the emollient after opening the blinded data. During the trial, eight families withdrew informed consent (two infants in the intervention group and six infants in the control group). The dermatologist withdrew an infant in the intervention group from the study because of having a hemangioma.

Among eight families who withdrew consent, two families in the intervention group said that it was difficult for them to visit the NCCHD. There were no infants from families that withdrew consent who had skin lesions. Adverse events caused by this emulsion-type emollient were not observed during this RCT. The mean daily amount of emulsion-type moisturizer used by the intervention group was 7.86 ± 4.34 g (0 g for the control group, excluding the two infants placed in the wrong group). The mean daily amount of petroleum jelly applied to the control group was 0.101 ± 0.286 g (mean frequency of use, 0.235 day/week).

During their first 32 weeks of life, 19 infants in the intervention group had AD/eczema compared with 28 infants in the control group. Calculation of cumulative incidence values for AD/eczema by using the Kaplan-Meier method showed that the intervention group maintained intact skin for a significantly longer period than the control group ($P = 0.012$, log-rank test; Fig. 23.1). Cox regression analysis showed the risk of AD/eczema to be significantly lower in the intervention group (hazard ratio, 0.48; 95% CI, 0.27–0.86) (Fig. 23.1).

In analyses of secondary outcomes (allergen-specific IgE concentrations), the serum levels of anti-egg white and anti-ovomucoid IgE in infants at 32 weeks were evaluated by using the diamond-like carbon [DLC] chip with high-density allergen immobilization and high sensitivity [29]. The proportions of infants who were sensitized by allergens were similar between the intervention and control groups, although the intervention group had significantly higher levels of stratum corneum hydration in the lower leg at weeks 12 and 24 compared with those seen in the control group (Fig. 23.2). A greater

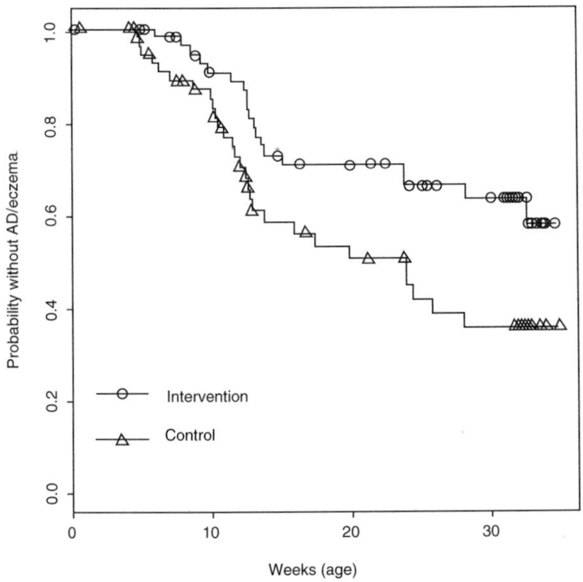

Fig. 23.1 Proportions of infants who did not have AD/eczema. Kaplan-Meier plots show the proportions of infants in the intervention (*circle*) and control (*triangle*) groups with AD/eczema during the first 32 weeks of life. The log-rank test indicated statistically significant differences between groups ($P = 0.012$)

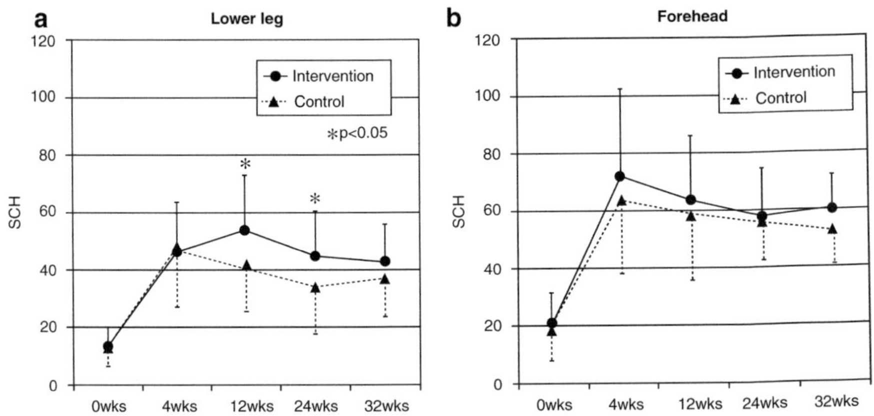

Fig. 23.2 Stratum corneum hydration (SCH) change in the lower leg (**a**) and forehead (**b**) in each group. Symbols (*circles* and *triangles*) and bars stand for means and SDs. SCH values were significantly higher for the lower leg in the intervention group at 12 weeks of age compared with those in the control group ($P < 0.05$, ANOVA)

proportion of infants with AD/eczema had allergic sensitization based on the serum levels of anti-egg white IgE than those without AD/eczema ($P = 0.043$, Table 23.1).

Loss-of-function mutations in FLG were detected in 6 of the 57 DNA samples from infants, but it was not able to demonstrate whether the development of AD/eczema correlates with the presence of mutations, probably because of the small sample size.

Table 23.1 Allergic sensitization at week 32

Level of specific IgE	With AD/eczema ($n = 43$)	Without AD/eczema ($n = 49$)	P values**
Egg white (kUA/L*)			
≥0.35	56% (24/43)	33% (16/49)	0.043
≥0.70	56% (24/43)	29% (14/49)	0.015
Ovomucoid (kUA/L*)			
>0.35	19% (8/43)	8.2% (4/49)	0.24
>0.70	12% (5/43)	6.1% (3/49) 0.57	0.57

*The levels of specific IgE (binding unit of IgE [BUe]/mL) measured with a DLC chip were converted into CAP-FEIA equivalents (kUA/L) [29]. Cutoff values for allergic sensitization were set at 0.35 or greater or 0.7 or greater

**The X^2 test was used to calculate the difference between the two study groups

23.6 Soap: A Specific Issue in Japanese Bathing as a Part of Skin Care

Skin care behavior consists of a body wash and emollient application. Western guidelines of AD advice patients not to use soap for a body wash [28, 30] since the pH of soap is alkaline which neutralizes skin pH and increases protease activity on the corneo-desmosome resulting in acceleration of epidermal barrier destruction [31], and limited use of nonsoap cleansers (that are neutral to low pH, hypoallergenic, and fragrance-free) is recommended [30].

Bathing system in Japan is different from that in the other countries. Typical way of Japanese bathing is composed of a body wash with bubbling soap at outside space of bathtub, washing away all bubbled soap from the body thoroughly with plenty of warm water before bathing, and soaking the cleared body in the warm water in the bathtub (bathing). Japanese way of bathing needs plenty of water to wash a body, and soap does not usually remain on the body surface.

Therefore, many Japanese patients do not mind using soap even if its pH is alkaline, and soap does not seem to damage their skin barrier as long as it is washed away thoroughly with plenty of warm water. Although this bathing way is effective to prevent infantile seborrheic eczema, babies are susceptible to dry skin if not applied with emollient after bathing, even in high humid climate in Japan. Many participants in the Japanese RCT for the prevention of AD washed their bodies with soap.

23.7 Prevention of Food Allergy and Atopic March by Skin Care for Atopic Dermatitis

Recent epidemiological studies support that AD is one of the strong risk factors for the onset of food allergy and other allergic diseases such as bronchial asthma and allergic rhinitis [32–37]. And basic cutaneous researches have been revealing complex mechanisms of epidermal sensitization to allergens [38–42]. Treatment with proactive therapy and skin care was routinely instructed for childhood AD patients in the hospital the author have been working.

A case-control study showed that food allergen-specific IgE levels of AD patients proactively treated for 2 years significantly decreased than those of patients reactively treated [43]. An RCT carried out for prevention of hen's egg allergy with early heated egg administration revealed that early intake of small doses of egg was effective for prevention of egg allergy but the two infants who failed to be prevented were not well controlled in their eczema [10]. Another RCT which compared proactive therapy with reactive therapy showed that proactively treated patients' house dust mite-specific IgE remains low, while those of reactively treated patients significantly increased [44]. Post hoc analysis of the Japanese study of preventive RCT revealed that even congenitally vulnerable infants with high transepidermal water loss from birth could be protected from the onset of AD by skin care treatment with emollients carried out from first week of life [45]. A recent birth cohort study revealed that the earlier eczema emerges the higher risk of food allergy follows [46].

Those findings suggest that keeping skin clear with attentive skin care treatment might be protective against food allergy and the progression of atopic march in genetically high-risk children. In the future, large-scale intervention studies for longer period and prospective observational studies are expected to show the effectiveness of long-term skin care treatment with emollients on the onset of eczema and early intervention of eczema on prognosis of AD and other allergic diseases.

References

1. Arshad SH, Matthews S, Gant C, Hide DW. Effect of allergen avoidance on development of allergic disorders in infancy. Lancet. 1992;339(8808):1493–7.
2. Horak F Jr, Matthews S, Ihorst G, Arshad SH, Frischer T, Kuehr J, et al. Effect of mite-impermeable mattress encasings and an educational package on the development of allergies in a multinational randomized, controlled birth-cohort study -- 24 months results of the Study of Prevention of Allergy in Children in Europe. Clin Exp Allergy. 2004;34:1220. 10.1111/j.1365-2222.2004.02024.x.
3. Woodcock A, Lowe LA, Murray CS, Simpson BM, Pipis SD, Kissen P, et al. Early life environmental control: effect on symptoms, sensitization, and lung function at age 3 years. Am J Respir Crit Care Med. 2004;170:433–9. doi:10.1164/rccm.200401-083OC.
4. Chan-Yeung M, Ferguson A, Watson W, Dimich-Ward H, Rousseau R, Lilley M, et al. The Canadian Childhood Asthma Primary Prevention Study: outcomes at 7 years of age. J Allergy Clin Immunol. 2005;116:49–55. doi:10.1016/j.jaci.2005.03.029.
5. Kramer MS, Kakuma R. Cochrane Database of Systematic Reviews 2012, 9:CD000133.
6. Snijders BEP, Thijs C, van Ree R, van den Brandt PA. Age at first introduction of cow milk products and other food products in relation to infant atopic manifestations in the first 2 years of life: the KOALA birth cohort study. Pediatrics. 2008;122:e115–22.
7. Koplin JJ, Osborne NJ, Wake M, Martin PE, Gurrin LC, Robinson MN, et al. Can early introduction of egg prevent egg allergy in infants? A population-based study. J Allergy Clin Immunol. 2010;126:807–13. doi:10.1016/j.jaci.2010.07.028.
8. Du Toit G, Roberts G, Sayre PH, Bahnson HT, Radulovic S, Santos AF, et al. Randomized trial of peanut consumption in infants at risk peanut allergy. N Engl J Med. 2015;372:803–13. doi:10.1056/NEJMoa1414850.
9. Ierodiakonou D, Garcia-Larsen V, Logan A, Groome A, Cunha S, Chivinge J, et al. Timing of allergenic food introduction to the infant diet and risk of allergic or autoimmune disease: a systematic review and meta-analysis. JAMA. 2016;316:1181–19. doi:10.1001/jama.2016.12623.
10. Natsume O, Kabashima S, Nakazato J, Yamamoto-Hanada K, Narita M, Kondo M, et al. Two-step egg introduction for prevention of egg allergy in high-risk infants with eczema(PETIT): a randomized double-blind placebo controlled trial. Lancet. 2017;389(10066):276–86. doi:10.1016/S0140-6736(16)31418-0.

11. Kalliomäki M, Salminen S, Arvilommi H, Kero P, Koskinen P, Isolauri E. Probiotics in primary prevention of atopic disease: a randomised placebo-controlled trial. Lancet. 2001;357(9262):1076–9. doi:10.1016/S0140-6736(00)04259-8.
12. Kalliomäki M, Salminen S, Poussa T, Arvilommi H, Isolauri E. Probiotics and prevention of atopic disease: 4-year follow-up of a randomised placebo-controlled trial. Lancet. 2003;361(9372):1869–71. doi:10.1016/S0140-6736(03)13490-3.
13. Panduru M, Panduru NM, Salavastru CM, Tiplica GS. Probiotics and primary prevention of atopic dermatitis: a meta-analysis of randomized controlled studies. J Eur Acad Dermatol Venereol. 2015;29:232–42. doi:10.1111/jdv.12496.
14. Tang ML. Probiotics and prebiotics: immunological and clinical effects in allergic disease. Nestle Nutr Workshop Ser Pediatr Program. 2009;64:219–51. doi:10.1159/000235793.
15. van der Aa LB, Heymans HSA, van Aalderen WMC, Sprikkelman AB. Probiotics and prebiotics in atopic dermatitis: review of the theoretical background and clinical evidence. Pediatr Allergy Immunol. 2010;21:e355–67. doi:10.1111/j.1399-3038.2009.00915.x.
16. Lee J, Seto D, Bielory L. Meta-analysis of clinical trials of probiotics for prevention and treatment of pediatric atopic dermatitis. J Allergy Clin Immunol. 2008;121:116–121.e11. doi:10.1016/j.jaci.2007.10.043.
17. Odhiambo JA, Williams HC, Clayton TO, Robertson CF, Asher MI. ISAAC Phase Three Study Group. Global variations in prevalence of eczema symptoms in children from ISAAC phase three. J Allergy Clin Immunol. 2009;124:1251–8.e23. doi:10.1016/j.jaci.2009.10.009.
18. Williams H, Stewart A, von Mutius E, Cookson W, Anderson HR, International Study of Asthma and Allergies in Childhood (ISAAC) Phase One and Three Study Groups. Is eczema really on the increase worldwide? J Allergy Clin Immunol. 2008;121:947–54.e15. doi:10.1016/j.jaci.2007.11.004.
19. Boguniewicz M, Leung DY. Atopic dermatitis: a disease of altered skin barrier and immune dysregulation. Immunol Rev. 2011;242:233–46. doi:10.1111/j.1600-065X.2011.01027.x.
20. Leung DY. New insights into atopic dermatitis: role of skin barrier and immune dysregulation. Allergol Int. 2013;62:151–61. doi:10.2332/allergolint.13-RAI-0564.
21. Brown SJ, McLean WH. One remarkable molecule: Filaggrin. J Invest Dermatol. 2012;132 (3 Pt 2):751–62. doi:10.1038/jid.2011.393.
22. Loden M. Role of topical emollients and moisturizers in the treatment of dry skin barrier disorders. Am J Clin Dermatol. 2003;4:771–88.
23. Wigger-Alberti W, Elsner P. Petrolatum prevents irritation in a human cumulative exposure model in vivo. Dermatology. 1997;194:247–50.
24. Ghali FE. Improved clinical outcomes with moisturization in dermatologic disease. Cutis. 2005;76(6 suppl):13–8.
25. Simpson EL, Berry TM, Brown PA, Hanifin JM. A pilot study of emollient therapy for the primary prevention of atopic dermatitis. J Am Acad Dermatol. 2010;63:587–93. doi:10.1016/j.jaad.2009.11.011.
26. Simpson EL, Chalmers JR, Hanifin JM, Thomas KS, Cork MJ, McLean WH, et al. Emollient enhancement of the skin barrier from birth offers effective atopic dermatitis prevention. J Allergy Clin Immunol. 2014;134(4):818–23. doi:10.1016/j.jaci.2014.08.005.
27. Horimukai K, Morita K, Narita M, Kondo M, Kitazawa H, Nozaki M, et al. Application of moisturizer to neonates prevents development of atopic dermatitis. J Allergy Clin Immunol. 2014;134:824–830.e6. doi:10.1016/j.jaci.2014.07.060.
28. Blume-Peytavi U, Cork M, Faergemann J, Szczapa J, Vanaclocha F, Gelmetti C. Bathing and cleansing in newborns from day 1 to first year of life: recommendations from a European round table meeting. J Eur Acad Dermatol Venereol. 2009;23:751–9. doi:10.1111/j.1468-3083.2009.03140.x.
29. Suzuki K, Hiyoshi M, Tada H, Bando M, Ichioka T, Kamemura N, et al. Allergen diagnosis microarray with high-density immobilization capacity using diamond-like carbon-coated chips for profiling allergen-specific IgE and other immunoglobulins. Anal Chim Acta. 2011;706:321–7. doi:10.1016/j.aca.2011.08.034.

30. Eichenfield LF, Tom WL, Berger TG, Krol A, Paller AS, Schwarzenberger K, et al. Guidelines of care for the management of atopic dermatitis Section 2. Management and treatment of atopic dermatitis with topical therapies. J Am Acad Dermatol. 2014;71:116–32. doi.org/10.1016/j.jaad.2014.03.023
31. Nelson HS. New perspectives on epidermal barrier dysfunction in atopic dermatitis: gene–environment interactions. J Allergy Clin Immunol. 2006;118:3–21. doi:10.1016/j.jaci.2006.04.012.
32. Not available.
33. Flohr C, Perkin M, Logan K, Marrs T, Radulovic S, Campbell LE, et al. Atopic dermatitis and disease severity are the main risk factors for food sensitization in exclusively breastfed infants. J Invest Dermatol. 2014;134(2):345–50. doi:10.1038/jid.2013.298.
34. Saunes M, Øien T, Dotterud CK, Romundstad PR, Storrø O, Holmen TL, et al. Early eczema and the risk of childhood asthma: a prospective, population-based study. BMC Pediatr. 2012;12:168. doi:10.1186/1471-2431-12-168.
35. Amat F, Saint-Pierre P, Bourrat E, Nemni A, Couderc R, Boutmy-Deslandes E, et al. Early-onset atopic dermatitis in children: which are the phenotypes at risk of asthma? Results from the ORCA cohort. PLoS One. 2015;10(6):e0131369. doi:10.1371/journal.pone.0131369.
36. Almqvist C, Li Q, Britton WJ, Kemp AS, Xuan W, Tovey ER, Marks GB, et al. Early predictors for developing allergic disease and asthma: examining separate steps in the 'allergic march'. Clin Exp Allergy. 2007;37(9):1296–302.
37. Tsakok T, Marrs T, Mohsin M, Baron S, du Toit G, Till S, et al. Does atopic dermatitis cause food allergy? A systematic review. J Allergy Clin Immunol. 2016;137(4):1071–8. doi:10.1016/j.jaci.2015.10.049.
38. Yoshida K, Kubo A, Fujita H, Yokouchi M, Ishii K, Kawasaki H, et al. Distinct behavior of human Langerhans cells and inflammatory dendritic epidermal cells at tight junctions in patients with atopic dermatitis. J Allergy Clin Immunol. 2014;134(4):856–64. doi:10.1016/j.jaci.2014.08.001.
39. Yokouchi M, Kubo A, Kawasaki H, Yoshida K, Ishii K, Furuse M, et al. Epidermal tight junction barrier function is altered by skin inflammation, but not by filaggrin-deficient stratum corneum. J Dermatol Sci. 2015;77(1):28–36. doi:10.1016/j.jdermsci.2014.11.007.
40. Kawasaki H, Nagao K, Kubo A, Hata T, Shimizu A, Mizuno H, et al. Altered stratum corneum barrier and enhanced percutaneous immune responses in filaggrin-null mice. J Allergy Clin Immunol. 2012;129(6):1538–46.e6. doi:10.1016/j.jaci.2012.01.068.
41. Amano W, Nakajima S, Kunugi H, Numata Y, Kitoh A, Egawa G, et al. The Janus kinase inhibitor JTE-052 improves skin barrier function through suppressing signal transducer and activator of transcription 3 signaling. J Allergy Clin Immunol. 2015;136(3):667–677.e7. doi:10.1016/j.jaci.2015.03.051.
42. Egawa G, Kabashima K. Multifactorial skin barrier deficiency and atopic dermatitis: essential topics to prevent the atopic march. J Allergy Clin Immunol. 2016;138(2):350–358.e1. doi:10.1016/j.jaci.2016.06.002.
43. Fukuie T, Nomura I, Horimukai K, Manki A, Masuko I, Futamura M, et al. Proactive treatment appears to decrease serum immunoglobulin-E levels in patients with severe atopic dermatitis. Br J Dermatol. 2010;163:1127–9. doi:10.1111/j.1365-2133.2010.09904.x.
44. Fukuie T, Hirakawa S, Narita M, Nomura I, Matsumoto K, et al. Potential preventive effects of proactive therapy on sensitization in moderate to severe childhood atopic dermatitis: a randomized, investigator-blinded, controlled study. J Dermatol. 2016;43:1283–92. doi:10.1111/1346-8138.13408.
45. Horimukai K, Morita K, Narita M, Kondo M, Kabashima S, Inoue E, et al. Transepidermal water loss measurement during infancy can predict the subsequent development of atopic dermatitis regardless of filaggrin mutations. Allergol Int. 2016;65:103–8. doi:10.1016/j.alit.2015.09.004.
46. Shoda T, Futamura M, Yang L, Yamamoto-Hanada K, Narita M, Saito H, et al. Timing of eczema onset and risk of food allergy at 3 years of age: a hospital-based prospective birth cohort study. J Dermatol Sci. 2016;84(2):144–8. doi:10.1016/j.jdermsci.2016.08.003.

Approach for Aggravating Factors in Atopic Dermatitis

24

Sakae Kaneko

Abstract

Atopic dermatitis (AD) is a chronic relapsing eczematous skin disease characterized by pruritus and inflammation and is accompanied by cutaneous physiological dysfunction (Saeki et al. J Dermatol 36: 563–577, 2009).

A wide variety of etiological and exacerbating factors has been proposed, with the importance level of each varying among individual patients. In addition, inflammation associated with this disease will be elucidated by both allergic and nonallergic mechanisms. Etiological and exacerbating factors vary among age groups. While the dominant factors in the first half of childhood include foods, sweating, physical irritation (including scratching), environmental factors, and microbes/fungi, the dominant factors in the second half of childhood to adulthood include environmental factors, sweating, physical irritation (including scratching), microbes/fungi, contact allergens, stress, and foods (Fig. 24.1) (Katayama et al. Allergology International 63: 377–398, 2014).

The detection of both atopic dermatitis (AD) aggravating factors and countermeasures is crucial. Additionally, the method of patient instruction relating to these countermeasures is an important aspect of AD management. We conducted a questionnaire-based survey (Kaneko et al. Nishinihon J Dermatol 73, 614–618, 2011; Kaneko et al. Japanese J Dermatol 123, 2091–2097, 2013; Kaneko et al. Arerugi 63, 1250–1257, 2014) on physicians, patients, and pharmacists, on the topic of instruction given to patients with AD on an outpatient basis, and our findings are summarized below.

S. Kaneko
Department of Dermatology, Faculty of Medicine, Shimane University, 89-1 Enya-cho, Izumo, Shimane 693-8501, Japan
e-mail: kanekos2@med.shimane-u.ac.jp

I. Katayama et al. (eds.), *Evolution of Atopic Dermatitis in the 21st Century*,
https://doi.org/10.1007/978-981-10-5541-6_24

Keywords
Aggravating factors • Management • Sweat • Itch-scratch cycle • Stress-scratch cycle • Instructions for patients

24.1 Aggravating Factors

24.1.1 Sweat

In daily clinical practice, patients often complain of aggravation of eruptions in conjunction with sweating. Sweat is an aggravating factor in atopic dermatitis (AD), regardless of age. This condition can be due to the direct stimulation of sweat, a type 1 allergic reaction against the components of sweat [6], reactions to environmental antigens in sweat (house dust antigens, mite antigens, fungal protein MGL_1304 [7], etc.), or the environment inducing the sweating; in other words, increased itching can be caused by increased body temperature. In contrast, in patients with AD, there can be a reduction in axon reflex sweating accompanying stimulation with acetylcholine [8], and reduced sweat responses can be due to heat stimulation [9]. This is thought to be due to a peripheral nerve disorder rather than a disorder of the sweat glands or ducts. Since sweat moisturizes the skin, has an antibacterial effect, and regulates body temperature, it is also possible that a sweat function abnormality is related to aggravation of AD. Prevention of sweating through regulation of body temperature is recommended, as is taking a shower after sweating to prevent aggravation of AD; alternatively, sweating through bathing for the purpose of recovery of sweat function is actively encouraged.

AD patients' negative impression of sweat might derive form crude personal experiences that are ordinarily linked to sweating. So the negative image must be resolved. Sweating plays key roles in skin homeostasis, antimicrobial [10] and moisturizing effects [8], and in skin surface pH regulation [11]. In the course of the sweat management instructions, it was fine to sweat profusely but additionally requested that patients do at least one of the following: (1) shower at least once during the day, (2) wash the affected areas of their skin with water, (3) apply wipes to irritated parts of their skin, and/or (4) change their clothes when they became soaked with sweat. The countermeasures for sweating were helpful and assured coaching. Sweat management instructions should be provided to patients, regardless of whether sweat (*Malassezia*) allergies or other factors are responsible for their adult AD.

24.1.2 Food

AD can be due to food allergies in childhood, and it is not uncommon for the elimination of a food allergen to lead to improvement in eczema. Allergen testing is conducted in cases in which the effect of normal treatment is insufficient or patient questioning results in a causal link being suspected between the intake of a specific

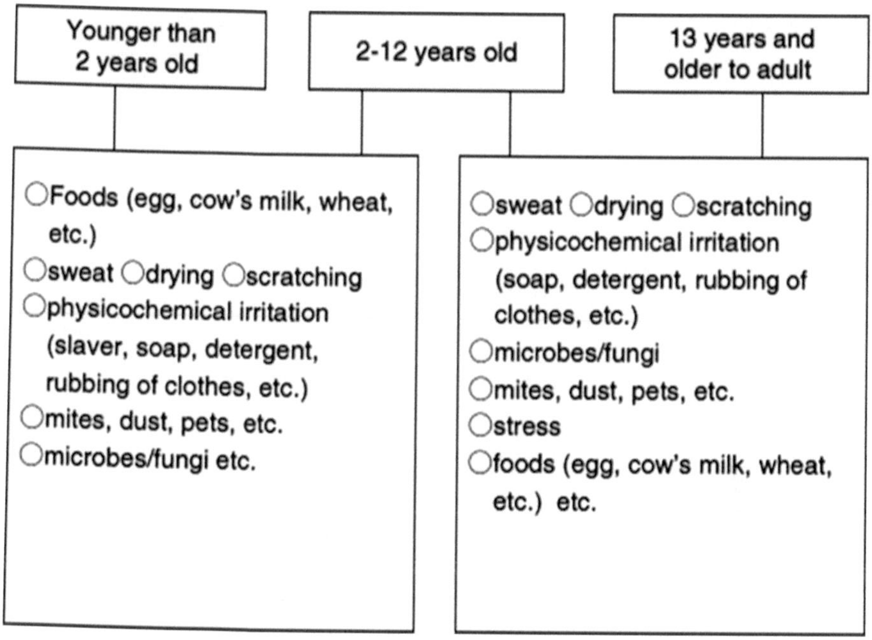

Fig. 24.1 Causes and exacerbating factors. Since causes and exacerbating factors vary among patients, care should be taken to identify them sufficiently for each patient before taking removal measures. Modified from Ministry of Health and Welfare, Japan. [Guidelines for the Treatment of Atopic Dermatitis 2008] (In Japanese)

food and the aggravation of symptoms. If a suspect allergen is detected, 1–2 weeks of allergen elimination and load testing are conducted for confirmation. If anaphylaxis is likely, load testing should always be conducted carefully with the patient admitted. Food allergen determination is conducted with a combination of these methods. Elimination should not continue indefinitely; however, while the patient is monitored, allergic reactions should be assessed by determining whether the ingestion of a food containing the allergen is possible (Fig. 24.1) [1].

24.1.3 Scratching

Scratching is a direct aggravating factor for AD skin lesions. An itch-scratch cycle (Fig. 24.2) develops, such that even after the elimination of other aggravating factors, the cycle can be a significant contributor to the continuation of skin rashes. There are various mechanisms of itching in AD, and it can involve histamine, non-histamine chemical mediators, direct stimulation of nerve fibers in the epidermis, involvement of the opioid system, neurogenic inflammation, and the effect of allergic inflammation. Since these mechanisms can combine to cause itching, it is necessary to comprehensively treat the patient with sufficient understanding of these mechanisms.

Fig. 24.2 Itch-scratch cycle

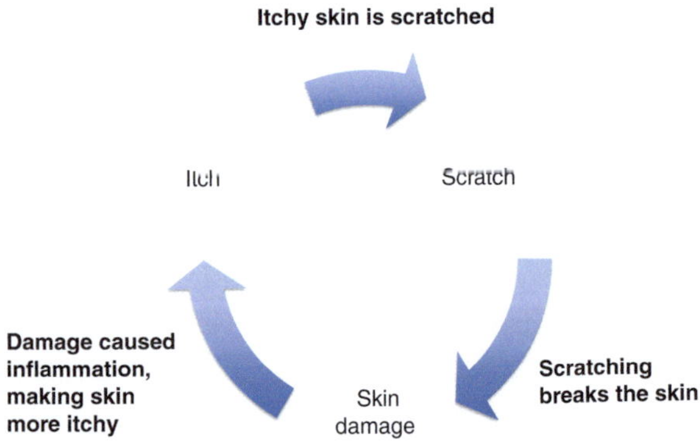

24.1.4 Environmental Factors

24.1.4.1 Mites

House dust mites have long been identified as an aggravating factor; when patients with AD relocate, their symptoms may either improve or become aggravated. There may be high sensitization to house dust mites, and many cases have a high RAST score for the mites. In 1988, Norris et al. [12] conducted a double-blind mite antigen-loading test on the forearm of patients with AD, and there was aggravation of the skin rash at the point of mite antigen loading. However there was no significant difference in the skin symptoms when countermeasures were taken, including a double-blind randomized trial [13] using high-density bed covers or a similar trial [14] in which an anti-mite spray was also used. For this reason, high-cost bedding is not recommended for AD alleviation. Converting homes to hard flooring, frequent vacuuming, and not using fabric sofas or soft toys can reduce mite numbers. However, there are reports both validating and invalidating the effectiveness of vacuuming more than usual for the removal of mites to benefit patients with AD.

24.1.4.2 Living Environment (Climate, Pollen)

Some patients with AD go through a repeated cycle of alleviation and aggravation depending on the season. For those with dry skin, winter is generally a time of aggravation for patients with AD; for those with contagious impetigo, summer is a time of aggravation. Furthermore, some patients experience aggravation from spring to summer, when they start to sweat.

Given that the rates of AD prevalence differ between Japan and other countries [15], it is suggested that there is some kind of link between climate/level of atmospheric pollution and the onset of AD. In a study of the epidemiology of AD in Tibet, there was no defined onset, perhaps due to the dry environment, in which barrier function was maintained. In addition, approximately 30% of patients with AD also had cedar pollen allergies, and dermatitis was aggravated by exposure to cedar pollen [16].

24.1.5 Bacteria/Fungi

There are a range of bacteria and fungi that can become aggravating factors. There is a two-sided link between infections and AD: (1) in the area of an AD rash, the skin's barrier function (including antibacterial peptide reduction [17]) is decreased and can become the site of an infection; (2) an immune response abnormality caused by an infection can alter the development and status of AD. Fungi such as *Candida* in the digestive tract or *Malassezia* on the skin have also been regarded as aggravating factors. This is owing to the fact that IgE antibodies against fungi are detected at a high frequency in patients with AD. In particular, in patients with severe symptoms on the head, face, and neck, it is said that specific IgE antibodies against *Malassezia* appear in high numbers. Furthermore, there is evidence that some patients with AD experience symptom alleviation with antifungal agents, supporting the idea that there is a link between fungal antigens and AD [18, 19].

24.1.6 Stress

Aggravation due to psychological stress is often seen in daily clinical practice. The stressors vary between age groups, and it is important to treat them appropriately so that the stress is effectively eliminated. Patients with AD have a two-phase distribution: the initial childhood phase, with a later peak around the age of 18 years. Therefore, it is logical that aggravating factors at this time include the stresses of university entrance exams, with associated sleep deprivation and chronic fatigue [20]. It is not yet sufficiently clear how stress becomes an aggravating factor for patients with AD. One theory states that a stress-scratch cycle (Fig. 24.3) develops, in which a psychogenic reaction occurs at times of stress, leading to addictive scratching and skin aggravation; this is followed by a sensation of itchiness in the aggravated skin, with more scratching and aggravation leading to further stress [21, 22]. This abnormal

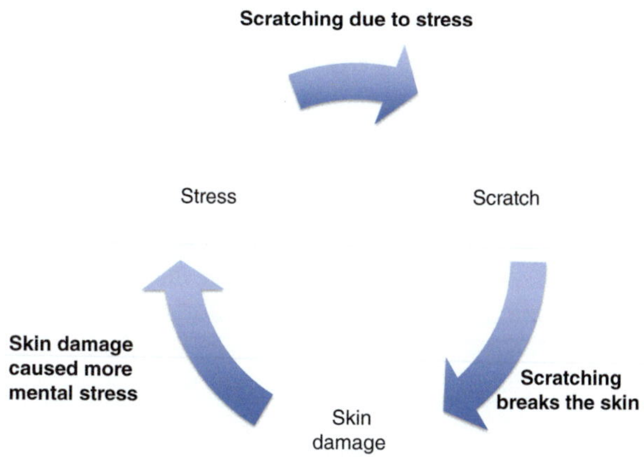

Fig. 24.3 Stress-scratch cycle

scratching is a type of behavioral abnormality induced by a psychological/social burden; in that situation, a psychiatric approach may be important.

24.1.7 Contact Antigens

Contact dermatitis is divided into allergic contact dermatitis, which occurs after sensitization, and primary irritation contact dermatitis, which can occur in anyone, depending on irritant concentration. Patients with AD are susceptible to both types of contact dermatitis, due to the decreased skin barrier function and long-term continuous use of topical applications. If any of the topical drugs used in AD treatment (steroids, nonsteroidal drugs, moisturizers, etc.) are used long term, contact dermatitis can develop [23, 24]. In addition, contact dermatitis is also not uncommon with use of home remedies, topical Chinese medicines, cosmetics, etc. If AD becomes aggravated, it is necessary to suspect the complication of contact dermatitis caused by these types of topical agents. For diagnosis, it is vital to perform a patch test to identify and eliminate the causative substance.

24.1.8 Physical Stimulation

The skin of patients with AD is, for the reasons stated above, susceptible to increased dryness and itchiness, because of exposure to stimulating substances in daily life (dishwashing liquid, residual laundry detergent on clothing, chlorine for disinfection in pools, nylon or wool clothing, etc.). It is best to avoid tight-fitting or poorly ventilated clothing, stiff fabrics, and mechanical stimuli such as poor stitching and to choose soft fabrics such as cotton and silk [25]. Since the rise in pH after the use of soap impairs the barrier function, it is best to use mild or alkaline soaps and to avoid over-washing the body or hair. In the epidemiology of AD in Tibet, bathing was performed twice a month, and there was no AD onset [26].

24.2 Instructions for Patients with AD

Here, we outline the points from our surveys of physicians, patients, and pharmacists on the instructions provided to patients with AD for topical management:

1. Instructions for patients with AD on an outpatient basis by dermatologists [3]

   In a survey of 779 dermatologists, the most important issue was instruction in the application of topical steroid drugs, identified by 655 physicians (84.1%). This shows that patients will not apply a topical drug if it is prescribed without instruction in use. In a comparison between dermatologists and general physicians, the proportion demonstrating treatment techniques was significantly higher among the dermatologists. Furthermore, in a comparison between private practice physicians and employed physicians, the former placed more importance on appropriate diagnosis/treatment; the private practice physicians managed acute symptoms and gave dietary instruction, while employed physicians placed importance on bathing instruction, education of the person in charge of treatment, instruction for moisturizing, etc. From the above, it became clear that there were differences between private practice and employed physicians in the treatment of AD on an outpatient basis and between dermatologists and general physicians in terms of importance placed on different treatments.

Many dermatologists believed that a relationship based on trust between patient and physician was important for treatment instruction.

2. Instructions for patients with AD treated on an outpatient basis [4]

We conducted a survey with essentially the same content as that given to the abovementioned physicians and received replies from 435 patients. Positive responses to instructions received mostly included: "I received the correct information about the disease" (261 people or 60%), followed by "I received an explanation about the prospects for treatment" (260 people, 59.8%) and "I received instruction on how to apply the moisturizer" (250 people, 57.5%). Thus, the survey of physicians and patients mostly yielded the same positive responses.

With cross aggregation, analysis was performed for the items answered by patients and between patient responses and physician responses. The most frequent responses regarding giving (physician side) or receiving (patient side) instructions were related to "the application of topical steroid drugs" and "instruction on the application of moisturizing drugs," with the same percentage on both physician and patient sides. The item with a high percentage on the patient side, however, a low percentage on the physician side was "I received the correct information about the disease," thereby indicating that the patient seemed to retain the information. In contrast, the items with a high percentage on the physician side but a low percentage on the patient side were "explanations of inappropriate treatments to avoid" and "explanations to dispel concern over steroid use." Therefore, it was thought that these instructions were difficult for patients to absorb. It was also thought important for instruction to be given with consideration for items in which gaps in communication between physician and patient can easily occur.

3. Results of questionnaire provided to pharmacists [5]

From the surveys [3, 4] of physicians and patients, it is clear that "instruction on the application of topical drugs" is important. We therefore conducted a survey on the instructions given by pharmacists, who have an important role in "instruction on the application of topical drugs." Upon analysis of 548 responses (response rate, 13.8%), it was found that the most commonly provided instruction on topical steroid drugs was "application site" (85.9%), followed by "frequency and timing" (68.2%). "The instruction of applying small amounts to prevent side effects" was selected by 45.8% of patients. With regard to tacrolimus ointment, the most frequent instruction was the side effect of "explanation about a tingling sensation" (52.0%); compared with topical drugs and moisturizers, most instructions were given "with a pamphlet" (27.4%). "Instruction on application with actual demonstration" was rarely conducted for any of the drugs. It became clear that pharmacists placed the most importance on instructions relating to directions for use and dosage of topical drugs.

From the survey of patients [4], if AD treatment guidelines were known, a significant range of instruction was given. From the survey of pharmacists [5], if AD treatment guidelines were known, it was clear that they gave patients a significant range of instruction. From the above, it is beneficial for patients and pharmacists to be familiar with AD treatment guidelines.

References

1. Saeki H, Furue M, Furukawa F, et al. Guidelines for management of atopic dermatitis. J Dermatol. 2009;36:563–77.
2. Katayama I, Kohno Y, Akiyama K, et al. Japanese guideline for atopic dermatitis 2014. Allergol Int. 2014;63:377–98.
3. Kaneko S, Sumikawa Y, Dekio I, et al. Questionnaire-based study on the knack of medical personnel with regard to providing directives to outpatients with atopic dermatitis. Nishinihon J Dermatol. 2011;73:614–8. [In Japanese]
4. Kaneko S, Kakamu T, Sumikawa Y, et al. Questionnaire-based study of the Doctor's Guidance for patients with atopic dermatitis. Jpn J Dermatol. 2013;123:2091–7. [In Japanese]
5. Kaneko S, Kakamu T, Matsuo H, et al. Questionnaire-based study on the key to the guidance to the patients with atopic dermatitis by pharmacist. Arerugi. 2014;63:1250–7. [In Japanese]
6. Hide M, Tanaka T, Yamamura Y, et al. IgE-mediated hypersensitivity against human sweat antigen in patients with atopic dermatitis. Acta Derm Venereol. 2002;82:335–40.
7. Hiragun T, Ishii K, Hiragun M, et al. Fungal protein MGL_1304 in sweat is an allergen for atopic dermatitis patients. J Allergy Clin Immunol. 2013;132:608–15.
8. Eishi K, Lee JB, Bas SJ, et al. Impaired sweating function in adult atopic dermatitis: results of the quantitative sudomotor axon reflex test. Br J Dermatol. 2002;147:683–8.
9. Murota H, Izumi M, Abd El-Latif MI, et al. Artemin causes hypersensitivity to warm sensation, mimicking warmth-provoked pruritus in atopic dermatitis. J Allergy Clin Immunol. 2012;130:671–82.
10. Rieg S, Steffen H, Seeber S, et al. Deficiency of dermcidin-derived antimicrobial peptides in sweat of patients with atopic dermatitis correlates with an impaired innate defense of human skin in vivo. J Immunol. 2005;174:8003–10.
11. Schmid-Wendtner MH, Korting HC. The pH of the skin surface and its impact on the barrier function. Skin Pharmacol Physiol. 2006;19:296–302.
12. Norris PG, Schofield O, Camp RD. A study of the role of house dust mite in atopic dermatitis. Br J Dermatol. 1988;118:435–40.
13. Gutgesell C, Heise S, Seubert S, et al. Double-blind placebo-controlled house dust mite control measures in adult patients with atopic dermatitis. Br J Dermatol. 2001;145:70–4.
14. Oosting AJ, de Bruin-Weller MS, Terreehorst I, et al. Effect of mattress encasings on atopic dermatitis outcome measures in a double-blind, placebo-controlled study: the Dutch mite avoidance study. J Allergy Clin Immunol. 2002;110:500–6.
15. Williams H, Robertson C, Stewart A, et al. Worldwide variations in the prevalence of symptoms of atopic eczema in the International Study of Asthma and Allergies in Childhood. J Allergy Clin Immunol. 1999;103:125–38.
16. Yokozeki H, Takayama K, Katayama I, et al. Japanese cedar pollen as an exacerbation factor in atopic dermatitis: result of atopy patch testing and histological examination. Acta Derm Venereol. 2006;86:148–51.
17. Kisich KO, Carspecken CW, Fieve S, et al. Defective killing of Staphylococcus aureus in atopic dermatitis is associated with reduced mobilization of human b-defensin-3. J Allergy Clin Immunol. 2008;12:62–8.

18. Morita E, Hide M, Yoneya Y, et al. An assessment of the role of candida albicans antigen in atopic dermatitis. J Dermatol. 1999;26:282–7.
19. Glatz M, Buchner M, Von Bartenwerffer A, et al. Malassezia spp.-specific immunoglobulin E level is a marker for severity of atopic dermatitis in adults. Acta Derm Venereol. 2015;95:191–6.
20. Takaki H, Ishii Y. Sense of coherence, depression, and anger among adults with atopic dermatitis. Psychol Health Med. 2013;18:725–34.
21. Higaki Y. Atopic dermatitis. Arerugi. 2010;59:82–90.
22. Amano H, Negishi I, Akiyama H, et al. Psychological stress can trigger atopic dermatitis in NC/Nga mice: an inhibitory effect of corticotropin-releasing factor. Neuropsychophamacology. 2008;33:566–73.
23. Halling-overgaard AS, Kezic S, Jakasa I, et al. Skin absorption through atopic dermatitis skin: a systematic review. Br J Dermatol. 2016; doi:10.1111/bjd.15065.
24. Takayama K. Japanese guideline for care of contact dermatitis; the guess and identification of the allergens. Arerugi. 2012;61:175–80.
25. Girsh CM, Peter AL. Comparison of dermatology and allergy guidelines for atopic dermatitis management. JAMA Dermatol. 2015;151:1009–13.
26. Sumikawa Y, Ueki Y, Miyoshi A, et al. Survey of atopic dermatitis and skin barrier functions in Japanese and Chinese school students. Arerugi. 2007;56:1270–5.

Impairment of Productivity in the Workplace/Classroom in Japanese Patients with Atopic Dermatitis

25

Hiroyuki Murota and Ichiro Katayama

Abstract

The burden of medical costs and impaired work productivity in patients with allergic diseases requires attention. The vicious cycle between the rise in medical expenses and decreased work productivity has a socioeconomic impact. Evaluation of work productivity has been conducted in Japanese patients with allergic diseases, and impaired productivity in workplace/classroom and decreased daily activity have been observed. The burdens of these factors can be improved by proper treatment. Thus, evaluation of work productivity could be an important endpoint to decide the efficacy of treatment provided. This chapter summarizes the characteristics of Japanese patients with allergic diseases and estimates the burden of medical costs to Japanese patients.

Keywords

Atopic dermatitis • Quality of life • Work productivity • Activity impairment • Questionnaire • Classroom productivity • Sedative antihistamine

25.1 Introduction

The diversified evaluations for quality of life (QOL) contribute to the understanding of the burden of disease on patients and inform the measures to maintain their wellness [1, 2]. There are several kinds of assessments to evaluate QOL, for example, QOL in general health, in specific disease, and in patients' families and productivity in the workplace/classroom [1, 3]. Work productivity is the indicator of productivity

H. Murota (✉) • I. Katayama
Department of Dermatology, Osaka University, Osaka, Japan
e-mail: h-murota@derma.med.osaka-u.ac.jp

I. Katayama et al. (eds.), *Evolution of Atopic Dermatitis in the 21st Century*,
https://doi.org/10.1007/978-981-10-5541-6_25

per 1 unit of workload or per laborer [4]. Workload can be calculated by taking working hours and number of laborers into consideration. Productivity represents the additional profit derived from labor [4]. The health condition of the laborer affects work productivity [3, 5]. Similarly, productivity in the classroom can be estimated from the outcome of examinations and will be affected by the health conditions of students.

Western countries have positively adopted assessing work productivity to evaluate the QOL of patients with allergies. For example, the European Union (EU) has focused on work productivity and medical expenses because this information can reveal the subjects, especially employees, with allergies that have not been treated properly. Therefore, these subjects can receive aid [6]. The impact of allergic symptoms on employees' performance may negatively impact work productivity [7, 8]. At same time, it has been reported that work productivity improves with proper treatment of the allergy [6, 9–11]. Thus, it can be speculated that improvement of employees' QOL and work productivity will promote better public welfare and have a favorable impact on the medical economy [6]. We must avoid the simplistic understanding that subjects with allergies are low performers. Meanwhile, clinicians should keep in mind that the improvement in patients' work productivity is the important outcome measure to be achieved.

25.2 Assessment of Impaired Productivity

Impaired productivity in the workplace/classroom can be assessed using two distinguishing domains: "absenteeism" and "presenteeism" [5, 8, 12] (Fig. 25.1). Absenteeism represents the loss of productivity due to an individual's absence from the workplace or classroom and includes loss of time or indirect costs (e.g., medical costs and transportation expenses to hospital) [8, 12]. Alternatively, symptoms related to the underlying disease may sometimes impair the patient's concentration or management abilities. Presenteeism represents losses resulting from the decreased ability to work despite being at the workplace or in the classroom [5, 12].

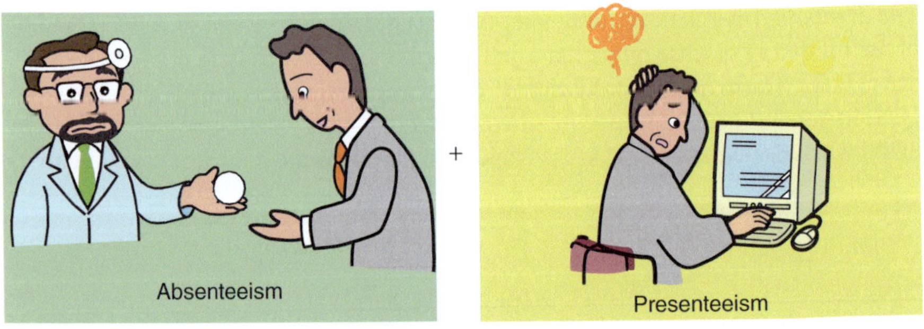

Fig. 25.1 Conceptual illustration of "absenteeism" and "presenteeism"

There are several assessment procedures for measuring patients' work productivity. Those procedures share core assessment domains with each other. The major shared domains are worktime missed (absenteeism), quality of work (presenteeism), work load, and personal factors including social, physical, and emotional aspects. All evaluation methods have distinctive and unique characteristics (Table 25.1). The Stanford/American Health Association Presenteeism Scale (SAHAPS) and Work Limitation Questionnaire (WLQ) consider personal factors and consist of a large number of questions about personal factors compared to work productivity. Almost all assessment procedures can evaluate presenteeism. An assessment procedure should be chosen by considering its distinctive characteristics and practical utility.

25.3 The Impact of Dermatoses on Work Productivity or Classroom Activity

In Japan, work productivity of patients with allergic rhinitis was assessed by the Work Productivity Activity Impairment Questionnaire-Allergy Specific (WPAI-AS), which consists of nine brief questions to evaluate productivity in the workplace, classroom, and daily life [12–14]. The results showed that productivity in these patients was impaired in approximately 39% of their innate ability [15]. It was also reported that the productivity of these subjects with allergic rhinitis was improved after therapeutic intervention [15].

Dermatoses also affect patients' performance in the workplace and classroom. Hand eczema is a representative dermatosis and has received the most attention as an occupational disease [14]. Urticaria also affects patients' QOL because of its spontaneous development and symptoms [9, 16]. Meanwhile, psoriasis severely impairs a patient's QOL because of its cosmetic effects and prolonged clinical course. Previously, work on impaired productivity in subjects with hand eczema, urticaria, and psoriasis was assessed by the Work *Productivity* and Activity Impairment Questionnaire (WPAI), and total work impairment percentages were 29%, 25%, and 15.5%, respectively [9, 11, 14, 17–19]. In urticaria patients, proper intervention with a less sedative antihistamine decreased the work impairment ratio, while sedative antihistamines failed to improve work productivity [9, 11]. Thus, the effect of treatment interventions on productivity in the workplace/classroom also should be investigated.

Itch is the major symptom of dermatoses and impairs patients' productivity in the workplace and classroom. Previous articles evaluated work productivity in Japanese subjects with itchy dermatoses and found severely impaired work productivity and daily activity [10, 11]. In that assessment, subjects who complained of itch and who consulted the dermatology clinic of a university hospital were asked to complete the WPAI, a self-administered questionnaire, before and after 1 month of treatment. The impairment ratio was assessed in patients with eczema/dermatitis, urticaria, atopic dermatitis, pruritus cutaneous, prurigo, and psoriasis (see below).

Table 25.1 Assessment of work productivity

Assessment tool	Health factors	Attendance at work	Quality of work	Workload/Work productivity	Individual traits (social, physical, and mental)	Others	
Work Productivity Short Inventory (WPSI)	General health Specific diseases	•		•			[23]
Work Limitations Questionnaire (WLQ)	General health	•	•	•	•	Work environment	[24]
World Health Organization Health and Work Performance Questionnaire	General health	•	•	•	•		[25]
Stanford Presenteeism Scale	General health			•	•	•	[26]
Endicott Work Productivity Scales (EWPS)	General health	•	•	•	•		[27]
Health and Labor questionnaire (HLQ)	General health, care management	•		•	•	•	[28]
Mac Arthur Health and Performance Questionnaire (MHPQ)	General health, disease prevention, health management	•	•	•	•	•	[29]
SF36	General health, care management		•	•		•	[30]

Stanford/American Health Association Presentation Scale (SAHAPS)	General health		•	•	•		[31]
Work Productivity and Activity Impairment-GeneralHealth(WPAI-GH)	General health	•		•		•	[12]
Work Productivity and Activity Impairment-AllergySpecific(WPAI-AS)	Care management	•		•		•	[13]

25.4 Work Impairment Ratio in Subjects with Atopic Dermatitis

Figure 25.2 shows the baseline impairment ratio for each of the dermatoses. WPAI measurement represents the overall impairment of productivity in the workplace/classroom and overall daily activity. The degree of overall work impairment ratio was higher in subjects with atopic dermatitis, eczema/dermatitis, and urticaria. The loss of time from work was more apparent in subjects with urticaria than those with the other dermatoses. In that study, subjects with a steady job comprised only approximately 20% of all laborers, and the loss of time from work was approximately 1.8% of total working hours. Loss of time from work for subjects without a steady job was approximately 5.3% of their total working hours. These results indicated that the impact of itchy dermatoses, such as atopic dermatitis, on attendance to workplace may differ by employment status.

In addition, impairment of daily activities was highest in subjects with atopic dermatitis, which is consistent with results in another Japanese study that used the WPAI assessment (Table 25.2) [20]. Moderate impairment of work productivity, with higher impairment of daily activities, was the unique characteristic of atopic dermatitis [11, 20]. At present, there have been no reports from other countries

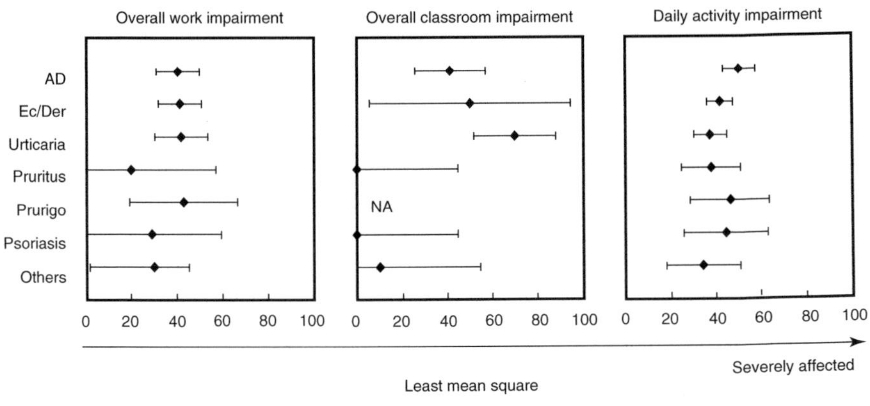

Fig. 25.2 Forest plots demonstrating that the degree of impairment in each disease at baseline was evaluated using a linear least-squares method. Horizontal lines represent 95% confidence intervals. The *rhomboid dot* on the center of *horizontal line* indicates the point estimate. *NA* not applicable. This figure was reprinted from ref. [11] with permission of Japanese Society of Allergology

Table 25.2 Assessment results of WPAI in Japanese patients with atopic dermatitis

	Work productivity impairment (%)	Work time missed (%)	Overall work productivity (%)	Activity impairment (%)
Murota et al. [11]	38.7 ± 26.3	4.9 ± 11.4	40.4 ± 26.8	50.2 ± 26.9
Yano et al. [20]	32.6 ± 23.5	0.5 ± 2.3	32.8 ± 23.7	4.29 ± 25.2

about the results of assessment of productivity using the WPAI in subjects with atopic dermatitis; thus, we could not judge whether this finding was unique to Japanese patients or not. At any rate, this phenomenon indicated that symptoms related to atopic dermatitis more severely impaired performance at home compared to the workplace. It was noteworthy that the daily activity impairment ratio was positively correlated to itch intensity. Itch frequently increases during evening to nighttime, when sympathetic nerve tone is weakened [21, 22]. Subjects are more likely to be home during this time period. Furthermore, disruptions to the usual daily schedule (e.g., staying up late at night) can also exacerbate the magnitude of itch [21, 22]. Thus, itch will be affected by subjects' lifestyles and can impair their daily activity.

25.5 Impact of Treatment Intervention on Work Productivity

Improvement in work productivity impairment should be the target of treatment for atopic dermatitis. The impact of antihistamines on work productivity was assessed by the WPAI in subjects with atopic dermatitis [10, 11]. Sedative and nonsedative antihistamines significantly decreased the magnitude of itch. Indeed, sedative antihistamines have frequently been prescribed to subjects with nighttime itch to induce drowsiness. However, the favorable effect on work/classroom productivity was more prominent with nonsedative antihistamines than with sedative antihistamines [10, 11]. This result indicated that improvement in work productivity will largely depend on what kind of treatment is chosen. In daily clinical practice, we should provide appropriate treatments/interventions by considering the patients' productivity in the workplace or classroom as an important outcome.

References

1. Bunn WB 3rd, Pikelny DB, Paralkar S, et al. The burden of allergies--and the capacity of medications to reduce this burden-in a heavy manufacturing environment. J Occup Environ Med. 2003;45:941–55.
2. Carr WW, Nelson MR, Hadley JA. Managing rhinitis: strategies for improved patient outcomes. Allergy Asthma Proc. 2008;29:349–57.
3. Guyatt GH, Feeny DH, Patrick DL. Measuring health-related quality of life. Ann Intern Med. 1993;118:622–9.
4. Cabinet office GoJ. Regional economy. 2015. http://www5.cao.go.jp/j-j/cr/cr15/chr150600.html
5. Goetzel RZ, Long SR, Ozminkowski RJ, et al. Health, absence, disability, and presenteeism cost estimates of certain physical and mental health conditions affecting U.S. employers. J Occup Environ Med. 2004;46:398–412.
6. Zuberbier T, Lotvall J, Simoens S, et al. Economic burden of inadequate management of allergic diseases in the European Union: a GA(2) LEN review. Allergy. 2014;69:1275–9.
7. Szeinbach SL, Seoane-Vazquez EC, Beyer A, et al. The impact of allergic rhinitis on work productivity. Prim Care Respir J. 2007;16:98–105.
8. Lamb CE, Ratner PH, Johnson CE, et al. Economic impact of workplace productivity losses due to allergic rhinitis compared with select medical conditions in the United States from an employer perspective. Curr Med Res Opin. 2006;22:1203–10.

9. Thompson AK, Finn AF, Schoenwetter WF. Effect of 60 mg twice-daily fexofenadine HCl on quality of life, work and classroom productivity, and regular activity in patients with chronic idiopathic urticaria. J Am Acad Dermatol. 2000;43:24–30.
10. Murota H, Kitaba S, Tani M, et al. Effects of nonsedative antihistamines on productivity of patients with pruritic skin diseases. Allergy. 2009;65(7):929–30. doi:10.1111/j.398-9995.2009.02262.x.
11. Murota H, Kitaba S, Tani M, et al. Impact of sedative and non sedative antihistamines on the impaired productivity and quality of life in patients with pruritic skin diseases. Allergol Int. 2010;59:345–54.
12. Reilly MC, Zbrozek AS, Dukes EM. The validity and reproducibility of a work productivity and activity impairment instrument. Pharmacoeconomics. 1993;4:353–65.
13. Reilly MC, Tanner A, Meltzer EO. Work, classroom and activity impairment instruments: validation studies in allergic rhinitis. Clin Drug Investig. 1996;11:278–88.
14. Reilly MC, Lavin PT, Kahler KH, et al. Validation of the dermatology life quality index and the work productivity and activity impairment-chronic hand dermatitis questionnaire in chronic hand dermatitis. J Am Acad Dermatol. 2003;48:128–30.
15. Okubo K, Gotoh M, Shimada K, et al. Fexofenadine improves the quality of life and work productivity in Japanese patients with seasonal allergic rhinitis during the peak cedar pollinosis season. Int Arch Allergy Immunol. 2005;136:148–54.
16. Hide M, Hiragun T, Japanese DA. Japanese guidelines for diagnosis and treatment of urticaria in comparison with other countries. Allergol Int. 2012;61:517–27.
17. Pearce DJ, Singh S, Balkrishnan R, et al. The negative impact of psoriasis on the workplace. J Dermatolog Treat. 2006;17:24–8.
18. Amatya B, Wennersten G, Nordlind K. Patients' perspective of pruritus in chronic plaque psoriasis: a questionnaire-based study. J Eur Acad Dermatol Venereol. 2008;22:822–6.
19. Fowler JF, Ghosh A, Sung J, et al. Impact of chronic hand dermatitis on quality of life, work productivity, activity impairment, and medical costs. J Am Acad Dermatol. 2006;54:448–57.
20. Yano C, Saeki H, Ishiji T, et al. Impact of disease severity on work productivity and activity impairment in Japanese patients with atopic dermatitis. J Dermatol. 2013;40:736–9.
21. Murota H, Katayama I. Exacerbating factors of itch in atopic dermatitis. Allergol Int. 2016;63:377.
22. Lavery MJ, Stull C, Nattkemper LA, et al. Nocturnal pruritus: prevalence, characteristics and impact on ItchyQoL in a chronic itch population. Acta Derm Venereol. 2016;97(4):513–5.
23. Goetzel RZ, Ozminkowski RJ, Long SR. Development and reliability analysis of the Work Productivity Short Inventory (WPSI) instrument measuring employee health and productivity. J Occup Environ Med. 2003;45:743–62.
24. Lerner D, Amick BC 3rd, Rogers WH, et al. The work limitations questionnaire. Med Care. 2001;39:72–85.
25. Kessler RC, Barber C, Beck A, et al. The World Health Organization health and work performance questionnaire (HPQ). J Occup Environ Med. 2003;45:156–74.
26. Koopman C, Pelletier KR, Murray JF, et al. Stanford presenteeism scale: health status and employee productivity. J Occup Environ Med. 2002;44:14–20.
27. Endicott J, Nee J. Endicott Work Productivity Scale (EWPS): a new measure to assess treatment effects. Psychopharmacol Bull. 1997;33:13–6.
28. van Roijen L, Essink-Bot ML, Koopmanschap MA, et al. Labor and health status in economic evaluation of health care. The health and labor questionnaire. Int J Technol Assess Health Care. 1996;12:405–15.
29. A new tool to measure the relationship between health-related quality of life and workforce productivity.
30. Jenkinson C, Coulter A, Wright L. Short form 36 (SF36) health survey questionnaire: normative data for adults of working age. BMJ. 1993;306:1437–40.
31. Lynch W, Riedel J, Institute for Health and Productivity Management. Measuring employee productivity. A guide to self-assessment tools. Denver, CO: William Mercer Inc.; 2001.

New and Future Therapies

26

Ken Igawa and Hiroo Yokozeki

Abstract

Atopic dermatitis (AD) is caused by a complex interrelationship of a variety of genetic and environmental factors, leading to the maintenance of the chronic inflammatory skin condition.

Most conventional treatments have been designed for the so-called average patient. However, because of recent advances in life science, a more precise diagnosis of individual patients can be made, and even among patients who have the same disease, detailed subgroup classification is presumably possible. The concept that treatment and prophylactic methods can be developed for each subgroup to deepen medical treatments is referred to as 'precision medicine'.

In recent years, many previously unknown points concerning the mechanisms of the pathogenesis of AD have been elucidated, and novel treatments in line with the pathological mechanisms or based on subgroup classifications have been developed.

It is presumed that the re establishment of medical care in the field of allergic diseases will also be based on the concept of 'precision medicine'. Herein, we describe how future treatment strategies for atopic dermatitis can be developed on the basis of the idea of 'precision medicine'.

Keywords

Atopic dermatitis • Precision medicine • Novel therapeutic approach • Nucleic acid drugs

K. Igawa, M.D., Ph.D. (✉)
Department of Dermatology, Dokkyo Medical University, 880 Kita-Kobayashi, Mibu-machi, Shimotsuga-gun, Tochigi 3210293, Japan
e-mail: igawa@dokkyomed.ac.jp

H. Yokozeki
Department of Dermatology, Tokyo Medical and Dental University, Tokyo, Japan

I. Katayama et al. (eds.), *Evolution of Atopic Dermatitis in the 21st Century*, https://doi.org/10.1007/978-981-10-5541-6_26

In recent years, 'precision medicine' has been proposed as a direction of medicine that should be aimed for.

Most conventional treatments have been designed for the so-called average patient. However, because of recent advances in life science, it has become possible to collect an extremely large quantity of data concerning individuals in comparison with the past; as a result, a more precise diagnosis of individual patients can be made, and even among patients who have the same disease, detailed subgroup classification is presumably possible. The concept that treatment and prophylactic methods can be developed for each subgroup to deepen medical treatments is referred to as 'precision medicine'; this concept is a step further from conventional 'personalised medicine'.

It is presumed that the re-establishment of medical care in the field of allergic diseases will also be based on this concept. Herein, we describe how future treatment strategies for atopic dermatitis can be developed on the basis of the idea of 'precision medicine'.

26.1 Introduction

Atopic dermatitis (AD) is defined as a 'disease in which a patient presents with a primary lesion of eczema with repeated exacerbation and remission; many patients have atopic diathesis in Japan (Japanese Dermatological Association). In either case, the current consensus concerning the concept of the disease is that the onset of the condition is caused by a complex interrelationship of a variety of genetic and environmental factors (acquired aggravating factors), leading to the maintenance of the chronic inflammatory skin condition.

AD classically develops during early childhood, and in most cases, spontaneous remissions occur along with age; however, in some cases, symptoms repeatedly disappear and reappear, leading to adult-type AD. It is possible to control skin symptoms in the majority of cases through the three pillars of treatment advocated from Japanese Dermatological Association (appropriate pharmacotherapy, removal of aggravating factors and skin care). However, it is certain that there are at least some patients for whom control of symptoms is difficult with the current target therapies. In recent years, many previously unknown points concerning the mechanisms of the pathogenesis of AD have also been elucidated; novel treatments in line with the pathological mechanisms or based on subgroup classifications have been developed (Fig. 26.1). In this review, therapeutic approaches targeting skin barrier protein, such as filaggrin and/or antimicrobial peptide (AMPs), are described in Sect. 26.2. Therapeutic or management approaches for AD from 'IgE antibody' aspect, such as anti-IgE antibody, are described in Sect. 26.3. Normalized or inhibitory procedures for an increased Th2-type immune status as therapeutic approaches for AD are described in Sects. 26.5 and 26.6. Promising novel biological drugs targeting IL-4, IL-31 and TSLP are now on the way to clinical trial and described in Sect. 26.6.

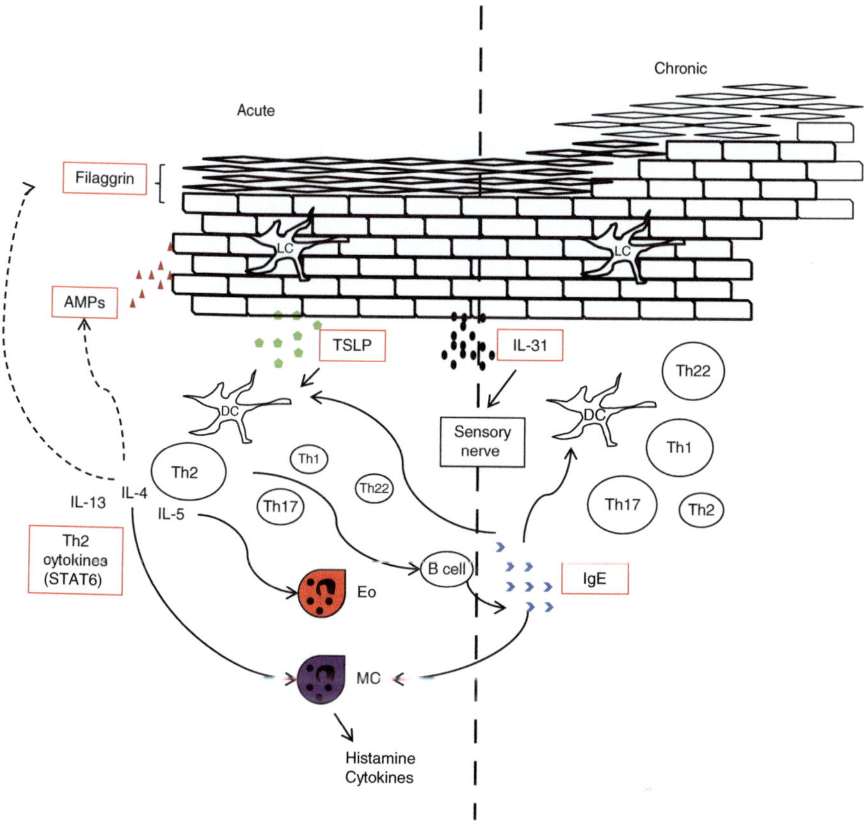

Fig. 26.1 Partial cellular and molecular immunological mechanisms in lesional skin of AD. Factors surrounded by *red square* are targets of therapeutic approaches described in this manuscript. 'Acute' shows acute phase of AD and 'Chronic' shows chronic phase of AD. In acute phase of AD skin lesion, Th2-type lymphocytes should be dominated and produce Th2-type cytokines, such as IL-4, IL5 and IL-13. In chronic phase of AD skin lesion, mixed-type Th lymphocytes (Th1, Th17, Th22 dominated and also Th2) should be infiltrated. *Solid arrows* show positive regulation, and *dotted arrows* show negative regulation. *AMPs* antimicrobial peptides, *TSLP* thymic stromal lymphopoietin, *Eo* eosinophils, *MC* mast cells, *LC*: Langerhans cells, *DC* dendritic cells

26.2 Approach from a 'Barrier Disorder'

26.2.1 Physical Barrier

As seen from the fact that one of the three pillars of AD treatment advocated by the Japanese Dermatological Association is 'skin care', skin barrier dysfunction has been widely recognised as an important element of the pathogenesis of AD, and various studies concerning the topic have been conducted [1, 2]. Since the relationship between filaggrin gene mutations and AD was reported in 2006, the examination of the pathology of AD from this aspect has gained further attention.

The following possible effects of filaggrin mutation on AD have been indicated. Because filaggrin is one of the important elements in skin barrier formation and when mutation is present, there is an increased possibility that at least the skin barrier function decreases, facilitating exogenous invasion and sustained intrusion of the allergen, which may contribute to the onset or exacerbation of AD.

This speculation is supported by data from research [3–6], and it appears that the actual conditions are reflected by these results; however, because many studies have reported that filaggrin gene mutations occur in ~30% of all AD cases and there are many individuals with filaggrin gene mutation who have normal traits, it may be safer to say that decreased filaggrin expression in the skin is one of the many factors that lead to the onset of AD.

However, the existence of a mutation in the filaggrin gene results in a certain degree of loss of skin barrier function in which the expression of filaggrin is reduced in the skin and as previously mentioned can be expected to be a possible risk factor for continued skin problem; it can be assumed that by screening filaggrin gene mutations, it will be possible to elucidate one of the multiple risk factors of AD.

Moreover, it was reported in 2014 that the onset of AD can be prevented by aggressive use of moisturising agents from infancy [7, 8]. From the standpoint of skin barrier dysfunction, these are important reports concerning the onset and exacerbation of AD.

26.2.2 Functional Barrier

As previously mentioned, the skin has both a so-called physical barrier, composed of filaggrin and other proteins, and a functional barrier that inhibits the infection or fixation of pathogenic microorganisms. Peptides that exhibit antibacterial or antiviral activities, which are collectively referred to as antimicrobial peptides (AMPs), are produced from epidermal keratinocytes and contribute to the primary biological defence of the skin surface [9–11]. Expression of LL-37 and human beta-defensin (hBD)-2 and hBD-3 that belong to AMPs has been reported to decrease in the local skin of patients with AD [12–14]. These findings suggest that it is one of the factors of bacterial fixation or infection in the skin surface of patients with AD that is commonly observed. It is often observed in the clinical practice that microbial infection of the skin exacerbates the symptoms of AD; even when infection is not present but fixation of pathogenic microorganisms has occurred, the possibility that the produced exotoxin may act as a superantigen and is involved in the exacerbation of the symptoms of AD by promoting the activation of nonspecific T cells has been indicated [15].

In this context, it has been reported that activated vitamin D3 increases the expression of AMPs in cultured keratinocytes [16]; in the case of some AMPs, vitamin D response elements in the promoter region of the gene [17, 18], elevated (recovered) AMP expression in the skin of patients with AD following oral vitamin D formulation administration and further amelioration of dermal symptoms have also been reported by other studies [19–22].

26.2.3 Others

There are in vitro data that reveal a reduction in the expression of proteins involved in the physical skin barrier (e.g. filaggrin) and AMPs (i.e. LL-37, hBD) involved in the functional skin barrier when the Th2 cytokine is present, even when there are no genetic mutations [12, 23, 24]. There are many patients with AD in which an abnormal increase in Th2-type immune response is thought to be a factor of the pathogenesis of the condition; based on these findings, it is possible that attempted treatments to correct the part of the abnormal enhancement of the Th2-type immune response in AD not only suppress the inflammatory reaction involved in this immune response but may also promote recovery of the skin barrier function.

26.3 Approach from Elevated Serum IgE Antibody Levels

As a result, the idea that increased Th2-type immune response, which may lead to increased production of IgE antibodies, is an onset or exacerbation factor of AD has long existed [25]. These findings form the basis for the examination of possible AD treatments targeting IgE antibodies.

In recent years, a subgroup with normal serum IgE antibody has been proposed [26], which is considered to be an effective method to categorise patients who are thought to have heterogeneous AD. However, such a group may not have treatment methods targeting IgE antibodies. Thus, by dividing AD into subgroups, it may be possible to discover specific treatments or management methods for each subgroup.

26.3.1 Anti-IgE Antibody (Omalizumab)

The fact that the subgroup with elevated serum IgE antibody levels comprise 80% of the total subgroup and the question of whether IgE antibodies are actively involved in the pathogenesis of AD remains, there are still concerns to discuss.

Regarding the findings that suggest the possibility that IgE antibodies are directly involved in the pathogenesis of AD, there are data that suggest that as a result of the presence of FcεRI-positive antigen-presenting cells in AD lesions, the antigen-presenting ability of the T cells of the antigen-presenting cells is dramatically enhanced, arising from intracellular signalling due to the presence of antigens and antigen-specific IgE antibodies [27]. These findings suggest the possibility of therapeutic effects of anti-IgE antibody (omalizumab) on AD. The treatment mechanism appears to be through trapping of the allergens by the immune complexes of the IgE antibody and omalizumab to prevent the activation of FcεRI-positive cells by the allergens [28].

However, several pilot and case studies have attempted to discover treatments for AD; of these, conflicting conclusions have been reported. It appears that therapeutic effects can be obtained through selection of target patients [29, 30], and the question whether clinical efficacy commensurate with the current cost can be obtained remains.

26.3.2 Intrinsic and Extrinsic ADs

Attempts were originally made to classify diseases as 'intrinsic' or 'extrinsic' starting with asthma [31]. This concept has similarly been utilised for AD, and so far, 'allergic' and 'non-allergic' types of AD have been reported. Also 'intrinsic' type of AD has been reported as 'atopiform dermatitis' [26, 32]. In all cases, it appears that antigen sensitisation by the IgE antibody does not occur, that is, there is a group in which nonspecific or antigen-specific IgE antibodies do not increase. It may be possible to classify this type as 'intrinsic AD' and all other types as 'extrinsic AD'.

When such group classifications are made, various examinations are performed to examine the characteristics of each group, in addition to IgE antibody values. Reports on intrinsic AD to date have shown the characteristics of late-onset AD in women, as well as low severity, whereas extrinsic AD had a strong relationship with barrier dysfunction, which is characterised by early onset and has a comparatively high severity [33].

In recent years, classification based on types in which Th2-type immune reaction is dominant and types in which it is not dominant (Th1, 17, 22 mixed types) has been proposed, regardless of high or normal IgE antibody levels. Thus, these attempts aim to classify AD, a disease that is considered a loose collection of heterogeneous diseases, into subgroups through reconfiguration of uniform multiple groups as much as possible, and it is expected that the so-called tailor-made therapy can be established for each group and these attempts lead to 'precision medicine'.

26.4 Approach from an Aim of 'Reducing Inflammation'

Although various factors and mediated pathways exist in AD cases, clinical findings reveal somewhat uniform chronic inflammatory responses in the skin. Therefore, when considering treatments for AD, the necessity of the examination of inflammation reduction is clear. In fact, the most popular current pharmacotherapies for AD, such as topical steroids and ointments containing immunosuppressive agents, are a result of this approach.

26.4.1 Proactive Therapy Utilising Topical Agents

As stated above, topical steroids and topical agents containing immunosuppressive agents have a reliable suppressing effect on inflammation and are currently the primary (topical) pharmacotherapies used for AD. It has been reported that when these agents (standard remission induction therapy, which is so-called reactive therapy) are used, exacerbation of symptoms is significantly inhibited by continued proactive therapy through external use twice per week after remission induction [34, 35]. Although topical agents are already widely used, it may be possible to obtain better therapeutic effects through application of the preparations. As a result, the question of how long proactive therapy should continue arises; however, recent guidelines issued in Germany recommend the treatments to be administered initially for 3 months [36]. However, much accumulation of data is needed concerning these findings.

Ointments containing immunosuppressive agents are currently used for the treatment of various skin diseases, including AD; however, since the beginning, there have been concerns about the use of such ointments with regard to the risk of onset of lymphomas and local malignant tumours. Systematic reviews in 2015 reported that there is no evidence that actively suggests the onset of malignant tumours following such use [37, 38]. Although a satisfactory conclusion has been reached, further long-term observations may be necessary.

26.4.2 Others

Biological drugs that are already used in the clinical treatment of psoriasis in dermatology in Japan are predicted to be used in the treatment of AD. Although these are case and open-label studies, there are many reports available [39, 40]. TNF inhibitors that are already used in Japan include those in self-injection forms; such drugs may be applied to AD treatment in the future. As in the case of psoriasis, it is necessary to consider the possibility of safety problems in using such treatments (i.e. easy to infect or so-called paradoxical reactions).

26.5 Attempts to Apply Nucleic Acid Drugs to the Treatment of AD

Drugs with functional molecules that utilise nucleic acids with a variety of functions and are widely applied as pharmaceutical products are referred to as 'nucleic acid drugs' [41]. Currently, various attempts are being made in several fields. For example, antisense DNA, MicroRNA and decoy oligodeoxynucleotides (decoy ODNs) have been developed to inhibit gene expression and are used for various purposes [41]. Here, we explain the decoy ODNs and small interfering RNAs (siRNAs) that we also examined.

In the transcriptional regulatory region that controls the gene expression of DNA, a DNA sequence that binds with a specific transcription factor is artificially synthesised to obtain a double-stranded DNA fragment. This is made into decoy ODNs. When administered intracellularly, the transcriptional regulatory factors are competitively trapped by the decoy ODNs, thereby exerting inhibitory effect of gene expression (Fig. 26.2).

RNA interference (RNAi) was originally a phenomenon discovered in nematodes, and a similar phenomenon was subsequently found to exist in various species. In short, when a double-stranded RNA is present, the phenomenon in which mRNA having a complementary base sequence is decomposed occurs [42]. Using this phenomenon to intracellularly introduce the artificially synthesised double-stranded RNA, the method of inhibiting the expression of a given gene has been established.

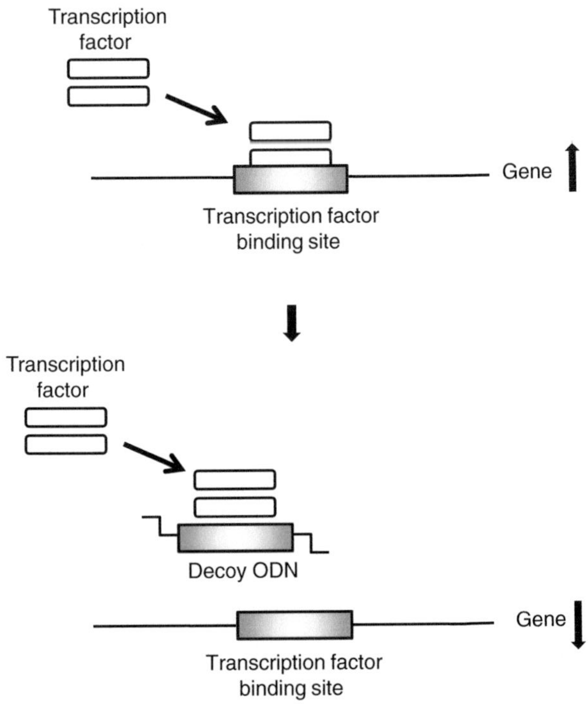

Fig. 26.2 Gene suppression mechanisms of decoy ODNs. A DNA sequence of binding site of transcription factor is artificially synthesised, and we used this as decoy ODNs. When administered intracellularly, the transcriptional factors are competitively trapped by the decoy ODNs, thereby exerting inhibitory effect of gene expression

26.5.1 NF-kappaB Decoy ODNs

Morishita et al. reported that the results of gene suppression using decoy ODNs that target NF-kappaB, a transcription regulatory factor, revealed an amelioration in the conditions in an animal model of ischaemic heart disease [43]. Therapeutic effects of NF-kappaB decoy ODNs were also noted in animal models of AD [44], and a clinical trial for severe AD using an ointment containing NF-kappaB decoy ODNs has been conducted.

26.5.2 Attempts at Utilising Nucleic Acid Drugs That Target the Signal Transducer and Activator of Transcription (STAT) 6 for the Treatment of AD

AD is considered an intractable condition with various causes in each patient; however, there appear to be several candidate background factors with shared mechanisms. Filaggrin gene mutations, which have attracted much attention in recent years, may have at least some relationship with epidermal barrier dysfunction [45]. Thus, it can be surmised that this is one of the factors contributing to the treatment resistance of AD.

However, the overproduction of IgE antibodies is a phenomenon often seen in AD, and it has been previously considered by some that increased Th2-type immune response may be an exacerbating factor of AD onset. Although classifications can be made on the basis of intrinsic AD or non-type 2 immune response AD (normal IgE antibody levels) or extrinsic AD or type 2 immune response AD (elevated IgE antibody levels) [33], the dominance of Th2-type immunity has also been observed in the locally inflamed skin in intrinsic AD [46], regardless of IgE antibody status; it can be considered that increased Th2-type immune response is involved to a certain degree in all patients with AD.

We have previously focused on the pathogenesis of AD, which is based on this increase in Th2-type immune response. In 2000, Yokozeki et al. reported the intracellular signal transduction of IL-4 and IL-13 cytokines; by focusing on STAT6, which plays an important role in Th2-type immune response as a transcriptional regulatory factor, an interesting result that a prominent inhibition of hapten-induced contact hypersensitivity in knockout mice was noted [47]. These results suggest that Th2-type immune response plays as an active positive factor of induction of skin allergy inflammatory reaction. It has been subsequently confirmed that the STAT6-mediated response pathway is also actively involved in the pathogenesis in a mouse model of various skin allergic inflammatory reactions [48, 49]; by inhibiting this pathway, skin allergic inflammatory reactions may be treated. Specifically, a decoy nucleic acid (STAT6 decoy ODNs) was used to inhibit the function of the target, STAT6. We examined the effects of STAT6 decoy ODNs starting from local injections to finally in topical preparations; however, we concluded that allergic skin inflammatory responses in a mouse model were clearly suppressed by the administration of STAT6 decoy ODNs [48, 49].

It has also been reported that by simultaneously stimulating human epidermal keratinocytes, fibroblasts or vascular endothelial cells with IL-4, eotaxin or enhanced production of cell adhesion factor is observed [50, 51]. Furthermore, there is an accumulation of data that suggests that Th2-type immune response is actively involved in the increase of the inflammatory reactions in the local skin in mice and humans.

On the basis of these study results, a pilot study to examine the therapeutic effects of the inhibition of Th2-type immune response on skin conditions in actual patients with AD was conducted. Patients with moderate to severe adult AD with facial or trunk erythema were selected as subjects; however, therapeutic effects were observed in all subjects following the use of ointments containing STAT6 decoy ODNs (Fig. 26.3) [52].

Furthermore, it was reported that by utilising RNAi that targets STAT6 (in this case, short interfering RNA; STAT6 siRNA was created), mouse skin or nasal allergic inflammation reactions could be suppressed [53]. Thus, the possibility ~Th2-type immune response has been clearly indicated additionally, the utility of nucleic acid drugs using decoy ODNs and siRNA has been demonstrated as a method of treatment. Furthermore, excessive Th2-type immune response had recently been reported to inhibit the production of molecules responsible for skin barrier function [23, 54], and it is the authors' opinion that our proposed concept of the treatment of AD by the inhibition of Th2-type immunity is a treatment method with higher specificity to pathology in comparison with conventional targeted therapies, such as topical steroids and topical agents containing immunosuppressive agents.

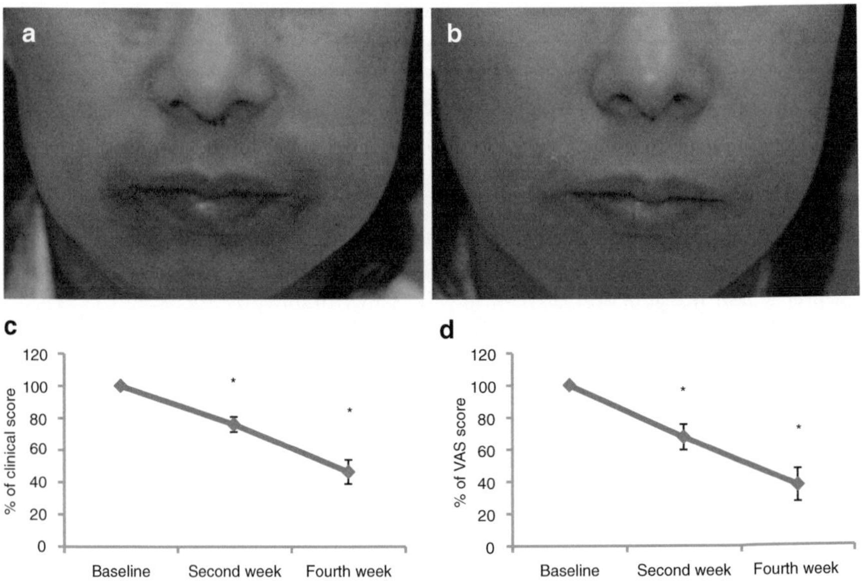

Fig. 26.3 Therapeutic trial of STAT6 decoy ODN ointment for AD. Clinical features of facial erythema in a representative case at baseline (**a**), at week 2 (**b**).The changes of clinical (**c**) and visual analogue score (VAS) scores for pruritus (**d**) for facial lesions. Data were expressed as average percentage of baseline scores ± SEM. *$p < 0.05$

When developing nucleic acid drugs that target STAT6 for clinical use, the most critical problem was the high molecular weight of the nucleic acid drugs (10,000–20,000 Da). The skin has a considerably strict barrier function, and the size of substances that can relatively freely penetrate the skin from the outside is no >500 Da. [32]. In fact, in clinical studies using the previously mentioned ointment containing STAT6 decoy ODNs, efficacy was not observed in all cases; one reason for this appeared to be the possible permeability problems of nucleic acids in the skin. Moreover, if the problem of permeability can be solved in terms of therapeutic effects and economic aspects considering commercialisation of the product (if efficacy with a small amount of nucleic acid can be achieved, costs can be reduced), its utility may be greatly improved. Thus, the use of novel technologies with high efficacy that can introduce highly polymerised compounds, such as STAT6 decoy ODNs into the cells that comprise the skin through horny layer permeability, is currently being examined, and research concerning the development of nucleic acid drugs targeting STAT6 is progressing.

26.6 Attempts at AD Treatments Using Novel Biological Drugs

As above mentioned, there is a wide range of factors responsible for the pathogenesis of AD, and each patient has a completely different clinical presentation. Nevertheless, the elements that comprise the pathogenesis of AD are also being elucidated gradually, and development of treatment methods targeting the elucidated elements that are shared by a comparatively large number of patients is progressing.

26.6.1 Antihuman IL-31RA Antibody

IL-31 is a comparatively novel cytokine that was cloned by Dillon et al. in 2004 [55]. Activated T cells, in particular, CD4-positive T cells of Th2-type, are considered the main production source. The receptor is a heterodimer consisting of IL-31RA and oncostatin M R (OSMR) and expressed by activated macrophages, eosinophils, basophils, epidermal keratinocytes and dorsal root ganglions, among other cells [55]. In IL-31 transgenic mice that were created at the same time, severe itchiness was induced; skin inflammatory response accompanied by hair loss was observed, and the skin lesion histology resembled that of AD [55]. Furthermore, Sonkoly et al. reported in 2006 that an examination of IL-31 mRNA expression in the local skin of human subjects with inflammatory skin diseases revealed that the expression of AD was noted in the local site of inflammation, whereas expression of AD was not noted in cases of psoriasis but was strongly noted in cases of nodular prurigo, which is well known to be a disease accompanied by severe itching [56].

It is well known that patients with AD often experience itchiness that is difficult to control even through the use of antihistamines [57]. It is possible that IL-31 may be a cause of this intractable itchiness in AD, and because dermal irritation was induced in a mouse model, it is a leading target for the development of novel therapeutic treatments of AD, as previously mentioned. As a result, humanised antihuman IL-31RA antibody to inhibit the action of IL-31 has been developed, and clinical trials targeting AD (phase I/Ib) have been conducted. In October 2015, the results were reported, and in comparison with the placebo group, clear inhibition of itching, amelioration of sleep disorders and reduction of topical steroid dose in the administration group were noted [58].

26.6.2 Anti-IL-4Rα Antibody

Concerning the concept in which the treatment of AD by correction of Th2-type immune response (as stated in the section of this paper concerning 'attempts at utilising nucleic acid drugs that target STAT6 for the treatment of AD') in comparison with conventional AD treatments, it is possible that the treatment in line with pathology can be administered. AD trials using fully human anti-IL-4 receptor chain antibody have been conducted in Europe, and the results of phase I/IIa trial [59] and IIb trial [60] were reported in 2014 and October 2015, respectively; it has been shown to cause no serious side effects and has favourable therapeutic effects on moderate to severe ADs.

26.6.3 Others

Thymic stromal lymphopoietin (TSLP) plays a major role in allergic inflammatory response. It is also believed to play an important role in AD, and it has been reported that its expression is elevated in locally inflamed skin of patients with AD [61]. Furthermore, the skin of genetically modified mice in which TSLP was overexpressed in epidermal keratinocytes had a similar presentation to that of AD [62].

Increased Th2-type cytokine and serum IgE antibody levels have also been observed in these mice [62]. Furthermore, it has been recently reported that TSLP directly acts on the neurons to induce itchiness [63] and it is possible that the inhibition of the TSLP pathway not only suppresses inflammatory reactions but may also be effective in inhibiting itchiness. Currently, an antibody clinical research targeting TSLP is progressing.

References

1. Berth-Jones J, Damstra RJ, Golsch S, et al. Twice weekly fluticasone propionate added to emollient maintenance treatment to reduce risk of relapse in atopic dermatitis: randomised, double blind, parallel group study. BMJ. 2003;326:1367.
2. Szczepanowska J, Reich A, Szepietowski JC. Emollients improve treatment results with topical corticosteroids in childhood atopic dermatitis: a randomized comparative study. Pediatr Allergy Immunol. 2008;19:614–8.
3. Fallon PG, Sasaki T, Sandilands A, et al. A homozygous frameshift mutation in the mouse Flg gene facilitates enhanced percutaneous allergen priming. Nat Genet. 2009;41:602–8.
4. Scharschmidt TC, Man MQ, Hatano Y, et al. Filaggrin deficiency confers a paracellular barrier abnormality that reduces inflammatory thresholds to irritants and haptens. J Allergy Clin Immunol. 2009;124:496–506. e1–6
5. Novak N, Baurecht H, Schäfer T, et al. Loss-of-function mutations in the filaggrin gene and allergic contact sensitization to nickel. J Invest Dermatol. 2008;128:1430–5.
6. Ross-Hansen K, Menné T, Johansen JD, et al. Nickel reactivity and filaggrin null mutations--evaluation of the filaggrin bypass theory in a general population. Contact Dermatitis. 2011;64:24–31.
7. Horimukai K, Morita K, Narita M, et al. Application of moisturizer to neonates prevents development of atopic dermatitis. J Allergy Clin Immunol. 2014;134:824–30.e6.
8. Simpson EL, Chalmers JR, Hanifin JM, et al. Emollient enhancement of the skin barrier from birth offers effective atopic dermatitis prevention. J Allergy Clin Immunol. 2014;134:818–23.
9. Schauber J, Dorschner RA, Yamasaki K, et al. Control of the innate epithelial antimicrobial response is cell-type specific and dependent on relevant microenvironmental stimuli. Immunology. 2006;118:509–19.
10. Hata TR, Gallo RL. Antimicrobial peptides, skin infections, and atopic dermatitis. Semin Cutan Med Surg. 2008;27:144–50.
11. Schauber J, Gallo RL. Antimicrobial peptides and the skin immune defense system. J Allergy Clin Immunol. 2009;124:R13–8.
12. Ong PY, Ohtake T, Brandt C, et al. Endogenous antimicrobial peptides and skin infections in atopic dermatitis. N Engl J Med. 2002;347:1151–60.
13. Nomura I, Goleva E, Howell MD, et al. Cytokine milieu of atopic dermatitis, as compared to psoriasis, skin prevents induction of innate immune response genes. J Immunol. 2003;171:3262–9.
14. Rieg S, Steffen H, Seeber S, et al. Deficiency of dermcidin-derived antimicrobial peptides in sweat of patients with atopic dermatitis correlates with an impaired innate defense of human skin in vivo. J Immunol. 2005;174:8003–10.
15. Macias ES, Pereira FA, Rietkerk W, et al. Superantigens in dermatology. J Am Acad Dermatol. 2011;64:455–72. quiz 73–4
16. Schauber J, Oda Y, Büchau AS, et al. Histone acetylation in keratinocytes enables control of the expression of cathelicidin and CD14 by 1,25-dihydroxyvitamin D3. J Invest Dermatol. 2008;128:816–24.
17. Wang TT, Nestel FP, Bourdeau V, et al. Cutting edge: 1,25-dihydroxyvitamin D3 is a direct inducer of antimicrobial peptide gene expression. J Immunol. 2004;173:2909–12.

18. Gombart AF, Borregaard N, Koeffler HP. Human cathelicidin antimicrobial peptide (CAMP) gene is a direct target of the vitamin D receptor and is strongly up-regulated in myeloid cells by 1,25-dihydroxyvitamin D3. FASEB J. 2005;19:1067–77.
19. Hata TR, Kotol P, Jackson M, et al. Administration of oral vitamin D induces cathelicidin production in atopic individuals. J Allergy Clin Immunol. 2008;122:829–31.
20. Javanbakht MH, Keshavarz SA, Djalali M, et al. Randomized controlled trial using vitamins E and D supplementation in atopic dermatitis. J Dermatolog Treat. 2011;22:144–50.
21. Sidbury R, Sullivan AF, Thadhani RI, et al. Randomized controlled trial of vitamin D supplementation for winter-related atopic dermatitis in Boston: a pilot study. Br J Dermatol. 2008;159:245–7.
22. Segaert S. Vitamin D regulation of cathelicidin in the skin: toward a renaissance of vitamin D in dermatology? J Invest Dermatol. 2008;128:773–5.
23. Howell MD, Kim BE, Gao P, et al. Cytokine modulation of atopic dermatitis filaggrin skin expression. J Allergy Clin Immunol. 2007;120:150–5.
24. Howell MD, Kim BE, Gao P, et al. Cytokine modulation of atopic dermatitis filaggrin skin expression. J Allergy Clin Immunol. 2009;124:R7–R12.
25. Grewe M, Bruijnzeel-Koomen CA, Schöpf E, et al. A role for Th1 and Th2 cells in the immunopathogenesis of atopic dermatitis. Immunol Today. 1998;19:359–61.
26. Novak N, Bieber T. Allergic and nonallergic forms of atopic diseases. J Allergy Clin Immunol. 2003;112:252–62.
27. Bieber T. Fc epsilon RI-expressing antigen-presenting cells: new players in the atopic game. Immunol Today. 1997;18:311–3.
28. Hsu CL, Shiung YY, Lin BL, et al. Accumulated immune complexes of IgE and omalizumab trap allergens in an in vitro model. Int Immunopharmacol. 2010;10:533–9.
29. Vigo PG, Girgis KR, Pfuetze BL, et al. Efficacy of anti-IgE therapy in patients with atopic dermatitis. J Am Acad Dermatol. 2006;55:168–70.
30. Belloni B, Ziai M, Lim A, et al. Low-dose anti-IgE therapy in patients with atopic eczema with high serum IgE levels. J Allergy Clin Immunol. 2007;120:1223–5.
31. Rackemann FM. Intrinsic Asthma. Bull N Y Acad Med. 1947;23:302–6.
32. Brenninkmeijer EE, Spuls PI, Legierse CM, et al. Clinical differences between atopic and atopiform dermatitis. J Am Acad Dermatol. 2008;58:407–14.
33. Tokura Y. Extrinsic and intrinsic types of atopic dermatitis. J Dermatol Sci. 2010;58:1–7.
34. Wollenberg A, Reitamo S, Girolomoni G, et al. Proactive treatment of atopic dermatitis in adults with 0.1% tacrolimus ointment. Allergy. 2008;63:742–50.
35. Peserico A, Städtler G, Sebastian M, et al. Reduction of relapses of atopic dermatitis with methylprednisolone aceponate cream twice weekly in addition to maintenance treatment with emollient: a multicentre, randomized, double-blind, controlled study. Br J Dermatol. 2008;158:801–7.
36. Werfel T, Heratizadeh A, Aberer W, et al. S2k guideline on diagnosis and treatment of atopic dermatitis--short version. J Dtsch Dermatol Ges. 2016;14:92–106.
37. Cury Martins J, Martins C, Aoki V, et al. Topical tacrolimus for atopic dermatitis. Cochrane Database Syst Rev. 2015; CD009864.
38. Legendre L, Barnetche T, Mazereeuw-Hautier J, et al. Risk of lymphoma in patients with atopic dermatitis and the role of topical treatment: a systematic review and meta-analysis. J Am Acad Dermatol. 2015;72:992–1002.
39. Jacobi A, Antoni C, Manger B, et al. Infliximab in the treatment of moderate to severe atopic dermatitis. J Am Acad Dermatol. 2005;52:522–6.
40. Buka RL, Resh B, Roberts B, et al. Etanercept is minimally effective in 2 children with atopic dermatitis. J Am Acad Dermatol. 2005;53:358–9.
41. Yokozeki H. A nucleic acid-based medication for allergic skin diseases. Jpn J Clin Immunol. 2012;35:107–11.
42. Hannon GJ. RNA interference. Nature. 2002;418:244–51.
43. Morishita R, Sugimoto T, Aoki M, et al. In vivo transfection of cis element "decoy" against nuclear factor-kappaB binding site prevents myocardial infarction. Nat Med. 1997;3:894–9.

44. Nakamura H, Aoki M, Tamai K, et al. Prevention and regression of atopic dermatitis by ointment containing NF-kB decoy oligodeoxynucleotides in NC/Nga atopic mouse model. Gene Ther. 2002;9:1221–9.
45. Palmer CN, Irvine AD, Terron-Kwiatkowski A, et al. Common loss-of-function variants of the epidermal barrier protein filaggrin are a major predisposing factor for atopic dermatitis. Nat Genet. 2006;38:441–6.
46. Suárez-Fariñas M, Dhingra N, Gittler J, et al. Intrinsic atopic dermatitis shows similar TH2 and higher TH17 immune activation compared with extrinsic atopic dermatitis. J Allergy Clin Immunol. 2013;132:361–70.
47. Yokozeki H, Ghoreishi M, Takagawa S, et al. Signal transducer and activator of transcription 6 is essential in the induction of contact hypersensitivity. J Exp Med. 2000;191:995–1004.
48. Yokozeki H, Wu MH, Sumi K, et al. In vivo transfection of a cis element 'decoy' against signal transducers and activators of transcription 6 (STAT6)-binding site ameliorates IgE-mediated late-phase reaction in an atopic dermatitis mouse model. Gene Ther. 2004;11:1753–62.
49. Sumi K, Yokozeki H, Wu MH, et al. In vivo transfection of a cis element 'decoy' against signal transducers and activators of the transcription 6 (STAT6) binding site ameliorates the response of contact hypersensitivity. Gene Ther. 2004;11:1763–71.
50. Miyazaki Y, Satoh T, Nishioka K, et al. STAT-6-mediated control of P-selectin by substance P and interleukin-4 in human dermal endothelial cells. Am J Pathol. 2006;169:697–707.
51. Igawa K, Satoh T, Hirashima M, et al. Regulatory mechanisms of galectin-9 and eotaxin-3 synthesis in epidermal keratinocytes: possible involvement of galectin-9 in dermal eosinophilia of Th1-polarized skin inflammation. Allergy. 2006;61:1385–91.
52. Igawa K, Satoh T, Yokozeki H. A therapeutic effect of STAT6 decoy oligodeoxynucleotide ointment in atopic dermatitis: a pilot study in adults. Br J Dermatol. 2009;160:1124–6.
53. Hosoya K, Satoh T, Yamamoto Y, et al. Gene silencing of STAT6 with siRNA ameliorates contact hypersensitivity and allergic rhinitis. Allergy. 2011;66:124–31.
54. Kim BE, Leung DY, Boguniewicz M, et al. Loricrin and involucrin expression is downregulated by Th2 cytokines through STAT-6. Clin Immunol. 2008;126:332–7.
55. Dillon SR, Sprecher C, Hammond A, et al. Interleukin 31, a cytokine produced by activated T cells, induces dermatitis in mice. Nat Immunol. 2004;5:752–60.
56. Sonkoly E, Muller A, Lauerma AI, et al. IL-31: a new link between T cells and pruritus in atopic skin inflammation. J Allergy Clin Immunol. 2006;117:411–7.
57. Ikoma A, Steinhoff M, Ständer S, et al. The neurobiology of itch. Nat Rev Neurosci. 2006;7:535–47.
58. Nemoto O, Furue M, Nakagawa H, et al. The first trial of CIM331, a humanized antihuman interleukin-31 receptor A antibody, in healthy volunteers and patients with atopic dermatitis to evaluate safety, tolerability and pharmacokinetics of a single dose in a randomized, double-blind, placebo-controlled study. Br J Dermatol. 2016;174:296–304.
59. Beck LA, Thaçi D, Hamilton JD, et al. Dupilumab treatment in adults with moderate-to-severe atopic dermatitis. N Engl J Med. 2014;371:130–9.
60. Thaçi D, Simpson EL, Beck LA, et al. Efficacy and safety of dupilumab in adults with moderate-to-severe atopic dermatitis inadequately controlled by topical treatments: a randomised, placebo-controlled, dose-ranging phase 2b trial. Lancet. 2016;387:40–52.
61. Soumelis V, Reche PA, Kanzler H, et al. Human epithelial cells trigger dendritic cell mediated allergic inflammation by producing TSLP. Nat Immunol. 2002;3:673–80.
62. Yoo J, Omori M, Gyarmati D, et al. Spontaneous atopic dermatitis in mice expressing an inducible thymic stromal lymphopoietin transgene specifically in the skin. J Exp Med. 2005;202:541–9.
63. Wilson SR, Thé L, Batia LM, et al. The epithelial cell-derived atopic dermatitis cytokine TSLP activates neurons to induce itch. Cell. 2013;155:285–95.

Part IX

Complications

Allergic Rhinitis and Pollinosis

27

Takahiro Tokunaga and Shigeharu Fujieda

Abstract

Atopic dermatitis (AD) is the first symptom in the allergic march in children. Thereafter, in some patients, the condition progresses to bronchial asthma and allergic rhinitis (AR) in adolescence and adult life. The percentage of patients with both AD and AR has been found to be 6–9% of children and adolescents in the entire population. Severe early-onset AD is associated with the development of AR, and, similarly, early-onset AR is associated with the development of AD. These facts suggest that the impairment of epithelial barrier function by AD in infants causes subsequent AR. Genome-wide association studies have shown several genes to be associated with both AD and AR. These genes hold the key to elucidating the mechanism of the development of allergic diseases. Furthermore, risk factors and protective factors for atopic diseases have been identified. Among these factors, probiotics might have potential in the remission of AD and AR. Specific immunotherapy is also a promising treatment, and it is expected to provide an option for interventions to prevent the allergic march.

Keywords

Allergic rhinitis • Allergic march • Genome-wide association study • Probiotics • Immunotherapy

T. Tokunaga • S. Fujieda (✉)
Division of Otorhinolaryngology - Head & Neck Surgery, Department of Sensory and Locomotor Medicine, Faculty of Medical Science, University of Fukui,
23-3, Matsuoka-Shimoaizuki, Eiheiji-cho, Yoshida-gun, Fukui 910-1193, Japan
e-mail: sfujieda@u-fukui.ac.jp

I. Katayama et al. (eds.), *Evolution of Atopic Dermatitis in the 21st Century*,
https://doi.org/10.1007/978-981-10-5541-6_27

27.1 Epidemiology

Atopic dermatitis (AD) is the first disease to develop in the allergic march. The allergic march affects the development of AD and concomitant sensitization to food and aeroallergens in early childhood, progressing to bronchial asthma and allergic rhinitis (AR) in later childhood and adult life [1, 2]. In the course of the allergic march, the preceding diseases often subside, and only the symptoms of AR remain. However, in some patients, the preceding disease is not ameliorated.

An epidemiological survey of 19,461 high school students in Japan showed that the incidence rate from birth to the present was 14.3% for AD and 22.6% for AR. In this survey, the percentage of patients who had AD complicated by AR was 38.3%, whereas in 23.8% of AR patients, AR was complicated by AD. The percentage of patients with both AD and AR was 6.0% of all students (Table 27.1) [3]. In a study on 31,209 Korean children, the prevalence of AD symptoms in the previous 12 months was 19.3% for 0–3-year-old children, 19.7% for 4–6-year-old children, 16.7% for 7–9-year-old children, and 14.5% for 10–13-year-old children. The prevalence rates of AR in these age groups were 28.5%, 38.0%, 38.5%, and 35.9%, respectively. The percentage of patients with both AD and AR was 8.7% of all children [4]. There was concordance between the results in Japan and those in Korea for the most part. However, there is large variation in the prevalence of allergic diseases depending on countries, races, and age. Moreover, it is noteworthy that the self-diagnosed prevalence of allergic disease in the open population and physician-diagnosed prevalence in general practice differ significantly [5].

Kurukulaaratchy RJ et al. conducted a cohort study identifying the heterogeneity of young adult rhinitis by cluster analysis. They divided rhinitis into four clusters (Table 27.2) [6], among which clusters 1 (moderate childhood-onset rhinitis) and 3 (severe earliest-onset rhinitis with asthma) tended to complicate AD. The Swedish Dampness in Buildings and Health Study [7] found that the risk factors for the development of bronchial asthma and AR were (1) severity of eczema in infants, (2) lower age at eczema development, and (3) retention of eczema symptoms. Early childhood eczema was strongly associated with the development of both bronchial asthma (odds ratio [OR], 3.07; 95% confidence interval [CI], 1.79–5.27) and AR

Table 27.1 Comorbidity of allergic diseases

	AD	AR	BA	FA
Number of patients	3068	4933	2060	1787
No complications	1320 (43.0%)	2976 (60.3%)	784 (38.1%)	623 (34.9%)
Complication				
AD	–	1174 (23.8%)	675 (32.8%)	714 (40.0%)
AR	1174 (38.3%)	–	862 (41.8%)	728 (40.7%)
BA	675 (22.0%)	862 (17.5%)	–	426 (23.8%)
FA	714 (23.3%)	728 (14.8%)	426 (20.7%)	–

Epidemiological survey of 19,461 high school students in Japan. The table shows the number and percentage of cases complicated by other allergic diseases (Tokunaga T et al. [3], modified table)
AD atopic dermatitis, *AR* allergic rhinitis, *BA* bronchial asthma, *FA* food allergy

Table 27.2 Heterogeneity of young adult rhinitis

	Cluster	BA	Atopy	Eczema	Total IgE	BDR	BHR	Perennial rhinitis
1	Moderate childhood-onset rhinitis	+	+++	+++	++	+	+	++
2	Mild adolescent-onset rhinitis	+	+	++	+	+	+	+
3	Severe earliest-onset rhinitis with asthma	+++	+++	+++	++	+++	+++	+++
4	Moderate childhood-onset male rhinitis with asthma	++	++	+	+++	++	+	++

Four clusters divided by seven factors. +, mild or low; ++, moderate; +++, severe or high (Kurukulaaratchy RJ et al. [6], modified table)
BA bronchial asthma, *BDR* bronchodilator reversibility, *BHR* bronchial hyperresponsiveness

(OR, 2.63; 95% CI, 1.85–3.73). This study also found that those with early-onset eczema, moderate-to-severe eczema, and persistent eczema had the highest odds of developing bronchial asthma and AR. Carlsten et al. [8] also showed that only early-onset persistent eczema was associated with all atopy-related phenotypes. Early-onset persistent eczema was associated with pediatric allergist-diagnosed bronchial asthma (OR, 7.48; 95% CI, 2.53–22.2), AR (OR, 3.47; 95% CI, 1.34–8.99), and food allergy (OR, 13.4; 95% CI, 2.94–61.4). This study was the first to provide clear evidence of an atopic march from AD to food allergy. There is a notable relation between early-onset rhinitis and severe AD. Children with moderate-to-severe AD have a 50% risk of developing asthma and a 75% risk of developing AR [9, 10].

It is well known that the impairment of epithelial barrier function by eczema or AD in infants causes the consequent bronchial asthma and AR. In vivo studies have shown that percutaneous allergen sensitization causes the symptoms of bronchial asthma and AR in mice [11, 12]. The mechanism of the induction of type 2 immune responses by percutaneous sensitization remains unclear. According to a study in a mouse model [13], thymic stromal lymphopoietin—which is produced by skin epithelial cells exposed to an allergen—activates basophils. Activated basophils localize to regional lymph nodes, and they induce naïve T cells to become Th2 cells as antigen-presenting cells (APCs) producing IL-4 [14]. Skin sensitization precedes airway sensitization to the same allergen and is one of the strongest predictors of the development of childhood asthma and allergic rhinitis [15]. Together, these findings suggest that interventions to improve barrier function, which is likely to minimize the ingress of allergens, could be an important measure to control the onset of the atopic march.

27.2 Genomic Factors

Genome-wide association studies (GWASs) have revealed genes associated with the development of allergic diseases [16]. Among these, filaggrin is an important gene involved in the development of both AD and AR [17]. Furthermore, the loci of chromosomes 11q13, 2q12, 16p13.3, and 17q21.32 were found to be associated with AD and other allergic diseases. These loci include genes involved in epithelial barrier function, innate immunity, regulatory T (Treg) cells, and the metabolic pathway of vitamin D, as well as the interleukin gene family. Among these genes, *IL1RL1*, *HLA*, *OR10A3-NLRP10*, *GLB1*, *IL-13*, and *C11orf30* were reported to be associated with AR [18].

The locus 11q13 was first reported by a GWAS in AD [19]. Subsequent GWASs showed that this locus is associated with bronchial asthma [20], eosinophilic esophagitis [21], and AR [22]. Interestingly, this locus is associated with not only the development of symptoms but also allergen sensitization [23]. The peaks of a single nucleotide polymorphisms (SNPs) associated with these allergic diseases exist between genes *C11orf30* and *LRRC32*. However, which gene is associated with these diseases has not been investigated in detail. *LRRC32* is expressed on the cell surface of Treg cells, and it acts as a latent receptor of TGF-β [24], which may be associated with the pathophysiology of allergy. The genes in loci associated with allergic diseases include the genes encoding epithelial cell-derived cytokines. The locus 2q12 includes *IL1RL1*, which is one of the candidate genes underlying allergic diseases. This locus was first reported by a GWAS of bronchial asthma [25]. This locus was shown to be associated with AD, peripheral eosinophilia, and allergen sensitization. *IL1RL1* and *IL1RAP* consist of a heterodimeric receptor of interleukin-33 (IL-33). IL-33, which is released by epithelial cell damage, affects type 2 innate lymphoid cells and mast cells and induces them to release Th2 cytokines. Sakashita M et al. reported that serum levels of IL-33 were significantly higher in patients with Japanese cedar pollinosis (JCP) than in control individuals, and polymorphisms of IL-33 were associated with JCP [26]. These genes identified by various GWASs may contribute to the mechanism of allergic disease development, but there is no evidence that these genes affect the relationship between AD and AR thus far.

27.3 Risk Factors and Protective Factors

Many risk factors and some protective factors have been identified for atopic diseases. Most of these determine the development of bronchial asthma. However, factors related to AD or AR have not been explored and reported in great detail.

The epidemiological survey of high school students in Japan showed the factors involved in the onset and remission of allergic diseases (Fig. 27.1) [3]. Family history of the same disease had the highest association with the development and remission of allergic symptoms. The genetic factors underlying AD and AR are described in Sect. 27.2 (genomic factors). Constipation was found to be associated with the development of AD and AR. In this survey, the prevalence of constipation was significantly higher in female participants (male subjects, 9.2%; female subjects, 35.3%). Although multivariate analysis showed the risk of development of AD and AR to be higher in male individuals, the prevalence of AD and AR was higher in female individuals. These results suggest that constipation is closely associated with the development of AD and AR.

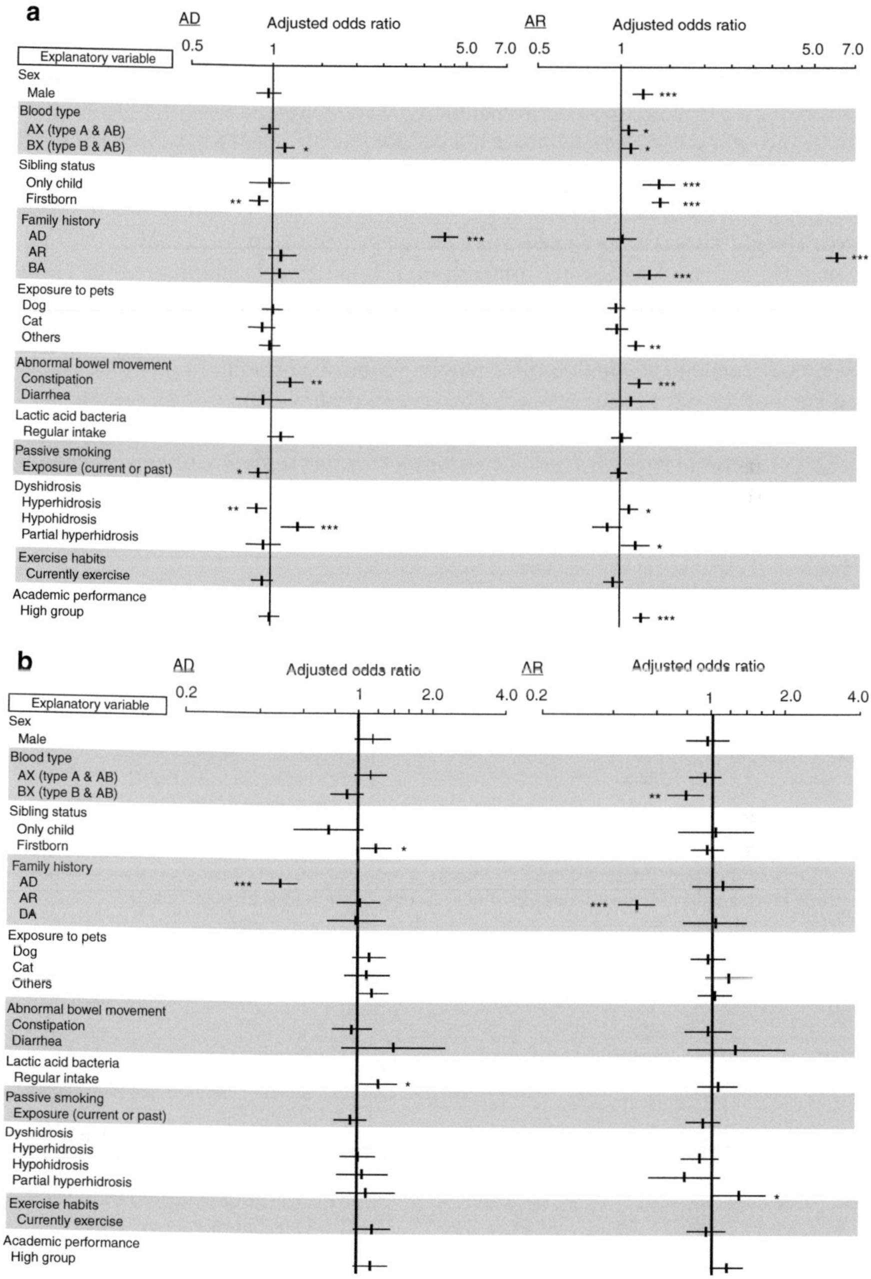

Fig. 27.1 (**a**) Analysis of factors involved in the onset of allergic diseases. (**b**) Analysis of factors involved in the remission of allergic diseases. Propensity score analysis using the inverse probability weighting method was performed. Error bars represent 95% confidence intervals (Tokunaga T et al. [3], modified figure). *, $p < 0.05$; **, $p < 0.01$; ***, $p < 0.001$. *AD* atopic dermatitis, *AR* allergic rhinitis, *BA* bronchial asthma

Regular intake of lactic acid bacteria was not linked to the development of allergic diseases, but it was responsible for the remission of AD. Intestinal microbiota may affect the development of allergic diseases. The anti-allergic mechanism of microbiota is attributed mainly to facultative anaerobes inhabiting the ileum, predominantly *Lactobacillus* spp. They induce the type 1 immune response by APCs (i.e., dendritic cells and macrophages) [27]. Several studies have evaluated the effect of probiotics in allergic diseases, among which AD has been investigated the most. The findings of randomized double-blind placebo-controlled studies of probiotics in the treatment of AD are summarized in Table 27.3. Probiotics may be effective for the treatment of AD, but according to a Cochrane review, sufficient evidence of the effectiveness of probiotics in the treatment of AD is not available [28]. On the other hand, randomized double-blind placebo-controlled studies of probiotics in the treatment of AR have been performed by several groups (Table 27.4). A systematic review suggested that probiotic therapy might be useful in AR, but such a treatment is not yet recommended because of variations in the study conditions, including

Table 27.3 Probiotics for the treatment of atopic dermatitis

Study	Age (years)	*Lactobacillus* probiotic	Result
Inoue Y et al. [35]	≥16	*L. acidophilus* strain L-92	Decreased SCORAD ($p = 0.002$)
Wang IJ et al. [36]	1–18	*L. paracasei*, *L. fermentum*, and their mixture	Decreased SCORAD ($p < 0.001$)
Han Y et al. [37]	0.5–13	*L. plantarum* CJLP133	Decreased SCORAD ($p = 0.004$)
Drago L et al. [38]	18–46	*L. salivarius* LS01	Decreased SCORAD ($p < 0.001$), improved DLQI ($p = 0.021$)
Moroi M et al. [39]	20–65	*L. paracasei* K71 (heat-killed)	Decreased skin severity score ($p < 0.01$)

Recently performed randomized, double-blind, placebo-controlled studies are listed
SCORAD scoring atopic dermatitis, *DLQI* dermatology life quality index

Table 27.4 Probiotics for the treatment of allergic rhinitis

Study	Age (years)	*Lactobacillus* probiotic	Result
Costa DJ et al. [40]	18–60	*L. paracasei* LP-33	Decreased RQLQ global score ($p = 0.026$)
Lin WY et al. [41]	6–13	*L. paracasei* HF.A00232	Decreased PRQLQ global score ($p < 0.01$)
Lin TY et al. [42]	6–12	*L. salivarius*	Decreased symptom and medication score ($p < 0.01$)
Lue KH et al. [43]	7–12	*L. johnsonii* EM1 (added to levocetirizine)	Decreased TSS ($p < 0.05$), no significant change in PRQLQ
Wassenberg J et al. [44]	18–35	*L. paracasei* ST11	Nasal congestion with NPT, decrease in VAS ($p < 0.05$)

Recently performed randomized, double-blind, placebo-controlled studies are listed
RQLQ rhinitis quality of life, *PRQLQ* pediatric rhinoconjunctivitis quality of life questionnaire, *TSS* total symptom score, *NPT* nasal provocation test, *VAS* visual analog scale

varied doses and intake periods, type and severity of the symptoms, and species and strains of the probiotics [29].

Immunotherapy is the only known treatment that alters the natural course of allergic diseases and induces long-term remission [30]. It acts, at least partly, through the induction of Treg cells and suppression of type 2 cytokine responses [31]. Several studies have reported the effect of immunotherapy in preventing allergen sensitization. Pajno GB et al. studied 134 asthmatic children (age range 5–8 years) who were monosensitized to the house dust mite (HDM). They divided children into those who received specific immunotherapy (SIT) and those who did not. In the 6-year follow-up, 75.4% and 33.3% of the children who did and did not receive SIT, respectively, had not developed new sensitivities ($p < 0.0002$) [32]. Moreover, in AR, SIT may prevent the onset of new sensitizations in children. Marogna M et al. performed an open randomized controlled study with 216 children with AR. In the 3-year follow-up, 3.1% and 34.8% of children who did and did not receive sublingual immunotherapy (SLIT), respectively, had developed new sensitivities (OR, 16.85; 95% CI, 5.73–49.13) [33]. Nevertheless, the clinical usefulness of SIT for AD remains controversial. Nahm DH et al. performed an observational cohort study with 251 patients with AD. The favorable clinical response to SIT was significantly higher in patients with severe AD (90.6%) than in those with mild to moderate AD (63.7%) ($p < 0.001$). Furthermore, patients with shorter disease duration had a significantly more favorable clinical response to SIT. A recent meta-analysis of randomized clinical trials on SIT with HDM preparation in patients with AD provided moderate-level evidence of the efficacy for AD [34]. Evidence of whether SIT is effective in preventing the allergic march remains insufficient. Further studies are needed to validate the effectiveness of SIT in preventing the allergic march.

27.4 Concluding Remarks

About one third of AD patients are accompanied with AR. Severe early-onset AD tends to progress to bronchial asthma and AR. Interventions to skin epithelial barrier dysfunction and intestinal microbiota may be effective to prevent allergic march in children with AD. Immunotherapy may be a treatment option of preventing allergic march.

References

1. Spergel JM. From atopic dermatitis to asthma: the atopic march. Ann Allergy Asthma Immunol. 2010;105(2):99–106 . quiz 107–9, 117. doi:10.1016/j.anai.2009.10.002.
2. Bantz SK, Zhu Z, Zheng T. The atopic march: progression from atopic dermatitis to allergic rhinitis and asthma. J Clin Cell Immunol. 2014;5(2):202. doi:10.4172/2155-9899.1000202.
3. Tokunaga T, Ninomiya T, Osawa Y, et al. Factors associated with the development and remission of allergic diseases in an epidemiological survey of high school students in Japan. Am J Rhinol Allergy. 2015;29(2):94–9. doi:10.2500/ajra.2015.29.4135.

4. Hong S, Son DK, Lim WR, et al. The prevalence of atopic dermatitis, asthma, and allergic rhinitis and the comorbidity of allergic diseases in children. Environ Health Toxicol. 2012;27:e2012006. doi:10.5620/eht.2012.27.e2012006.
5. Pols DHJ, Wartna JB, Moed H, van Alphen EI, Bohnen AM, Bindels PJE. Atopic dermatitis, asthma and allergic rhinitis in general practice and the open population: a systematic review. Scand J Prim Health Care. 2016;34(2):143–50. doi:10.3109/02813432.2016.1160629.
6. Kurukulaaratchy RJ, Zhang H, Patil V, et al. Identifying the heterogeneity of young adult rhinitis through cluster analysis in the Isle of Wight birth cohort. J Allergy Clin Immunol. 2015;135(1):143–50. doi:10.1016/j.jaci.2014.06.017.
7. von Kobyletzki LB, Bornehag C-G, Hasselgren M, Larsson M, Lindström CB, Svensson Å. Eczema in early childhood is strongly associated with the development of asthma and rhinitis in a prospective cohort. BMC Dermatol. 2012;12:11. doi:10.1186/1471-5945-12-11.
8. Carlsten C, Dimich-Ward H, Ferguson A, et al. Atopic dermatitis in a high-risk cohort: natural history, associated allergic outcomes, and risk factors. Ann Allergy Asthma Immunol. 2013;110(1):24–8. doi:10.1016/j.anai.2012.10.005.
9. Thomsen SF. Epidemiology and natural history of atopic diseases. Eur Clin Respir J. 2015;2:1–6. doi:10.3402/ecrj.v2.24642.
10. van der Hulst AE, Klip H, Brand PLP. Risk of developing asthma in young children with atopic eczema: a systematic review. J Allergy Clin Immunol. 2007;120(3):565–9. doi:10.1016/j.jaci.2007.05.042.
11. Akei HS, Brandt EB, Mishra A, et al. Epicutaneous aeroallergen exposure induces systemic TH2 immunity that predisposes to allergic nasal responses. J Allergy Clin Immunol. 2006;118(1):62–9. doi:10.1016/j.jaci.2006.04.046.
12. Spergel JM, Mizoguchi E, Brewer JP, Martin TR, Bhan AK, Geha RS. Epicutaneous sensitization with protein antigen induces localized allergic dermatitis and hyperresponsiveness to methacholine after single exposure to aerosolized antigen in mice. J Clin Invest. 1998;101(8):1614–22. doi:10.1172/JCI1647.
13. Muto T, Fukuoka A, Kabashima K, et al. The role of basophils and proallergic cytokines, TSLP and IL-33, in cutaneously sensitized food allergy. Int Immunol. 2014;26(10):539–49. doi:10.1093/intimm/dxu058.
14. Yoshimoto T, Yasuda K, Tanaka H, et al. Basophils contribute to T(H)2-IgE responses in vivo via IL-4 production and presentation of peptide-MHC class II complexes to CD4+ T cells. Nat Immunol. 2009;10(7):706–12. doi:10.1038/ni.1737.
15. Lodge CJ, Lowe AJ, Gurrin LC, et al. House dust mite sensitization in toddlers predicts current wheeze at age 12 years. J Allergy Clin Immunol. 2011;128(4):782–788.e9. doi:10.1016/j.jaci.2011.06.038.
16. Portelli MA, Hodge E, Sayers I. Genetic risk factors for the development of allergic disease identified by genome-wide association. Clin Exp Allergy. 2015;45(1):21–31. doi:10.1111/cea.12327.
17. Imoto Y, Enomoto H, Fujieda S, et al. S2554X mutation in the filaggrin gene is associated with allergen sensitization in the Japanese population. J Allergy Clin Immunol. 2010;125(2):498–500.e2. doi:10.1016/j.jaci.2009.10.062.
18. Hirota T, Takahashi A, Kubo M, et al. Genome-wide association study identifies eight new susceptibility loci for atopic dermatitis in the Japanese population. Nat Genet. 2012;44(11):1222–6. doi:10.1038/ng.2438.
19. Esparza-Gordillo J, Weidinger S, Fölster-Holst R, et al. A common variant on chromosome 11q13 is associated with atopic dermatitis. Nat Genet. 2009;41(5):596–601. doi:10.1038/ng.347.
20. Ferreira MAR, Matheson MC, Duffy DL, et al. Identification of IL6R and chromosome 11q13.5 as risk loci for asthma. Lancet. 2011;378(9795):1006–14. doi:10.1016/S0140-6736(11)60874-X.
21. Sleiman PMA, Wang M-L, Cianferoni A, et al. GWAS identifies four novel eosinophilic esophagitis loci. Nat Commun. 2014;5:5593. doi:10.1038/ncomms6593.

22. Ramasamy A, Curjuric I, Coin LJ, et al. A genome-wide meta-analysis of genetic variants associated with allergic rhinitis and grass sensitization and their interaction with birth order. J Allergy Clin Immunol. 2011;128(5):996–1005. doi:10.1016/j.jaci.2011.08.030.
23. Bønnelykke K, Matheson MC, Pers TH, et al. Meta-analysis of genome-wide association studies identifies ten loci influencing allergic sensitization. Nat Genet. 2013;45(8):902–6. doi:10.1038/ng.2694.
24. Edwards JP, Fujii H, Zhou AX, Creemers J, Unutmaz D, Shevach EM. Regulation of the expression of GARP/latent TGF-β1 complexes on mouse T cells and their role in regulatory T cell and Th17 differentiation. J Immunol. 2013;190(11):5506–15. doi:10.4049/jimmunol.1300199.
25. Moffatt MF, Gut IG, Demenais F, et al. A large-scale, consortium-based genomewide association study of asthma. N Engl J Med. 2010;363(13):1211–21. doi:10.1056/NEJMoa0906312.
26. Sakashita M, Yoshimoto T, Hirota T, et al. Association of serum interleukin-33 level and the interleukin-33 genetic variant with Japanese cedar pollinosis. Clin Exp Allergy. 2008;38(12):1875–81. doi:10.1111/j.1365-2222.2008.03114.x.
27. Shida K, Nanno M, Nagata S. Flexible cytokine production by macrophages and T cells in response to probiotic bacteria: a possible mechanism by which probiotics exert multifunctional immune regulatory activities. Gut Microbes. 2011;2(2):109–14. doi:10.4161/gmic.2.2.15661.
28. Boyle RJ, Bath-Hextall FJ, Leonardi-Bee J, Murrell DF, Tang ML. Probiotics for treating eczema. Cochrane Database Syst Rev 2008;(4):CD006135. doi:10.1002/14651858.CD006135.pub2.
29. Das RR, Singh M, Shafiq N. Probiotics in treatment of allergic rhinitis. World Allergy Organ J. 2010;3(9):239–44. doi:10.1097/WOX.0b013e3181f234d4.
30. Bousquet J, Lockey R, Malling HJ. Allergen immunotherapy: therapeutic vaccines for allergic diseases. A WHO position paper. J Allergy Clin Immunol. 1998;102(4 Pt 1):558–62. doi:10.1016/S0091-6749(98)70271-4.
31. Francis JN, Till SJ, Durham SR. Induction of IL-10+CD4+CD25+ T cells by grass pollen immunotherapy. J Allergy Clin Immunol. 2003;111(6):1255–61. doi:10.1067/mai.2003.1570.
32. Pajno GB, Barberio G, De Luca F, Morabito L, Parmiani S. Prevention of new sensitizations in asthmatic children monosensitized to house dust mite by specific immunotherapy. A six-year follow-up study. Clin Exp Allergy. 2001;31(9):1392–7. http://www.ncbi.nlm.nih.gov/pubmed/11591189
33. Marogna M, Tomassetti D, Bernasconi A, et al. Preventive effects of sublingual immunotherapy in childhood: an open randomized controlled study. Ann Allergy Asthma Immunol. 2008;101(2):206–11. http://www.ncbi.nlm.nih.gov/pubmed/18727478
34. Bae JM, Choi YY, Park CO, Chung KY, Lee KH. Efficacy of allergen-specific immunotherapy for atopic dermatitis: a systematic review and meta-analysis of randomized controlled trials. J Allergy Clin Immunol. 2013;132(1):110–7. doi:10.1016/j.jaci.2013.02.044.
35. Inoue Y, Kambara T, Murata N, et al. Effects of oral administration of Lactobacillus acidophilus L-92 on the symptoms and serum cytokines of atopic dermatitis in Japanese adults: a double-blind, randomized, clinical trial. Int Arch Allergy Immunol. 2014;165(4):247–54. doi:10.1159/000369806.
36. Wang I-J, Wang J-Y. Children with atopic dermatitis show clinical improvement after Lactobacillus exposure. Clin Exp Allergy. 2015;45(4):779–87. doi:10.1111/cea.12489.
37. Han Y, Kim B, Ban J, et al. A randomized trial of Lactobacillus plantarum CJLP133 for the treatment of atopic dermatitis. Pediatr Allergy Immunol. 2012;23(7):667–73. doi:10.1111/pai.12010.
38. Drago L, Iemoli E, Rodighiero V, Nicola L, De Vecchi E, Piconi S. Effects of Lactobacillus salivarius LS01 (DSM 22775) treatment on adult atopic dermatitis: a randomized placebo-controlled study. Int J Immunopathol Pharmacol. 2011;24(4):1037–48. http://www.ncbi.nlm.nih.gov/pubmed/22230409
39. Moroi M, Uchi S, Nakamura K, et al. Beneficial effect of a diet containing heat-killed Lactobacillus paracasei K71 on adult type atopic dermatitis. J Dermatol. 2011;38(2):131–9. doi:10.1111/j.1346-8138.2010.00939.x.

40. Costa DJ, Marteau P, Amouyal M, et al. Efficacy and safety of the probiotic Lactobacillus paracasei LP-33 in allergic rhinitis: a double-blind, randomized, placebo-controlled trial (GA2LEN Study). Eur J Clin Nutr. 2014;68(5):602–7. doi:10.1038/ejcn.2014.13.
41. Lin W-Y, Fu L-S, Lin H-K, Shen C-Y, Chen Y-J. Evaluation of the effect of Lactobacillus paracasei (HF.A00232) in children (6-13 years old) with perennial allergic rhinitis: a 12-week, double-blind, randomized, placebo-controlled study. Pediatr Neonatol. 2014;55(3):181–8. doi:10.1016/j.pedneo.2013.10.001.
42. Lin T-Y, Chen C-J, Chen L-K, Wen S-H, Jan R-H. Effect of probiotics on allergic rhinitis in Df, Dp or dust-sensitive children: a randomized double blind controlled trial. Indian Pediatr. 2013;50(2):209–13. http://www.ncbi.nlm.nih.gov/pubmed/22728633
43. Lue K-H, Sun H-L, Lu K-H, et al. A trial of adding Lactobacillus johnsonii EM1 to levocetirizine for treatment of perennial allergic rhinitis in children aged 7-12 years. Int J Pediatr Otorhinolaryngol. 2012;76(7):994–1001. doi:10.1016/j.ijporl.2012.03.018.
44. Wassenberg J, Nutten S, Audran R, et al. Effect of Lactobacillus paracasei ST11 on a nasal provocation test with grass pollen in allergic rhinitis. Clin Exp Allergy. 2011;41(4):565–73. doi:10.1111/j.1365-2222.2011.03695.x.

Food Allergy

28

Reiko Kishikawa and Akiko Sugiyama

Abstract

Infantile FA is most common which is onset preceded atopic dermatitis (AD) in "allergic march" with comorbidity in various allergic disease. The frequency of food allergy (FA) was most infantile under 1-year-old of all and has decreased in growing up by natural history. Recently the dysfunction of skin barrier, such a filaggrin protein, has been sometimes reported as etiology of "allergic march." It is said adult patients with FA have also some relations to AD.

Peculiar forms of FA, pollen-food syndrome (PFS)/oral allergic syndrome (OAS), latex fruit syndrome (LFS), and food-dependent exercise-induced anaphylaxis (FDEIA) occurred to adolescent and adult people and sometimes related to occupational food allergy involving AD symptoms.

The diagnosis and treatment of FA help in the understanding of medical workers and should be attentive to allergic patients with not only infant FA but also adult patients with latent FA.

If it happened the natural disaster, it should be necessary to supply FA patients with the specific food and AD patients with the shower facilities as soon as possible.

R. Kishikawa (✉)
Department of Allergology, National Hospital Organization Fukuoka Hospital, 4-39-1 Yakatabaru Minami-ku Fukuoka, Fukuoka, Japan
e-mail: kishi@mfukuoka2.hosp.go.jp

A. Sugiyama
Department of Dermatology, National Hospital Organization Fukuoka Hospital, 4-39-1 Yakatabaru Minami-ku Fukuoka, Fukuoka, Japan

I. Katayama et al. (eds.), *Evolution of Atopic Dermatitis in the 21st Century*, https://doi.org/10.1007/978-981-10-5541-6_28

Keywords
Atopic dermatitis and food allergy • Atopic (allergic) march • Adult food allergy and atopic dermatitis • Guidelines for food allergy • Disaster and food allergy/atopic dermatitis

28.1 Introduction

Food allergy (FA) is "a phenomenon in which adverse reactions are caused through antigen-specific immunological mechanisms after exposure to given food" [1, 2].

In this chapter, we will describe atopic dermatitis (AD), a complication of IgE-mediated FA, and outline FA according to the 2016 Japanese Guideline for The Diagnosis and Treatment of Allergic Disease. FA places both individual and social burdens [3] on allergic infants, children, adolescents, and adults.

28.2 Food Allergy Symptoms and Anaphylaxis

28.2.1 General Symptoms of Food Allergy [1, 2, 4, 5]

The general symptoms of FA, which are variable, affect many target organs and can be divided into immediate type (occurring within 2 h) and delayed type (occurring after 2 or more hours). The skin, mucosal membrane, airway, gastrointestinal tract, nervous system, cardiovascular, and systemic symptoms vary (Table 28.1).

Anaphylaxis is defined as general symptoms affecting >2 target organs without hypotension, whereas anaphylactic shock is defined as anaphylaxis with hypotension and unconsciousness. Anaphylaxis and anaphylactic shock are life-threatening events for which early responses and treatments are needed.

Table 28.1 Symptoms of food allergies [1, 2]

Organ	Symptoms
Skin	Erythema, urticaria, angioedema, pruritus, burning, sensation, eczema
Mucous membrane	Eye symptoms: Conjunctival hyperemia and edema, pruritus, lacrination, blepharedema
	Nasal symptoms: Rhinorrhea, nasal congestion, sneezing
	Oral symptoms: Discomfort/swelling of the oral cavity, lips, or tongue
Respiratory organs	Discomfort/itch/tightness in the pharynglolarynx, hoarseness, dysphagia, coughing, wheezing, retractive breathing, feeling of chest tightness, dyspnear, cyanosis
Digestive organs	Nausea, vomiting, abdominal pain, diarrhea, hematochezia
Nerve	Headach, lowed vigor, urrest, impaired consciousness
Circulatory organs	Decreased blood pressure, tachycardia, bradycardia, arrythmia, coldness of limbs, pallo(peripheral circulatory failure)
Systemic	Anaphylaxis and anaohylactic shock

Table 28.2 Severity of anaphylactic clinical symptoms [6]

Organs	1 (Mild)	2 (Moderate)	3 (Severe)
Skin	Lovalized urticaria, exanthema, wheal pruitus, Swallen, eye lid or lip	Generalized urticaria exthanthema, wheal pruritus	(–)
		Swollen face	(–)
Gastrointestinal tract	Pruritus of the throat or oral cavity,	Throat pain	(–)
	Mild abdominal pain	Moderate abdominal pain	Cramps
	Nausea, emesis, diarrhea	Recurrent emesis, diarrhea	Continuous emesis, loss of bowed control
Respiratory tract	Intermittent cough, nasal congestion, sneezing rhinorrhea	Recurrent cough	Persistent cough hoarseness, "barking" cough
		Chest tightness, wheezing detectable via auscultation	Audible wheezing, dyspnea, cyanosis, saturation < 92%, awallowing or speaking difficultics, throat tightness, respiratory arrest
Cardiovascular	(–)	Pale face, mild hypotension, tachycardia (increase >15 beats/min)	Hypotension, dysrthythmia, severe bradycardia, cardiac arrest
Neurological	Change in activity level, tiredness	Light-headedness, feeling of "pending doom", sommunolence, headache	Confusion, loss of consciousness, incontinence

Hypotension: ~1 Y-O < 70 mmHg, 1~10Y-O < [70mmHg + (2 × Age)], 11 Y-O ~Adult < 90 mmHg
Mild Hypo: ~1 Y-O < 80 mmHg, 1~10 Y-O < [80 mmHg + (2 × Age)], 11 Y-O~Adult < 100 mmHg

28.2.2 Anaphylaxis [1, 2, 4–6]

Anaphylaxis is defined as a strong, life-threatening whole-body reaction caused by internal exposure to a specific antigen. The sources of these antigens include food, drug, insect venom, latex, and transfused blood and can cause IgE- or non-IgE-mediated reactions. Table 28.2 presents the grades of anaphylaxis according to the Japanese Society Academy of Allergy (Table 28.2). In Japan, shock-related deaths are mainly attributable to drugs and insect venom. However, common anaphylaxis occurs most frequently in the context of FA. Hen's egg, cow's milk, wheat flour, shellfish, and soybeans are the main causative agents in Japan. However, peanut, tree nuts, fish and shellfish, hen's egg, and cow's milk are the main causative agents in Europe.

28.2.3 Epidemiology

A 2012 large-scale Japanese investigation reported the following FA prevalence rates: infants (<1-year-old), 5–10%; 1–6-year-old children, approximately 5%; and 6–12-year-old children, 1.5–3%. In other words, infants were most likely to exhibit

FA, and the prevalence tended to decrease with aging. In Japan, hen's egg, cow's milk, and wheat flour are the main causes of FA. In older children, shellfish, fruits, and buckwheat have been identified as causative agents [1, 2, 5, 7].

In contrast, the prevalence of FA among adults has seldom been investigated in Japan. Recently, however, reports of adult FA cases have increased. In addition, self-reports of FA have been investigated on websites. The overall prevalence was 1.9–10%, and shellfish was the most frequent causative agent. Additional larger-scale investigations are needed in the future [8]. In Western countries, the following FA prevalence rates have been reported: children, 1.4–5.5% [9–11]; adults, 0.8–3.2%; and all age groups, 1.4–3.6% [12, 13]. The prevalence rates detected during the double-blind placebo-controlled food challenge (DBPCFC) [9–14] were lower than those determined using other types of diagnosis [11]. In adult patients with FA, inadequate attention to a genuine food allergy sometimes would be risk factors for anaphylaxis/anaphylaxis shock [15].

On the other hand, Japan reported a moderate and severe AD rate comorbidity rate of 35–45% among infants with FA, similar to the rates in Western countries [1, 2, 16, 17].

28.3 Atopic Dermatitis and Food Allergy in Infants

28.3.1 Clinical Features of Food Allergy

28.3.1.1 Neonatal and Infantile Gastrointestinal Allergy [1, 2]

GI tract allergy is a type of FA. However, the symptoms of vomiting, bloody stool, and diarrhea are caused by IgE-independent mechanisms. Cow's milk was the most prevalent cause.

Many affected patients will naturally outgrow this disease.

28.3.1.2 Infantile Atopic Dermatitis Associated with Food Allergy [1, 2, 16–19]

The onset of this type of FA is most commonly observed in infants and is preceded by AD. Avoidance of the causative food generally leads to improvements in skin symptoms [19]. Additionally, FA symptoms tend to decrease naturally with age [16–18, 20]. Hen's egg, cow's milk, and soybean are the main causative agents of FA-related AD in Japan [1, 2]. Comorbid FA and AD occur at a high frequency. Generally, AD is considered the first step in the "allergic march" [1–3] and is followed by asthma, allergic rhinitis (AR), and FA in approximately 50% of cases. Furthermore, up to 80% of children with AD will reportedly develop AR or asthma later in childhood [1, 2, 16, 20].

Tupker et al. suggested [21] that inhalation of house dust mites (i.e., respiratory route) could induce dermatitis episodes in patients with AD. The authors concluded that a causal relationship might link bronchial and skin reactions.

We have experienced the same situation in clinical practice.

Allergic (Atopic) March and Food Allergy

In infants, various allergic diseases, including FA, AD, asthma, and AR, occur sequentially as part of the natural progression known as the "allergic (atopic) march." AD precedes FA, and other allergic diseases will develop over a period of several years [1, 2, 16, 22, 23]. Recently, dysfunction in filaggrin, a skin barrier component protein, has been reported as a cause of onset for various allergic diseases (i.e., "allergic (atopic) march") [24, 25]. Recently dysfunction of thymic stromal lymphopoietin (TSLP) in epidermal barrier on atopic march progression has also been reported [26].

Filaggrin Function and Food Allergy [27–30]
Filaggrin plays an important role as a skin barrier component. Filaggrin loss-of-function (FLG-LOF) mutations have been identified as a risk factor for allergic sensitization, atopic eczema, AR, and asthma. These mutations also lead to epidermal barrier dysfunction and increased trans-epidermal water losses (TEWLs). Increased TEWL can lead to clinical AD in patients at a high risk of atopy.

A combination of FLG-LOF mutation and allergic sensitization in childhood increases the risk of eczema. Recently, an association between FLG-LOF and food allergy has been investigated in many studies. FLG-LOF mutations have been reported to associate with FA in older children through mechanisms involving eczema and food allergen sensitization (FAS). Specifically, FLG-LOF leads to eczema, which in turn leads to early childhood FAS; this latter condition increases the risk of FA in later life.

Immediate-Type Food Allergy [1, 2, 4, 5]
These symptoms occur immediately (i.e., within 2 h). Infant FA without AD may develop, as the foods that commonly cause AD, including hen's egg, cow's milk, and wheat flour, often cause the preceding FA; furthermore, buckwheat, peanuts, fish, shellfish, and fruit become involved with age. Generally, it is difficult to outgrow this condition.

Adult Food Allergy
Adult patients with FA often exhibit immediate-type disease, are less likely to have a history of infant FA, and seldom exhibit continuous symptoms since childhood [1.2]. These patients generally consult the Department of Allergology/Dermatology for the first time after a sudden onset of skin and mucus membrane symptoms after a meal or may be referred from the emergency department (ED) immediately after treatment for anaphylaxis/anaphylactic shock. Wheat flour, shellfish, fresh fruits and vegetables, and, occasionally, *Anisakis* [31] are the main causes of allergic symptoms; however, the etiology is often unknown because patients only consult the hospital for a single event. These patients exhibit not only FA but also a comorbid allergic disease. Patients with a particular type of FA, such as food-dependent exercise-induced anaphylaxis (FDEIA), secondary pollen fruit syndrome after pollinosis, latex fruit syndrome (LFS), and other occupational FA, which involve airway and cutaneous sensitization to low concentrations of biological antigens, often consult the hospital.

A family history of various allergic diseases is an important risk factor for young adult with current AD and multiple atopic diseases. In addition, severe seasonal reactions are observed in patients with rhinoconjunctivitis and asthma [32–34]. During 3 months, elimination of causative foods, cheese, yogurt, and chocolate improves more or less some of AD symptoms [35].

28.3.2 Particular Food Allergy

28.3.2.1 Pollen-Food Syndrome, Oral Allergic Syndrome

Pollen-food syndrome (PFS) is a type I IgE-dependent FA that is generally localized to the oral mucosal membrane. The main causative agent is fresh vegetables or fruit. Patients with PFS often have complicating pollinosis; accordingly, PFS is also called pollen-associated syndrome [36, 37].

Patients with birch pollinosis in Hokkaido manifest a type I FA reaction after eating fruits from the rose family, which exhibit cross-reactivity with birch pollen antigen. Mild oral symptoms are common, although life-threatening anaphylaxis may occur, especially during the pollination season. Approximately one third of patients with PFS have concomitant AD. Therefore, asymptomatic individuals with AD may experience an exacerbation of AD even after eating cooked antigens [38, 39]. In Japan, rose family fruits are the most common cause of PFS [40].

28.3.2.2 Food-Dependent Exercise-Induced Anaphylaxis

FDEIA is induced in response to a combination of intake of a particular food and exercise; either alone will not induce anaphylaxis. IgE-mediated anaphylactic symptoms are induced within 2 h after eating the causative food and performing exercise. FDEIA is not common; it occurs in some adolescent and young adult patients in response to exercise and the intake of mainly wheat flour and shellfish, or occasionally fruit. More intense exercise and/or a larger quantity of causative food correlate with more severe symptoms [41–44]. Moreover, the use of nonsteroidal anti-inflammatory drugs (NSAIDs) exacerbates the severity of anaphylaxis [45, 46]. In Japan, many researchers have reported on FDEIA but not FDEIA-related AD [47]. Measurement-specific IgE antibodies to $\omega - 5$ gliadin are useful for the diagnosis of wheat-dependent exercise-induced anaphylaxis [48, 49].

28.3.2.3 Accidental Hydrolyzed Wheat-Dependent Exercise Anaphylaxis

In Japan, the presence of hydrolyzed wheat protein in facial soap and consequent induction of wheat allergy responses, including wheat-dependent exercise-induced anaphylaxis (WDEIA), has become a social issue. People who used the affected soaps experience wheat anaphylaxis caused by transdermal or transmucosal sensitization to the hydrolyzed wheat proteins. Some reports suggest that surfactants might aggravate skin permeability. This case suggested that we should understand the risk of skin sensitization to non-dietary food antigens [50–54]. Oatmeal for skin product for AD has occurred anaphylaxis accidentally, too [55].

28.3.2.4 Latex Fruit Syndrome (LFS)

Approximately 30–50% of patients with latex allergy will exhibit concomitant type I FA symptoms after the intake of fresh and/or processed fruits with cross-reactivity to latex, such as chestnuts, bananas, and kiwifruit. Anaphylaxis, asthma attack, urticaria, and oral allergy syndrome may be induced. This allergic reaction is known as LFS. Medical workers with individual atopic reactions, patients with spina bifida who undergo recurrent procedures involving latex, and workers who use latex gloves occupationally are at a high risk of LFS [56–58]. Although patients with AD are considered high-risk, a recent report suggests that these patients are less likely to be sensitized to latex and consequently develop LFS [59]. On the other hand, a case report described a patient with AD and concomitant FDEIA who quickly became sensitized to latex and developed a delayed-type latex allergy [60]. Medical advice regarding the use of latex leads to improved AD symptoms in affected patients. Generally, AD patients could potentially develop various allergic symptoms. LFS is a frequent type of FA and an important risk factor for occupational allergy [61].

28.3.2.5 Occupational Food Allergy

Some patients with "bakery asthma" develop secondary WDEIA and/or wheat flour FA, similar to workers who develop an occupational latex allergy. Workers with atopic factors are at a high risk of developing allergic disease following sensitization to even low concentrations of occupational food antigens [62]. In particular, AD may cause patients to change their occupation [63]. We must understand the social and individual burdens of AD and consider the quality of life related to health.

28.4 Diagnosis [1, 2, 64–68]

1. *Medical interview*: suspicious types of food, intake, induced symptoms, exercise, NSAIDs, recurrent symptoms, individual life habits and circumstances, occupation, environment are checked.
2. *Differential diagnoses* (e.g., contact dermatitis, collagen disease) must be eliminated.
3. *Skin test (in vivo)*: The skin prick test, which is safe and accurate, is recommended for both infants and adults. For patients with AD, an atopy patch test for food allergens is available. Medical treatment must be stopped for several days before the skin prick test. A prick-by-prick test, which directly pricks patients with food juices, is used for OAS patients. Even if the SPT is negative, allergic symptoms are occasionally induced.
4. *Serum specific IgE antibody (in vitro)*: This diagnostic test is commonly used for both infants and adults to quantitatively measure FA-specific IgE. A positive result indicates sensitization to a specific food allergen, although this does not always correspond to actual allergic symptoms. For some food allergens, specific IgE levels correlate with clinical symptoms.
5. *Basophil histamine release test (in vitro)*: This specific diagnostic test measures the concentration of histamine released from peripheral eosinophil blood cells and reflects strong reactions to specific food allergens in vivo. As for SPT, medical treatment must be stopped before HRT. HRT should not be performed more than 1 month after an episode of anaphylaxis.
6. *Elimination test*: Suspected foods are eliminated for approximately 2 weeks to determine the effect on allergic symptoms (e.g., improvement). Nursing mothers of affected infants should also eliminate the suspected foods.
7. *Oral food challenge test*: This is the most reliable diagnostic test for FA. However, some risk factors induce severe allergic symptoms, including anaphylaxis; therefore, we must ensure official notification and attain standard procedures for the challenge test.

(a) *Safety*: This test must be conducted under the guidance of professional medical doctors and nurses who are prepared to provide emergency care.
(b) *Administration method*: (1) *Open challenge test* is a diagnostic test method in which both the patient (subject) and tester are aware of the administered food. This is most common in Japan. (2) *Single-blind food challenge (SBFC)*: The tester knows about the administered food, but the patient (subject) is not informed. The tester provides the suspected food in combination with other foods. (3) *Double-blind placebo-controlled food challenge (DBPCFC)*: This is the international gold-standard test. Neither the tester nor patient (subject) is aware of the administered food. This test requires a controller to prepare the challenge and placebo foods. Unfortunately, this method is not suitable for many patients with FA in Japan, except those in university pediatrics departments, because of the complicated methodology and considerable time requirement.
(c) *Practice of challenge test*: (1) *The administered foods* are divided into 3–6 steps and challenged with incremental increases. (2) *The intake interval* is generally 15–30 min. (3) *Observation time after last challenge*: Sixty to 120 min for immediate-type responses and 24 h for delayed-type reactions are needed; therefore, the observations require a day or 1 night and 2 days.

8. *Food-exercise challenge test*: This method is used to diagnose FDEIA. During 2/3 nights and 3/4 days, the exercise challenge test only, food challenge test only, and combined food and exercise challenge are conducted. Negative results for the exercise-only and food-only challenges are important for a diagnosis of FDEIA. Ergometers and/or treadmills are often used for the exercise challenge. In adults, their life and safety are ensured.

28.5 Treatment and Prevention [1, 2, 69, 70]

1. *Diet therapy*: (a) *The avoidance of only the most suspicious foods* is effective even for individuals with FA. For both infant and adult AD patients with FA, the avoidance of SPT-positive foods for 3 months effectively improves skin symptoms. In particular, AD symptoms in infants improve remarkably after avoidance. (b) *Reduced allergenicity by cooking*: Heating renders allergenic proteins inactive. High-pressure cooking changes the structures of allergenic protein. (c) *Commercial low-allergen foods*: Low-allergen rice, wheat flour, bread, and other products are already sold in some specialty stores. These foods are available to the public nearly everywhere in Japan.
2. *Correspondence for emergencies*: (a) *Causative foods that are accidentally consumed* must be eliminated immediately from the oral cavity. Foods ingested into the stomach must be expelled by being headfirst position and/or striking back strongly and gargling with water. All antigens must be eliminated from the body. To prevent symptoms of shock, the head must be lowered to delay unconsciousness. (b) *Medication*: The Epipen® (generally infants, 15 mg; adults, 30 mg), available from EDs, must be injected by oneself or a bystander; subsequently, the patient must be transported to the ED as soon as possible. Medical doctors in the ED can immediately provide curative treatment. One Epipen® is provided per prescription in Japan.

3. *For mild symptoms and prevention*: Antihistamines and steroids are effective against urticarial and some allergic symptoms that occur after the accidental intake of causative foods.
   When necessary, the patient must be transported to the ED as soon as possible and given an Epipen® injection.

28.6 Prognosis and Natural History

Infants with FA often naturally acquire permanent oral tolerance and desensitization as they grow up. However, we must direct the patient's dietary therapy to avoid the excessive elimination of causative foods. Self-care (apart from parents) is also important for those with infant FA who have suffered from long-term, continuous symptoms. Recently, antigen-specific oral immunotherapy has been considered an active therapy. Adult patients with FA rarely exhibit a natural cessation of disease, and avoidance and medication are the primary measures used to avoid FA symptoms. However, the careful elimination of causative foods will decrease the related specific IgE antibody levels, thus allowing patients to eat some of the causative foods if they wish [1–3, 71]. Recent discussions have considered the early normalization of filaggrin dysfunction for halting the atopic march and onset of AD, FA, and other allergic diseases as a potential novel approach [72].

28.7 Preparing for Disasters

Recently, we experienced calamitous earthquakes and/or tsunamis in the Hansin district in 2005, Tohoku district in 2011, and Kumamoto district in 2016, among others, and expect that in the future, similar overwhelming disasters will occur here and in other countries. Minoura et al. reported [73] that it was necessary to supply FA patients with specific food-elimination diet and AD patients with shower facilities as soon as possible after a natural disaster. We emphasize that at a medical site, clean water is as important as anything else [74].

References

1. Japanese Society of Allergology. Japanese guideline for the diagnosis and treatment of allergic disease. Kyowa-Kikaku Tokyo. 2016; 400–431, 434–448, 450–484, 486–506.
2. Urisu, A. et al. on behalf of the Committee for Japanese Pediatrics Guideline for Food Allergy, Japanese Society of Pediatric Allergy and Clinical Immunology, and Japanese Society of Allergology. Japanese guideline for food allergy 2014. Allergologyint. 2014; 63(3), 399–419. doi: 10.2332/allergoint.14-RAI-0770.
3. Thomsen, S. F. Epidemiology and natural history of atopic diseases. Eur Clin Respir J. 2015; 24, 2.doi: 10.3402/ecrj, [pii] v2.24642.eCollection2015.
4. Sampson HA. Chapter 14 Anaphylaxis and food allergy. In: Metcalfe DD, Sampson HA, Simon RA, Lack G, editors. Food allergy, adverse reaction to foods and food additive. 5th ed. New York, NY: Wiley Blackwell; 2014. p. 178–91.

5. Ebisawa M. Chapter 9 Food-induced anaphylaxis and food associated exercise-induced anaphylaxis. In: James JM, Burks W, Eigenmann PA, editors. Expert consult food allergy. Philadelphia, PA: Elsevier Saunders; 2012. p. 113–28.
6. Yanagida N, Okada Y, Sato S, Ebisawa M. New approach for food allergy management using low-dose oral food challenges and low-dose oral immunotherapies. Allergol Int. 2016;65:135–40.
7. Imai T. Provision against food allergy in the school lunch program in Japan. Arerugi. 2005;54(10):1197–202.
8. Hasegawa M, et al. Prevalence of adult food allergy in Japan by internet investigation. Arerugi. 2013;62(9, 10):1336.
9. Kristjansson I, et al. Adverse reactions to food and food allergy in young children in Iceland and Sweden. Scand J Prim Health Care. 1999;17(1):30–4.
10. Osterballe M, Hansen TK, Mortz CG, Høst A, Bindslev-Jensen C. The prevalence of food hypersensitivity in an unselected population of children and adults. Pediatr Allergy Immunol. 2005;16(7):567–73.
11. Venter C, et al. Incidence of parentally reported and clinically diagnosed food hypersensitivity in the first year of life. J Allergy Clin Immunol. 2006;117(5):1118–24.
12. Jansen JJ, Kardinaal AF, Huijbers G, Vlieg-Boerstra BJ, Martens BP. Prevalence of food allergy and intolerance in the adult Dutch population. J Allergy Clin Immunol. 1994;93(2):446–56.
13. Pénard-Morand C, et al. Prevalence of food allergy and its relationship to asthma and allergic rhinitis in schoolchildren. Allergy. 2005;60(9):1165–71.
14. Zuberbier T, et al. Prevalence of adverse reactions to food in Germany—a population study. Allergy. 2004;59(3):338–45.
15. Seitz CS, Pfeuffer P, Raith P, Bröcker EB, Trautmann A. Food allergy in adults: an over- or underrated problem? Dtsch Arztebl Int. 2008;105(42):715–23. doi:10.3238/arztebl.2008.0715.
16. Perry TT, Becton DB, Jones SM. Chapter 5 Atopic dermatitis and food allergy. In: James JM, Burks W, Eigenmann PA, editors. Expert consult food allergy. Philadelphia, PA: Elsevier Saunders; 2012. p. 61–73.
17. Hauk PJ. The role of food allergy in atopic dermatitis. Curr Allergy Asthma Rep. 2008;8(3):188–94.
18. Welfel T, Breuer K. Role of food allergy in atopic dermatitis. Curr Opin Allergy Clin Immunol. 2004;4(5):379–85.
19. Uenishi T, Sugiura H, Tanaka T, Uehara M. Role of foods in irregular aggravation of skin lesions in children with atopic dermatitis. J Dermatol. 2008;35(7):407–12. doi:10.1111/j.1346-8138.2008.00494.x.
20. Schneider L, et al. Study of the atopic march: development of atopic comorbidities. Pediatr Dermatol. 2016;33(4):388–98. doi:10.1111/pde.12867.
21. Tupker RA, de Monchy JG, Coenraads PJ. House-dust mite hypersensitivity, eczema, and other non-pulmonary manifestations of allergy. Allergy. 1998;53(48 Suppl):92–6.
22. Greenhawt M. The role of food allergy in atopic dermatitis. Allergy Asthma Proc. 2010;3185:392–7. doi:10.2500/aap.2010.31.3393.
23. Dharmage SC, Lowe AJ, Matheson MC, Burgess JA, Allen KJ. Atopic dermatitis and the atopic march revisited. Allergy. 2014;69(1):17–27. doi:10.1111/all.12268.
24. Shaker M. New insights into the allergic march. Curr Opin Pediatr. 2014;26(4):516–20. doi:10.1097/MOP.0000000000000120.
25. Egawa G, Kabashima K. Multifactorial skin barrier deficiency and atopic dermatitis: essential topics to prevent the atopic march. J Allergy Clin Immunol. 2016) . e1;138(2):350–8. doi:10.1016/j.jaci.2016.06.002.
26. Li M. Current evidence of epidermal barrier dysfunction and thymic stromal lymphopoietin in the atopic march. Eur Respir Rev. 2014;23(133):292–8. doi:10.1183/09059180.00004314.
27. Palmer CN, et al. Common loss-of-function variants of the epidermal barrier protein filaggrin are a major predisposing factor for atopic dermatitis. Nat Genet. 2006;38:441–6.
28. Flohr C, et al. Filaggrin loss-of-function mutations are associated with early-onset eczema, eczema severity and transepidermal water loss at 3 months of age. Br J Dermatol. 2010;163:1333–6.

29. Venkataraman D, et al. Filaggrin loss-of-function mutations are associated with food allergy in childhood and adolescence. J Allergy Clin Immunol. 2014;134(4):876–82.
30. Ziyab AH, et al. Interplay of filaggrin loss-of-function variants, allergic sensitization, and eczema in a longitudinal study covering infancy to 18 years of age. PLoS One. 2012;7:e32721.
31. Heffler E, et al. High prevalence of Anisakis simplex hypersensitivity and allergy in Sicily, Italy. Ann Allergy Asthma Immunol. 2016;116(2):146–50. doi:10.1016/j.anai.2015.12.014.
32. Mattila L, et al. Food hypersensitivity among Finnish university students: association with atopic diseases. Clin Exp Allergy. 2003;33(5):600–6.
33. Woods RK, Thien F, Raven J, Walters EH, Abramson M. Prevalence of food allergies in young adults and their relationship to asthma, nasal allergies, and eczema. Ann Allergy Asthma Immunol. 2002;88(2):183–9.
34. Kijima A, et al. Prevalence and impact of past history of food allergy in atopic dermatitis. Allergol Int. 2013;62(1):105–12. doi:10.2332/allergolint.12-OA-0468.
35. Uenishi T, Sugiura H, Uehara M. Role of foods in irregular aggravation of atopic dermatitis. J Dermatol. 2003;30(2):91–7.
36. Mari A, Ballmer-Weber BK, Vieths S. The oral allergy syndrome: improved diagnostic and treatment methods. Curr Opin Allergy Clin Immunol. 2005;5:267.
37. Sampson HA, et al. Food allergy: a practice parameter update-2014. J Allergy Clin Immunol. 2014;134:1016.
38. Yamamoto T, Asakura K, Kataura A. Hypersensitivity to apple pulp among patients with birch pollinosis in Hokkaido. Arerugi. 1993;42:1701–6. (in Japanese)
39. Ono E, et al. Clinical features of oral allergy syndrome to plant foods allergens in Kanto regions. Arerugi. 2007;56(6):587–92.
40. Kondo Y, Urisu A, Tokuda R. Identification and characterization of allergens of tomato fruit by immunoblotting. Int Arch Allergy Immunol. 2001;126:294–9.
41. Sheffer AL, Austen KF. Exercise-induced anaphylaxis. J Allergy Clin Immunol. 1984;73:699.
42. Dohi M, et al. Food-dependent, exercise-induced anaphylaxis: a study on 11 Japanese cases. J Allergy Clin Immunol. 1991;87:34.
43. Hanakawa Y, et al. Food-dependent exercise-induced anaphylaxis: a case related to the amount of food allergen ingested. Br J Dermatol. 1998;138:898.
44. Brockow K, et al. Using a gluten oral food challenge protocol to improve diagnosis of wheat-dependent exercise-induced anaphylaxis. J Allergy Clin Immunol. 2015;135:977.
45. Harada S, et al. Aspirin enhances the induction of type I allergic symptoms when combined with food and exercise in patients with food-dependent exercise-induced anaphylaxis. Br J Dermatol. 2001;145:336.
46. Aihara M, et al. Food-dependent exercise-induced anaphylaxis: influence of concurrent aspirin administration on skin testing and provocation. Br J Dermatol. 2002;146:466.
47. Aihara Y, et al. Frequency of food-dependent, exercise-induced anaphylaxis in Japanese junior-high-school students. J Allergy Clin Immunol. 2001;108:1035.
48. Pastorello EA, et al. Wheat-dependent exercise-induced anaphylaxis caused by a lipid transfer protein and not by ω-5 gliadin. Ann Allergy Asthma Immunol. 2014;112:386.
49. Shibata R, Nishima S, Tanaka A, Borres MP, Morita E. Usefulness of specific IgE antibodies to ω-5 gliadin in the diagnosis and follow-up of Japanese children with wheat allergy. Ann Allergy Asthma Immunol. 2011;107(4):337–43.
50. Fukutomi Y, et al. Rhinoconjunctival sensitization to hydrolyzed wheat protein in facial soap can induce wheat-dependent exercise-induced anaphylaxis. J Allergy Clin Immunol. 2011;127:531–3.
51. Yokooji T, et al. Characterization of causative allergens for wheat-dependent exercise-induced anaphylaxis sensitized with hydrolyzed wheat proteins in facial soap. Allergol Int. 2013;62(4):435–45.
52. Hiragun M, et al. The sensitivity and clinical course of patients with wheat-dependent exercise-induced anaphylaxis sensitized to hydrolyzed wheat protein in facial soap—secondary publication. Allergol Int. 2013;62(3):351–8.
53. Chinuki Y, Morita E. Wheat-dependent exercise-induced anaphylaxis sensitized with hydrolyzed wheat protein in soap. Allergol Int. 2012;61(4):529–37.

54. Sugiyama A, et al. Clinical aspects of 41 cases performed challenge test with immediate-type wheat allergy due to hydrolyzed wheat protein (HWP-IWA). Arerugi. 2014;63:775–86. (in Japanese)
55. Radhakirishna N, et al. Anaphylaxis to oats after cutaneous sensitization by oatmeal in skin products used for the treatment of atopic dermatitis. J Allergy Clin Immunol Pract. 2016;4(1):152–3. doi:10.1016/j.jaip. 2015.07005.
56. Brehler R, Theissen U, Mohr C, Luger T. "Latex-fruit syndrome": frequency of cross-reacting IgE antibodies. Allergy. 1997;52:404.
57. Blanco C, et al. Latex allergy: clinical features and cross-reactivity with fruits. Ann Allergy. 1994;73:309.
58. Yagami T, Haishima Y, Nakamura A, Osuna H, Ikezawa Z. Digestibility of allergens extracted from natural rubber latex and vegetable foods. J Allergy Clin Immunol. 2000;106:752–62.
59. Ohsuna H, et al. Atopic dermatitis and latex allergy. Arerugi. 1998;47(2, 3):192.
60. Sugiura K, Sugiura M. A case of atopic dermatitis with food-dependent exercise-induced anaphylaxis (fdeia) and latex delayed-type hypersensitivity. Sci Dermatol. 2008;7(2):120–5.
61. Chen YH, Lan JL. Latex allergy and latex-fruit syndrome among medical workers in Taiwan. J Formos Med Assoc. 2002;101(9):622–6.
62. Catier A, et al. Chapter 19 Occupational reactions to food allergens. In: Metcalfe DD, Sampson HA, Simon RA, Lack G, editors. Food allergy, adverse reaction to foods and food additives. 5th ed. New York, NY: Wiley Blackwell; 2014. p. 245–65.
63. Drucker AM, et al. The burden of atopic dermatitis: summary of a report for the National Eczema Association. J Invest Dermatol. 2016; doi: 10.1016/j.jid.2016.07.012. pii: S0022-202X(16)32120-0.
64. Bindslev JC, et al. Standardization of food challenges in patients with immediate reactions to foods–position paper from the European Academy of Allergology and Clinical Immunology. Allergy. 2004;59(7):690–7.
65. Bock SA. Chapter 13 In vivo and in vitro diagnostic methods in the evaluation of food allergy. In: James JM, Burks W, Eigenmann PA, editors. Expert consult food allergy. Philadelphia, PA: Elsevier Saunders; 2012. p. 175–84.
66. Bock SA, Atkins FM. Patterns of food hypersensitivity during sixteen years of double-blind, placebo-controlled food challenges. J Pediatr. 1990;117(4):561–7.
67. Muraro A, et al. EAACI food allergy and anaphylaxis guidelines: diagnosis and management of food allergy. Allergy. 2014;69:1008.
68. Asero R, Femandez-Rivas M, Knulst AC, Bruijnzeel-Koomen CA. Double-blind, placebo-controlled food challenge in adults in every clinical practice; a reappraisal of their limitations and real indications. Curr Opin Allergy Clin Immunol. 2009;9(4):379–85. doi:10.1097/ACI.0b013e32832d9049.
69. Wassenberg J, Eingenmann P. Chapter 15 Management of food allergy and development of an anaphylaxis. In: James JM, Burks W, Eigenmann PA, editors. Expert consult food allergy. Philadelphia, PA: Elsevier Saunders; 2012. p. 205–18.
70. Rowlands D, Tofte SJ, Hanfin JM. Does food allergy cause dermatitis? Food challenge testing to dissociate eczematous from immediate reactions. Dermatol Ther. 2006;19(2):97–103.
71. Sicherer, S. H., Uris, A. Chapter 18 Natural history and prevention of food allergy, John M. James, Wesley Burks, Philippe A Eigenmann, Expert consult food allergy, Elsevier Saunders, Philadelphia, PA, 251–264 (2012).
72. Simpson EL, Eichenfield LF, Ellis CN, Mancini AJ, Paller AS. Current issues in atopic comorbidities and preventing the atopic march. Semin Cutan Med Surg. 2012;31(3 Suppl):S6–9. doi:10.1016/j.sder.2012.08.001.
73. Minoura T, Yanagida N, Watanabe Y, Yamaoka A, Miura K. The effects of great East Japan earthquake on patients with food allergy in Miyagi Prefecture. Arerugi. 2012;61(5):642–51.
74. Matsumura T, et al. Water supply facility damage and water resource operation at disaster base hospitals in miyagi prefecture in the wake of the Great East Japan Earthquake. Prehosp Disaster Med. 2015;30(2):193–8. doi:10.1017/S1049023X15000084.

Part X

Clinical Questions

Clinical Questions: Lifestyle of Japan and Atopic Dermatitis

29

Takeshi Nakahara

Abstract

Although the etiology and pathogenesis of atopic dermatitis (AD) are not fully understood, genetic and environmental factors are apparently involved in the onset and exacerbation of AD in a mutually interactive manner.

AD had become a very common skin disease from the 1950s through the 1970s in Japan. The incidence of AD in the Japanese population demonstrated an increase up to the 1990s but appeared to level off thereafter. These changes coincide with an era of rapid economic growth and have been attributed to the adoption of elements of a "Western" lifestyle such as diet or housing. Meanwhile, the Japanese also have specific traditions such as bathing. In addition, unpredictable climate change is occurring not only in Japan but also around the world.

What exactly are the lifestyle and other environmental ingredients that are responsible for the changing incidence of AD in Japan? This chapter reviewed selected environmental and lifestyle factors characterized in terms of the most significant influence on the prevalence and course of AD, especially in Japan.

Keywords

Atopic dermatitis • Climate • Air pollution • Bath • Diet

T. Nakahara
Division of Skin Surface Sensing, Department of Dermatology, Graduate School of Medical Sciences, Kyushu University, Fukuoka, Japan
e-mail: nakahara@dermatol.med.kyushu-u.ac.jp

I. Katayama et al. (eds.), *Evolution of Atopic Dermatitis in the 21st Century*,
https://doi.org/10.1007/978-981-10-5541-6_29

29.1 Introduction: Atopic Dermatitis and Environmental Factors

Atopic dermatitis (AD) is a common, chronic or chronically relapsing, severely pruritic, eczematous skin disease. The incidence of AD is generally considered to be increasing worldwide. Standardized questionnaire data from almost a million children aged 6–7 years and 13–14 years in the International Study of Asthma and Allergies in Childhood (ISAAC) suggest that AD is not a problem confined only to developed countries, with a high prevalence being found in many developing cities undergoing rapid demographic change [1]. Although the etiology and pathogenesis of AD are not fully understood, recent studies demonstrate that it involves a complex interaction of skin barrier dysfunction, exposure to external allergens or microbes, Th2-prone immune response, and itch-scratch behavior. Allergic reactions in AD are considered multifactorial, heterogeneous disorders caused by an interaction of environmental and genetic factors.

Genetic and environmental factors appear to be involved in the onset and exacerbation of AD in a mutually interactive manner. In 1993, Schultz Larsen et al. reported that the pairwise concordance rate of AD in monozygotic twins was 72%, while it was only 23% in their dizygotic counterparts [2]. Interestingly, the results of a similar study from the same country published in 2007 indicated that the concordance rate seemed to be affected by environmental factors even in genetically identical twins. In the 11,515 pairs of twins, the pairwise concordance rate of AD was 57% and 21% in the monozygotic and dizygotic twins, respectively [3]. AD-inducing environmental factors, as yet unknown, had shown increased effects in industrialized and developing countries and seemed to trigger the onset of AD in almost all individuals who were genetically predisposed to the disease.

Recent data regarding the burden of AD suggest that the picture in the developing world may soon resemble that of wealthier nations, in which AD affects over 20% of children. In the case of Japan, AD had become a very common skin disease from the 1950s through the 1970s. The incidence of AD in the Japanese population demonstrated an increase up to the 1990s, but appeared to level off thereafter [4, 5]. These changes coincide with an era of rapid economic growth and have been attributed to the adoption of a "Western" lifestyle. However, what exactly are the lifestyle and other environmental ingredients that are responsible for the changing incidence of AD? The objective of this chapter was to review selected environmental and lifestyle factors characterized in terms of the most significant influence on the prevalence and course of AD in Japan.

29.2 What Are the Factors in Climate that Have Effects on AD?

29.2.1 Temperature and Humidity

Climate can have a major impact on symptoms of AD. Many published data show that cold and dry weather increase the prevalence and risk of flares in patients with AD [6–10]. An ecological analysis was conducted using information on long-term climatic conditions in the different study areas from the World Weather Guide [6]. Among latitude, altitude, average outdoor temperature, and relative outdoor humidity, AD symptoms correlate positively with latitude and negatively with annual outdoor temperature, but correlations were not observed with any of the other factors. In a cross-sectional population-based survey of schoolchildren from ten Spanish centers in three different climatic regions, AD was positively associated with precipitation and humidity and was negatively associated with temperature and the number of sunny hours [7]. In a study of Taiwanese schoolchildren, no associations were found for the highest monthly means of temperature, whereas the annual means and the lowest monthly means of temperature were negatively related to flexural eczema but only in girls [8]. These results show that AD is significantly dependent on meteorological conditions. Studies that have researched flare factors in established AD support this notion, as lower outdoor temperatures, especially in combination with skin irritants, can contribute to the worsening of disease, whereas indoor climate seems less important [9]. However, the relationship between outdoor climate and disease flares is complex, with some children reporting worsening in the summer and others in winter, and the effects of outdoor temperature, ultraviolet (UV) light, and humidity are likely to interact. Engebretsen KA et al. reviewed the literature regarding the effect of environmental humidity and temperature on skin barrier function and dermatitis and conclude that low humidity and low temperatures lead to a general decrease in skin barrier function and increased susceptibility toward mechanical stress [10].

In Japan, yearly average temperature and humidity differ from region to region. The national yearly average temperature and humidity are 15.8 °C and 69%, respectively. The yearly average temperature and humidity of Hokkaido, Tokyo, and Okinawa are 9.8 °C/69%, 16.9 °C/61%, and 23.1 °C/74%, respectively. A cross-sectional study of the prevalence of AD conducted by the Japanese Ministry of Health, Labour and Welfare actually confirmed that the lowest prevalence of AD was found in Okinawa, where the highest temperature occurred. Hayashi et al. reported that the prevalence of AD in Gifu, with a temperate climate (15.8 °C/64%), was significantly higher than that in Itoman (in Okinawa), with a subtropical climate [11]. Significantly lower rates of current AD in the Ogasawara Islands (23.3 °C/78%), which are located away from mainland Japan and belong to a subtropical area, were also observed compared to previous reports from Japan [12]. In our population-based survey of children aged 5 years and younger on Ishigaki Island, Okinawa, Japan (Kyushu University Ishigaki Atopic Dermatitis Study: KIDS), the AD prevalence on Ishigaki Island was apparently lower than that reported by a research team of the Japanese Ministry of Health, Labour and Welfare [13]. They reported that the national mean prevalence of AD was 12.8% in individuals aged 4 months, 9.8% in those aged 18 months, 13.2% in those aged 3 years, 11.8% in those aged 6–7 years, 10.6% in those aged 12–13 years, and 8.2% in those aged 18 years. The AD prevalence on Ishigaki Island (6.3%) was approximately half that of children of corresponding ages in mainland Japan. In addition, although five types of loss-of-function mutations in the filaggrin (*FLG*) gene isolated in previous Japanese *FLG* mutation studies were identified, the frequency of *FLG* loss-of-function mutation in children of the KIDS cohort was not significantly different between the AD and non-AD groups (7.9% and 6.1%, respectively, $p = 0.174$), suggesting that *FLG* loss-of-function mutations are not always a predisposing factor for AD prevalence [14]. There are many possible explanations for this, such as different pathogens, dietary habits, or flora. However, we believe that the high tem perature (24.4 °C) and humidity (73.1%) of Ishigaki Island might reduce the incidence of AD, presumably reducing the onset of AD in those who have *FLG* mutations or a defect in enzymes that digest filaggrin. This study definitively showed that the involvement of the interaction of environmental and genetic factors in AD onset differs from region to region. Extremes of climate might suppress the effects of genetic factors.

29.2.2 Season

Although it has been generally accepted that seasonal aggravation of skin symptoms is a basic feature of AD, recent studies have suggested a decrease in the seasonal dependence of the dermatosis in European countries [15]. In Japan, the difference in climate in each of the four seasons is fairly clear-cut. Uenishi et al. examined the incidence of seasonal deterioration of AD in Japanese subjects. Of 682 patients aged 3–30 years with AD, 452 (66%) showed a seasonal aggravation of skin symptoms, and 230 (34%) experienced perennial deterioration. The overall incidences of exacerbation in spring, summer, autumn, and winter were 25%, 19%, 11%, and 36%, respectively [16]. In 1967, Masuda reported that the incidences of deterioration in spring, summer, autumn, and winter were 22%, 38%, 13%, and 34%, respectively [17]. Considering these results makes it evident that a real decrease in the incidence of seasonal aggravation of AD has occurred in Japan and that the incidence of summer deterioration has greatly decreased. The authors speculated that an important cause of the decrease in summer deterioration of AD may be a change in attitudes regarding the use of soap for bathing. In the 1960s, dermatologists in Japan prohibited patients with AD from using soap. As a result, the bodies of these patients were covered with sweat, scales, crusts, and debris of medicaments. Subsequently, however, several studies have demonstrated that such unclean skin is accompanied by severe pruritus, especially during the summer months when it is hot and humid in Japan [18, 19]. Therefore, most dermatologists now recommend that patients with AD use skin cleansing agent (i.e., soaps, detergent, cleanser) while bathing to keep both involved and uninvolved skin areas clean. Instead of the decrease in seasonal deterioration, perennial deterioration of the symptoms of AD has increased. Although it is not clear what factors are responsible for the increase in the occurrence of perennial worsening, the increase could be attributable to changes in environmental factors. For example, housing in Japan has generally changed from houses with open wooden structures to airtight homes made of concrete and synthetic materials. As a result, many patients with AD are perennially exposed to house dust and molds, which may provoke aggravation of the disease. In another study performed to investigate the relationship between residential environments and AD, 1378 elementary school children were examined by dermatological specialists in October 1994 (first series) and April 1995 (second series). Half of the children with AD showed symptoms in only one of the two seasons, either the autumn or spring, so the drifting of symptoms of AD occurred largely by season. Multiple logistic regression analysis showed that more children who were diagnosed positive for AD twice (AD(+,+)) lived in damp and moldy homes than did children who were diagnosed negative for AD twice (AD(−,−)). Thus, damp and moldy houses may be risk factors for the occurrence of AD [20].

In a study that evaluated the relationship between month of birth and prevalence of AD, individuals born in autumn showed the highest (7.5%), and those born in spring showed the lowest (5.5%), prevalence of AD [21]. These findings lead us to speculate that the climate to which one is exposed in early infancy affects the condition of the skin and that those born in autumn have dry skin in early infancy, which may ultimately result in a higher prevalence of AD among young schoolchildren. In fact, a recent study showed that skin barrier function measured through transepidermal water loss (TEWL) of the forehead during the first week of life is associated with the development of AD [22].

29.3 Does Air Pollution Exacerbate Symptoms of AD?

A systematic review of 26 studies suggested that there was good evidence of a higher disease burden in cities compared with the countryside, suggesting that place of residence may have a role in the pathogenesis of AD. One theory to explain this rise in AD is an increase in exposure to air pollution [23]. Air pollution became a social concern in the era of rapid economic growth in Japan. Nowadays, air pollution continues to increase in East Asia, particularly in China, and is considered to cause health problems in Japan. Studies on the association between outdoor pollution and AD from Sweden and East Germany found that AD risk increased with living close to heavy traffic [24, 25]. In a more recent population-based cross-sectional survey among more than 300,000 Taiwanese schoolchildren, objective measurement of traffic-related air pollutants, including nitrogen dioxide (NO_2) and carbon monoxide (CO), suggested that air pollution may contribute to the risk of AD [8]. Similarly, a cohort study among 3000 schoolchildren in West Germany with repeat objective pollutant measurements reported that NO_2 exposure was positively associated with physician-diagnosed AD at age 6 [26]. In a study involving 4907 French children (9–11 years of age) residing at their current address for 3 years or longer, lifetime eczema was significantly associated with 3-year average concentrations of PM10, NO2, NOx, and CO; adjusted odds ratios (ORs) were 1.13, 1.23, 1.06, and 1.08, respectively [27].

In addition to its effects on the prevalence of AD, outdoor air pollution also influences the skin symptoms in AD patients. In a prospective study, the concentrations of outdoor PM10, PM2.5, toluene, and total volatile organic compounds were higher on days when the patients had symptoms of AD than on days when they reported no symptoms [28]. PM is a mixture of solid and liquid particles of different origins with various chemical and physical properties, including pollen grains and mold spores. PM with a diameter of 10 μm or less is known as PM10, and particulate matter with a diameter of 2.5 μm or less is known as PM2.5. Diesel exhaust particulate (DEP) accounts for most of the airborne PM in the atmosphere in large cities. A study found that an increase in the concentration of outdoor PM10 of 1 $\mu g/m^3$ was significantly associated with a 0.44% increase in AD symptoms on the following day. The effect of PM on AD was also investigated in a study of 41 schoolchildren aged between 8 and 12 years [29]. In the study, daily symptom scores and daily PM concentrations were measured. The results showed that the pruritus score was significantly associated with the concentrations of PM with a diameter <0.1 μm, but not larger particles. In Japan, the very stringent restrictions on emission sources have resulted in a low level of PM2.5 mass concentration. Therefore, pollutants originating in China and arriving via long-range transport have a significant impact on the PM2.5 concentration. In the future, PM from China might be one of the major factors that exacerbate AD symptoms in Japan.

29.4 Do Bathing Habits Matter in AD?

29.4.1 Bathing Habits in Japan

Bathing is an important behavior for keeping the body clean and is one of the habits of Japanese daily life. Bathing styles involve a full bath (body immersed in water in bathtub) or whole-body bathing (shower bath). Japanese individuals are known for their "specific" bathing habits. People in Japan usually take a bath every day, and a full bath (with or without shower) is the most common type of home bathing in Japan. Many Japanese individuals like high water temperatures, and some take baths of a long duration. Most people use "skin cleansing agent (i.e., soaps, detergent, cleanser)," and some, particularly elderly individuals, enjoy scrubbing their skin when they wash and dry their body. For many Japanese people, bathing is not only for cleaning the body but also for relieving fatigue and attaining a relaxed state of mind.

In a recent report about bathing habits among 189 Japanese healthy people, 128 participants (67.7%) took ≥7 baths per week. The most common water temperature was 40–41 °C, reported by 70 participants (40.2%). The mean water temperature was 40.14 ± 1.14 °C. The most common bath duration was 10–15 min, reported by 58 participants (30.9%). The mean bathing duration was 11.95 ± 9.03 min. In terms of water level, 167 participants (83.3%) took a full bath [30]. Nishioka et al. previously reported the bathing habits of Japanese people with various skin diseases. About 80% of the participants took a bath every day, and the most common bath duration was 10–20 min. Over 80% took a full bath (with or without shower). Most of them used soap or detergent, and 85% used a towel when washing the body [31]. Hattori et al. also reported that about 85% of patients who have various skin diseases use implements such as towels or gauze, and 56.4% scrub their skin when they wash their body [32]. These data remind us of traditional bathing habits in Japanese daily life. Another report regarding bathing habits in Okinawa found that 36% of people bathe more than twice a day in the summer season. Interestingly, 81% of these individuals take only a shower bath [33].

29.4.2 Studies in Favor of Bathing

Although most dermatologists agree that the skin of patients with AD should be kept clean, there is no unanimity of opinion or good evidence regarding bathing technique or proper use of soap or detergent.

In a prospective trial of 58 schoolchildren with moderate to severe AD in Japan, daily showers vs. no shower were compared over a 4-week period. The authors found that showers were more effective in significantly improving scores on the SCORing Atopic Dermatitis (SCORAD), in cases of the most severe disease [34]. These results were replicated in two subsequent studies in the Japanese population: one involving 53 children over a 6-week period and another involving 11 children over a 4-week period. AD severity scores improved significantly with daily showers. These studies demonstrated that keeping the skin of patients with AD clean is very important in the management of the symptoms of AD [35, 36].

Additional studies from countries other than Japan have also shown results in favor of frequent bathing. In a prospective study comparing daily bathing with less than daily bathing, 81 patients with AD and their parents were instructed to bathe once daily from 10 to 15 min in warm water with a mildly acidic cleanser. After bathing, the parents were instructed to dry the children by dabbing with towels and to apply emollients within 3 min of towel drying. Topical corticosteroids (TCSs) were not allowed during the study period. Then, the investigators compared the good compliance group A (daily bathing) with the poor compliance group B (less than daily bathing) and found that the mean change in the SCORAD at 2 weeks was greater in group A than in group B [37]. In a recent retrospective review of subjects with moderate to severe AD whose symptoms were resistant to high potency corticosteroid or systemic therapy, daily bathing for 15–20 min, followed by application of a TCS, was associated with a high response rate, with most patients exhibiting almost clear or mild levels of severity [38].

29.4.3 Studies Against Bathing

As Hanifin and Tofte stated, bathing followed by evaporation causes stratum corneum contracture and fissures, thereby drying out the skin and impairing the epidermal barrier [38].

Some clinicians believe that water avoidance is the appropriate way to avoid further irritation of the skin and increased evaporative water losses. Furthermore, frequent bathing is often combined with overuse of skin cleaning agents (i.e., soaps). Other factors that could lead to AD flares include high water temperature and physical irritation from excess towel washing and drying or scrubbing of the skin. Regarding the water avoidance, however, Hanifin also proposed that bathing, if followed by the application of a moisturizer within 3 min, could hydrate the skin and keep the epidermal barrier soft and flexible. In the case of Japanese individuals, bathing frequency is not an issue because almost all Japanese people bathe every day. Thus, the relevant concerns are overuse of skin cleaning agents, high water temperature, and physical irritation from excess towel washing and drying or scrubbing of the skin, which might lead to symptoms of AD flares.

29.4.4 Skin Cleansing Agents (i.e., Soaps, Detergents, Cleansers)

Skin cleansing is an essential part of skin care as described above. Its primary function is to remove dirt, sweat, scales, crusts, sebum, other environmental pollutants, bacteria, and debris of medicaments from the skin. However, it is paradoxical that the act of cleansing typically leads to a weakening of the barrier; many skin cleansing agents are based on surfactants that interact detrimentally with the proteins and lipids of the stratum corneum (SC) [39–41]. In addition, many skin cleansing agents (i.e., soaps) can contribute to skin barrier breakdown by increasing the pH of the SC [42]. Therefore, it appears that, for most skin disorders, "excess" cleansing with "strong detergent" skin cleansing agents may lead to an exacerbation of symptoms.

However, in two pilot studies for infants, wash using a wash product was noninferior to water alone in terms of TEWL [43, 44]. In another study from Japan, 130 patients with AD, who had used no soap for at least a month, were allowed to use common toilet soaps when showering to keep the skin clean. Immediately after bathing, the skin lesions and areas of dry skin were treated with topical medications. When soap was used in this way, topically applied medications were found to be more effective before the use of soap. After 1 week, 119 (91.5%) of the 130 patients showed considerable improvement of the skin lesions. After 5 weeks, most patients experienced progressive improvement of eczema. Deterioration of eczema or dry skin did not occur [19]. In another study, water alone was identified as an ineffective cleanser, as it fails to remove fat-soluble substances such as feces and sebum [45]. Thus, water alone is not recommended for cleaning. Considering that the melting point of sebum is around 30 °C [46], dirt may be removed, to some extent, only by warm water. The use of skin cleansing agents is recommended in consideration of the situation, such as season, body region, age, and sensation of irritation.

29.4.5 Does Warmth Induce Itch?

Members of the transient receptor potential (TRP) family are temperature sensors, and TRPV1, V3, and V4 are expressed in epidermal keratinocytes [47]. TRPV1 is activated by various stimuli including heat (above approximately 42 °C), capsaicin, ATP, prostaglandins, and protons and is involved in the induction of histaminergic-related itch responses [48]. A subset of TRPV1-expressing sensory neurons, also known as pruritoceptive neurons, play an important role in the development of itch. Thus, TRPV1 protein has been linked to itch and heat sensations. In addition, the barrier recovery of human skin was accelerated at temperatures between 36 and 40 °C compared with the area at 34 °C, whereas it was delayed at 34 or 42 °C. TRPV1 activation by capsaicin regulates the epidermal permeability barrier in vivo. Thus, water temperatures above 42 °C might induce itch and barrier dysfunction through TRPV1 activation. In a recent study, 104 patients with AD were surveyed to determine whether there was a relationship between AD severity and bathing frequency and duration. The authors found that longer bathing duration was associated with greater AD severity (20–30 min > 10–20 min). They did not mention the water temperature; bathing duration might be related to warming the skin [49].

29.4.6 What Are the Most Appropriate Washing and Bathing Routines for Patients with AD?

The optimal practice methods of bathing might differ from patient to patient. Unfortunately, there is not enough evidence to support optimal bathing frequency, washing, types of skin cleaning agents, or water temperature. However, at a minimum, the skin of patients with AD should be kept clean by bathing. It is recommended that patients choose "not too strong detergent" skin cleaning agents and wash and dry gently. When deciding on the use of skin cleaning agents, various factors such as age, season, and regions should be considered. The application of an emollient after the bath is required to avoid evaporation, which causes dry skin. A water temperature around 38–40 °C is suitable to not induce itch or barrier dysfunction.

29.5 What Kind of Diet Is Preferred?

The Japanese diet rapidly changed after World War 2 from one mainly consisting of grains, vegetables, seaweed, and fish to a high-protein, high-lipid, high-carbohydrate diet, which contains large amounts of meat, fat and fatty oil, and sugar. Considering how uncommon AD and other allergies still are in most developing nations, consumption of a "Western" affluent diet might lead to an increase in AD risk. In a survey performed in England, wheezing and hypersensitivity were less frequently observed in children who had Asian-type eating habits, while the risks of hypersensitivity and AD were significantly higher in children who had Western-type eating habits, suggesting that Asian-type eating habits with rice as the principal food may have benefits in prevention of allergic disease including AD [50]. In ISAAC Phase Three, frequent consumption of fresh fruits was found to have a protective effect on AD risk, whereas the opposite was true for fast-food consumption [51]. An ecological analysis based on the ISAAC data set came to similar conclusions, showing a consistent inverse association between AD prevalence and per capita consumption of vegetables, protein from cereal and nuts, and all fresh and frozen fish. Similar risk reductions have been described in children with a high intake of fish during late infancy. These results have been attributed to fish's rich content of anti-inflammatory $n-3$ polyunsaturated fatty acids ($n-3$ PUFA). Western diets have become low in $n-3$ PUFAs over the past decades, with a corresponding increase in pro inflammatory $n-6$ PUFAs, such as linoleic acid. Consistent with this theory, maternal intake of $n-6$ PUFAs during pregnancy has been associated with an increased AD risk in Japanese children at 2 years of age [52]. In the study, the authors concluded that maternal intake of alpha-linolenic acid and docosahexaenoic acid during pregnancy may be preventive against infantile wheeze. Maternal intake of $n-6$ PUFAs, especially linoleic acid, during pregnancy may increase the risk of childhood eczema. In addition, case-control studies have demonstrated that AD sufferers have higher blood levels of linoleic acid ($n-6$ PUFA precursor) and lower levels of $n-3$ PUFAs. The changes in eating habits of the Japanese population might contribute to the increased prevalence of AD during the era of rapid economic growth.

An analysis of a cross-sectional nationwide survey of 5202 Korean young adults showed that obesity was positively related to the presence of AD in women [53]. A recently published meta-analysis of epidemiological studies from North America and Asia on the association between AD and obesity showed that obesity is associated with an increased prevalence of AD in children and adults [54]. In a recent case-control study of Chinese adults, the prevalence of obesity was 6.7% in healthy controls and 15.6% in patients with AD [55]. These data can be used as statistical evidence of a significant association between obesity and AD. However, the data also suggests that obesity is not present in 84.4% of patients with AD and cannot function as a causal factor in the majority of patients with AD. Thus, a careful interpretation of the currently available epidemiological reports and clinical experience indicates that the association between AD and obesity must be an epiphenomenon. The significant association between obesity and AD also supports the idea that environmental and lifestyle factors responsible for the development of obesity, including unhealthy dietary habits and lack of physical activity, could also be responsible for the development of AD.

Conclusions

From the twentieth century to the twenty-first century, through a period of high economic growth, elements of the Japanese lifestyle and environment such as dietary habits, housing, and air pollution have changed dramatically. In addition, the climate is changing unpredictably not only in Japan but also around the world. Meanwhile, there are also unchanged "traditional" Japanese lifestyle factors such as daily bathing habits. It is highly likely that many of these factors are involved differently in the pathogenesis of AD by region in Japan or by country, in addition to genetic factors. Management of AD that takes various lifestyle and environmental factors into consideration is necessary in the future.

References

1. Williams H, Stewart A, von Mutius E, Cookson W, Anderson HR. Is really on the increase worldwide? J Allergy Clin Immunol. 2008;121:947–54.
2. Larsen S. Atopic dermatitis: a genetic-epidemiologic study in a population-based twin sample. J Am Acad Dermatol. 1993;28:719–23.
3. Thomsen F, Ulrik S, Kyvik O, et al. Importance of genetic factors in the etiology of atopic dermatitis: a twin study. Allergy Asthma Proc. 2007;28:535–9.
4. Sugiura H, Umemoto N, Deguchi H, et al. Prevalence of childhood and adolescent atopic dermatitis in a Japanese population: comparison with the disease frequency examined 20 years ago. Acta Derm Venereol. 1998;78(4):293–4.
5. Yura A, Shimizu T. Trends in the prevalence of atopic dermatitis in school children: longitudinal study in Osaka Prefecture, Japan, from 1985 to 1997. Br J Dermatol. 2001;145(6):966–73.
6. Weiland SK, Husing A, Strachan DP, et al. Climate and the prevalence of symptoms of asthma, allergic rhinitis, and atopic eczema in children. Occup Environ Med. 2004;61:609–15.
7. Suarez-Varela MM, Garcia-Marcos Alvarez L, Kogan MD, et al. Climate and prevalence of atopic eczema in 6- to 7-year-old school children in Spain. ISAAC phase III. Int J Biometeorol. 2008;52:833–40.
8. Lee YL, Su HJ, Sheu HM, Yu HS, Guo YL. Traffic-related air pollution, climate, and prevalence of eczema in Taiwanese school children. J Invest Dermatol. 2008;128:2412–20.
9. Langan SM, Silcocks P, Williams HC. What causes flares of eczema in children? Br J Dermatol. 2009;161:640–6.
10. Engebretsen KA, Johansen JD, Kezic S, Linneberg A, Thyssen JP. The effect of environmental humidity and temperature on skin barrier function and dermatitis. J Eur Acad Dermatol Venereol. 2016;30(2):223–49.
11. Hayashi T, Kawakami N, Kondo N, et al. Prevalence of and risk factors for allergic diseases: comparison of two cities in Japan. Ann Allergy Asthma Immunol. 1995;75:525–9.
12. Okada Y, Kumagai H, Morikawa Y, Akasawa A. Epidemiology of pediatric allergic diseases in the Ogasawara Islands. Allergol Int. 2016;65(1):37–43.
13. Takeuchi S, Esaki H, Furusyo N, et al. Incidence, serum IgE and TARC/CCL17 levels in atopic dermatitis associated with other allergic diseases: an update from the Ishigaki cohort. Acta Derm Venereol. 2015;95(4):480–4.
14. Sasaki T, Furusyo N, Shiohama A, et al. Filaggrin loss-of-function mutations are not a predisposing factor for atopic dermatitis in an Ishigaki Island under subtropical climate. J Dermatol Sci. 2014;76(1):10–5.
15. Young E. Seasonal factors in atopic dermatitis and their relationship to allergy. Acta Derm Venereol. 1980;92:111–2.
16. Uenishi T, Sugiura H, Uehara M. Changes in the seasonal dependence of atopic dermatitis in Japan. J Dermatol. 2001;28(5):244–7.
17. Masuda T. Atopic dermatitis [in Japanese]. Nihon-Hifuka-Zensho, III-1-2. Tokyo: Kanehara Shuppan Co; 1967. p. 301–401.
18. Sasaki K, Sugiura H, Uehara M. Patch test reactions to the acetone-soluble fraction of human dander in atopic dermatitis. Dermatology. 1994;189:58–61.
19. Uehara M, Takada K. Use of soap in the management of atopic dermatitis. Clin Exp Dermatol. 1985;10(5):419–25.
20. Kimura Y, Kanazawa Y, Kida K, Mita R, Nishizawa Y, Hashimoto I. A study of Atopic dermatitis in elementary school children in Hirosaki city, Aomori prefecture, Japan. Environ Health Prev Med. 1998;3(3):141–5.
21. Kusunoki T, Asai K, Harazaki M, Korematsu S, Hosoi S. Month of birth and prevalence of atopic dermatitis in schoolchildren: dry skin in early infancy as a possible etiologic factor. J Allergy Clin Immunol. 1999;103(6):1148–52.
22. Horimukai K, Morita K, Narita M, et al. Transepidermal water loss measurement during infancy can predict the subsequent development of atopic dermatitis regardless of filaggrin mutations. Allergol Int. 2016;65(1):103–8.

23. Schram ME, Tedja AM, Spijker R, Bos JD, Williams HC, Spuls PI. Is there a rural/urban gradient in the prevalence of eczema? A systematic review. Br J Dermatol. 2010;162:964–73.
24. Montnemery P, Nihlen U, Goran Lofdahl C, Nyberg P, Svensson A. Prevalence of self-reported eczema in relation to living environment, socio-economic status and respiratory symptoms assessed in a questionnaire study. BMC Dermatol. 2003;3:4.
25. Schafer T, Vieluf D, Behrendt H, Kramer U, Ring J. Atopic eczema and other manifestations of atopy: results of a study in East and West Germany. Allergy. 1996;51:532–9.
26. Morgenstern V, Zutavern A, Cyrys J, Brockow I, Koletzko S, Kramer U, et al. Atopic diseases, allergic sensitization, and exposure to traffic-related air pollution in children. Am J Respir Crit Care Med. 2008;177:1331–7.
27. Penard-Morand C, Raherison C, Charpin D, et al. Long-term exposure to close-proximity air pollution and asthma and allergies in urban children. Eur Respir J. 2010;36:33–40.
28. Kim J, Kim EH, Oh I, et al. Symptoms of atopic dermatitis are influenced by outdoor air pollution. J Allergy Clin Immunol. 2013;132:495–8.
29. Song S, Lee K, Lee M, et al. Acute health effects of urban fine and ultrafine particles on children with atopic dermatitis. Environ Res. 2011;111:394–9.
30. Ishizawa T, Watanabe S, Yano S, et al. Relationship between Bathing Habits and Physical and Psychological State. J Jpn Soc Balneol Climatol Phys Med. 2012;75:227.
31. Nishioka K, Arai M. Questionnaire research about bathing habit in Japan [in Japansese]. Pract Dermatol. 1997;19:1137–42.
32. Hattori A, Tamura T. Bathing frequency and use of soap [in Japansese]. Pract Dermatol. 1999;21:360–4.
33. Hagiwara K, Nonaka K. Questionnaire research about bathing habit in Okinawa [in Japanese]. Pract Dermatol. 1999;21:350–9.
34. Kameyoshi Y, Tanaka T, Mochizuki M, et al. Taking showers at school is beneficial for children with severer atopic dermatitis [in Japanese]. Arerugi. 2008;57:130–7.
35. Mochizuki H, Muramatsu R, Tadaki H, Mizuno T, Arakawa H, Morikawa A. Effects of skin care with shower therapy on children with atopic dermatitis in elementary schools. Pediatr Dermatol. 2009;26:223–5.
36. Murota H, Takahashi A, Nishioka M, et al. Showering reduces atopic dermatitis in elementary school students. Eur J Dermatol. 2010;20:410–1.
37. Kim H, Ban J, Park MR, et al. Effect of bathing on atopic dermatitis during the summer season. Asia Pac Allergy. 2012;2(4):269–74.
38. Hajar T, Hanifin JM, Tofte SJ, Simpson EL. Prehydration is effective for rapid control of recalcitrant atopic dermatitis. Dermatitis. 2014;25(2):56–9.
39. Rhein LD, Robbins CR, Kernee K, Cantore R. Surfactant structure effects on swelling of isolated human stratum corneum. J Soc Cosmet Chem. 1986;37:125–39.
40. Wilhelm KP, Cua AB, Wolff HH, Maibach HI. Predicting surfactant induced stratum corneum hydration in vivo prediction of the irritation potential of anionic surfactants. J Invest Dermatol. 1994;101:310–5.
41. Wihelm KP, Wolff HH, Maibach HI. Effects of surfactants on skin hydration. In: Elsner P, Berardesca E, Maibach HI, editors. Bioengineering of the skin: water and the stratum corneum. Boca Raton, FL: CRC Press; 1994. p. 257–74.
42. Ananthapadmanabhan KP, Moore DJ, Subramanyan K, Misra M, Meyer F. Cleansing without compromise: the impact of cleansers on the skin barrier and the technology of mild cleansing. Dermatol Ther. 2004;17(Suppl 1):16–25.
43. Lavender T, Bedwell C, O'Brien E, Cork MJ, Turner M, Hart A. Infant skin-cleansing product versus water: a pilot randomized, assessor-blinded controlled trial. BMC Pediatr. 2011;11:35. doi:10.1186/1471-2431-11-35.
44. Lavender T, Bedwell C, Roberts SA, et al. Randomized, controlled trial evaluating a baby wash product on skin barrier function in healthy, term neonates. J Obstet Gynecol Neonatal Nurs. 2013;42(2):203–14.
45. Gelmetti C. Skin cleansing in children. J Eur Acad Dermatol Venereol. 2001;15:12–5. Review

46. Nicolaides N. Skin lipids. IV. Biochemistry and function. J Am Oil Chem Soc. 1965;42(8):708–12.
47. Denda M, Sokabe T, Fukumi-Tominaga T, Tominaga M. Effects of skin surface temperature on epidermal permeability barrier homeostasis. J Invest Dermatol. 2007;127(3):654–9.
48. Ho JC, Lee CH. TRP channels in skin: from physiological implications to clinical significances. Biophysics (Nagoya-shi). 2015;11:17–24.
49. Koutroulis I, Pyle T, Kopylov D, Little A, Gaughan J, Kratimenos P. The Association Between Bathing Habits and Severity of Atopic Dermatitis in Children. Clin Pediatr (Phila). 2016;55(2):176–81.
50. Carey OJ, Cookson JB, Britton J, Tattersfield AE. The effect of lifestyle on wheeze, atopy, and bronchial hyperreactivity in Asian and white children. Am J Respir Crit Care Med. 1996;154 (2 Pt 1):537–40.
51. Ellwood P, Asher MI, Garcia-Marcos L, et al. Do fast foods cause asthma, rhinoconjunctivitis and eczema? Global findings from the International Study of Asthma and Allergies in Childhood (ISAAC) Phase Three. Thorax. 2013;68:351–60.
52. Miyake Y, Sasaki S, Tanaka K, Ohfuji S, Hirota Y. Maternal fat consumption during pregnancy and risk of wheeze and eczema in Japanese infants aged 16-24 months: the Osaka Maternal and Child Health Study. Thorax. 2009;64:815–21.
53. Nahm DH. Associations of atopic dermatitis with obesity and unmarried status in young adults: evidence for atopic dermatitis as a life-style disorder with high social impact. Allerg Asthma Immunol Res. 2016;8(2):89–91.
54. Zhang A, Silverberg JI. Association of atopic dermatitis with being overweight and obese: a systematic review and metaanalysis. J Am Acad Dermatol. 2015;72(4):606–16.
55. Luo X, Xiang J, Dong X, Cai F, Suo J, Wang Z, et al. Association between obesity and atopic disorders in Chinese adults: an individually matched case-control study. BMC Public Health. 2013,13.12.

Erratum to: Senile Atopic Dermatitis

Ryoji Tanei

Erratum to:
Chapter 18 in: Ichiro Katayama/ Hiroyuki Murota / Takahiro Satoh (eds), Evolution of Atopic Dermatitis in the 21st Century
https://doi.org/10.1007/978-981-10-5541-6_18

The correction in page-239 was inadvertently missed and published. This has now been updated. The first reference citation in "18.2.6 Epidemiology" section was published incorrectly. This has also been updated now.

The updated online version of the original chapter can be found at https://doi.org/10.1007/978-981-10-5541-6_18

R. Tanei, M.D., Ph.D.
Department of Dermatology, Tokyo Metropolitan Geriatric Hospital and Institute of Gerontology, 35-2 Sakaecho, Itabashi, Tokyo 173-0015, Japan
e-mail: rtanei@aol.com; rtanei@tmghig.jp

I. Katayama et al. (eds.), *Evolution of Atopic Dermatitis in the 21st Century*,
https://doi.org/10.1007/978-981-10-5541-6_30

MIX
Papier aus verantwortungsvollen Quellen
Paper from responsible sources
FSC® C105338
FSC
www.fsc.org

If you have any concerns about our products,
you can contact us on
ProductSafety@springernature.com

In case Publisher is established outside the EU,
the EU authorized representative is:
Springer Nature Customer Service Center GmbH
Europaplatz 3, 69115 Heidelberg, Germany

Printed by Libri Plureos GmbH
in Hamburg, Germany